BRONCHIAL ASTHMA – EMERGING THERAPEUTIC STRATEGIES

Edited by **Elizabeth Sapey**

Bronchial Asthma – Emerging Therapeutic Strategies
Edited by Elizabeth Sapey

Published by InTech
Janeza Trdine 9, 51000 Rijeka, Croatia

Publishing Process Manager Silvia Vlase

Technical Editor Teodora Smiljanic

Cover Designer InTech Design Team

Additional hard copies can be obtained from orders@intechopen.com

Bronchial Asthma – Emerging Therapeutic Strategies, Edited by Elizabeth Sapey
p. cm.
ISBN 978-953-51-0140-6

For EU product safety concerns:
IN TECH d.o.o., Prolaz Marije Krucifikse Kozulić 3, 51000 Rijeka, Croatia,
info@intechopen.com or visit our website at intechopen.com.

Meet the editor

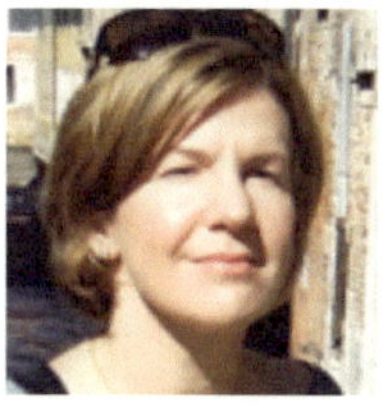

Dr Elizabeth Sapey gained her first science degree from the University of London (BSci Medical Science, 1st Class Honours), and went on to qualify as a Physician from the Royal London and St Bartholomew's School of Medicine and Dentistry. She specialized in Respiratory Medicine in 2001, and has been involved in research since then, focusing upon the inflammatory basis of chronic disease, with particular emphasis on neutrophilic inflammation and lung disease. She worked as a Clinical Fellow, and now is employed as a Clinical Lecturer after gaining her PhD at the University of Birmingham, UK, where she is involved in the management of difficult asthma. Dr Sapey is well published in international peer reviewed journals and has contributed to many books, focusing on chronic inflammation in the lung.

Contents

Preface XI

Part 1 Asthma – Diagnosis, Prevalence and Progression 1

Chapter 1 **The Natural History of Asthma 3**
Elizabeth Sapey and Duncan Wilson

Chapter 2 **Bronchial Challenge Testing 19**
Lutz Beckert and Kate Jones

Chapter 3 **Determination of Biomarkers in Exhaled Breath Condensate: A Perspective Way in Bronchial Asthma Diagnostics 37**
Kamila Syslová, Petr Kačer, Marek Kuzma, Petr Novotný and Daniela Pelclová

Part 2 Immunological Mechanisms in the Development and Progression of Asthma 75

Chapter 4 **Immune Mechanisms of Childhood Asthma 77**
T. Negoro, Y. Yamamoto, S. Shimizu, A. H. Banham, G. Roncador, H. Wakabayashi, T. Osabe, T. Yanai, H. Akiyama, K. Itabashi and Y. Nakano

Chapter 5 **Allergic Asthma and Aging 89**
Gabriele Di Lorenzo, Danilo Di Bona, Simona La Piana, Vito Ditta and Maria Stefania Leto-Barone

Chapter 6 **Airway Smooth Muscle: Is There a Phenotype Associated with Asthma? 117**
Gautam Damera and Reynold A. Panettieri, Jr.

Chapter 7 **Fluoride and Bronchial Smooth Muscle 139**
Fedoua Gandia, Sonia Rouatbi, Badreddine Sriha and Zouhair Tabka

Part 3 The Management of Asthma – Emerging Treatment Strategies 147

Chapter 8 **Management of Asthma in Children 149**
Abdulrahman Al Frayh

Chapter 9 **Mechanisms of Reduced Glucocorticoid Sensitivity in Bronchial Asthma 193**
Yasuhiro Matsumura

Chapter 10 **Antioxidant Strategies in the Treatment of Bronchial Asthma 217**
Martin Joyce-Brady, William W. Cruikshank and Susan R. Doctrow

Chapter 11 **Rehabilitation and Its Concern 231**
Ganesan Kathiresan

Preface

Asthma is a common, chronic and potentially debilitating disease. It is diagnosed currently on clinical grounds with a combination of symptoms (intermittent breathlessness, wheeze and cough) associated with variable airflow obstruction, which is classically reversible (by bronchodilation).

The heterogeneity of asthma clinically is likely to be due to differences in the cause and the inflammatory signal present in individual groups of patients. Predisposing environmental factors (where known) vary between individuals and across countries, depending on antigenic load. However, not all patients with asthma demonstrate atopy or allergy, and other immune responses are thought important in some patient groups.

It is becoming more recognised that there are specific patient phenotypes in asthma that are associated with differing patterns of disease progression, varying responses to treatment and these are likely to be driven by different genetic susceptibility factors leading to specific inflammatory outputs. Our current understanding of such factors is limited.

This book focuses on emerging theories of the immunological drivers of asthma, how these relate to different patient phenotypes, and how these can be utilised to diagnose asthma more accurately and treat asthma more effectively.

The editors would like to thank the authors for their contributions and we very much hope this book increases the interest in asthma research.

Dr Elizabeth Sapey
Centre for Translational Inflammation Research
University of Birmingham
United Kingdom

Part 1

Asthma – Diagnosis, Prevalence and Progression

1

The Natural History of Asthma

Elizabeth Sapey and Duncan Wilson
University of Birmingham
UK

1. Introduction

As our understanding of underlying mechanisms evolve disease definitions are adapted and refined. For example, until recently, one of the main distinctions between the definition of asthma and COPD was the presence or absence of reversible airflow obstruction. As greater advances are made in understanding pathology, newer and better definitions encompass the overlap that exists between these two conditions and the recognition that chronic inflammation underlies both.

Despite greater understanding of the inflammatory processes that drive asthma, there remains a lack of consensus regarding a definition and standards for diagnosis. Asthma is a clinical syndrome and currently there is no single test that confirms its presence. This has hampered studies of asthma epidemiology, as different investigators have used differing inclusion criteria to identify cases of disease.

As well as identifying the presence of disease, there is a need to understand the natural history of asthma in order to identify which therapeutic interventions are most likely to be beneficial at any given time. A growing body of evidence suggests that although several current treatment strategies are effective in controlling symptoms, none change the natural course of the illness. It is, therefore, crucial to identify risk factors for the development of asthma and triggers for asthma symptoms in order to develop effective primary and secondary prevention strategies.

This chapter will discuss how asthma is diagnosed, its incidence and prevalence, the associated healthcare utilization, and morbidity and mortality. It will also outline the clinical phenotypes associated with the onset, remission and progression of asthma, over time..

2. Definitions

Most definitions of asthma have emphasized the variable nature of symptoms, the presence of airflow obstruction and the reversible nature of the airflow obstruction, at least in the early stages of disease [1,2]. As the pathophysiology of asthma has become clearer, definitions have changed to include a statement of pathology. The latest definition to be widely embraced is a description of asthma as:

"A chronic inflammatory disorder of the airways in which many cells and cellular elements play a role. The chronic inflammation is associated with airway hyper-responsiveness that leads to recurrent episodes of wheezing, breathlessness, chest tightness and coughing; particularly at night or in the early morning. These episodes are usually associated with widespread but variable airflow obstruction within the lung that is often reversible either spontaneously or with treatment" [1].

In keeping with current theories, this definition implies that asthma is one disorder, rather than multiple complex disorders and syndromes [3] without detracting from its variable clinical presentation and course. This definition may encompass the spectrum of disease present and its inflammatory basis, but it is clinically unwieldy, as it does not provide a clear set of diagnostic criteria from which to identify patients. A more clinically relevant definition of asthma will not come into being until the pathogenesis of this condition is understood and a diagnostic biomarker is identified.

3. An overview of inflammation

Currently asthma is understood as being a chronic inflammatory disease where gene-environment interactions (often with different sensitizing agents) lead to the release of inflammatory mediators, the recruitment of specific cell populations, and airflow obstruction. The airflow limitation may range from being completely reversible to being fixed. Historically, there has been difficulty differentiating between COPD and asthma. These conditions can co-exist, so the clinical picture can reflect both, which may complicate the diagnostic process and alter responses to treatment. However, while symptoms and the results of forced respiratory maneuvers can be similar, there is increasing recognition that there are differences in the pulmonary inflammatory profile of patients with asthma and COPD that can help to differentiate between the two conditions [4]. An overview of the inflammatory cascade in asthma and COPD is provided in figure 1.

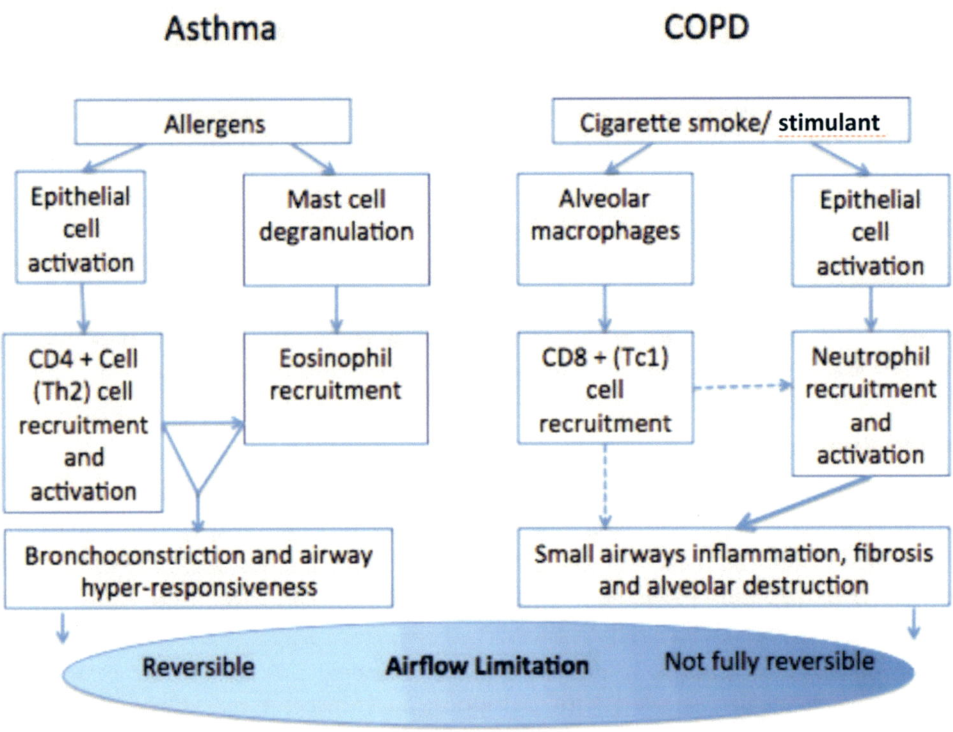

Fig. 1. **A broad overview of pulmonary inflammation in asthma and COPD** (adapted from [5]).

There are also differences in the pathology and immunology of mild to moderate and severe asthma, which can also complicate diagnosis. It is increasingly recognized that while mild and moderate asthma is a disease of eosinophils, severe asthma is associated with an influx of neutrophils[6]. It is hypothesized that that this difference in cell types may explain in part the increased resistance seen to corticosteroids with severe asthma, as neutrophilic inflammation is classically less responsive to this form of therapy [7]. It is unclear, however, whether neutrophils are causally related to severe asthma, or whether their presence is secondary to the frequent use of corticosteroids and unrelated to the natural history of the disease. Table 1 highlights differences in pulmonary inflammation in Asthma, Severe asthma and COPD.

	ASTHMA	SEVERE ASTHMA	COPD
Predominant Cells present in the lungs	Eosinophils Macrophages CD4+ T Cells (TH2)	Neutrophils Macrophages CD4+ T Cells (Th2)	Neutrophils Macrophages CD8+ T Cells (Tc1)
Key mediators in lung secretions and lung biopsies	Eotaxins IL-4, IL-5, IL-13 Nitric oxide	IL-8, IL-5, IL-13 Nitric Oxide	IL-8, TNF-alpha, IL-1 beta, LTB4, IL-6
Site of Disease	Proximal airways	Proximal airways and peripheral airways	Peripheral airways, lung parenchyma, pulmonary vessels
Pathological features	Fragile epithelium Mucous metaplasia Thickening of the basement membrane Oedema Bronchoconstriction	Fragile epithelium Mucous metaplasia Thickening of the basement membrane Oedema Bronchoconstriction	Squamous metaplasia, mucous metaplasia, small airway fibrosis, destruction of parenchyma.
Response to treatment	Large response to bronchodilators. Good response to steroids	Smaller or no bronchodilator response and reduced response to steroids	Small bronchodilator response, but this can alter with repeated testing, poor response to steroids

Adapted from [5].

Table 1. Differences in pulmonary inflammation asthma, severe asthma and COPD.

4. Severity classifications and asthma control

International guidelines stratify asthma by severity, using symptoms, exacerbations and markers of airflow obstruction (FEV_1 or peak expiratory flow). Severity classifications are Intermittent, Mild persistent, Moderate Persistent and Severe Persistent (table 2.) These scoring systems were only meant to be applied to patients not receiving inhaled corticosteroids [5] since this therapy can dramatically alter disease control. Despite this, it was widely recognized that this severity classification was often erroneously applied to patients already on treatment [8] and that the usefulness of such a system was limited. Severe Persistent asthma can become Mild or Intermittent Asthma if it is suitably controlled with medication, however, this change in severity classification may not reflect the severity of asthma present initially, nor the difficulty with which control was achieved [9]. Currently this classification system is limited to research studies only.

In light of these factors there has been a move to classify the severity of asthma by its clinical expression - characterizing symptomatic control [10]. This provides clear targets for physicians and patients and an easily recognized trigger mechanism to increase or decrease therapeutic regimes. Table 3 describes how asthma control is currently characterized.

Intermittent Symptoms less than once a week Nocturnal symptoms not more than twice a month Brief exacerbations FEV_1 or PEF > 80% predicted FEV_1 or PEF variability < 20%
Mild Symptoms more than once a week but less than once a day Nocturnal symptoms more than twice a month Exacerbations may affect activity and sleep FEV_1 or PEF > 80% predicted FEV_1 or PEF variability < 20 - 30%
Moderate Persistent Symptoms daily Nocturnal symptoms more than once a week Exacerbations may affect activity and sleep Daily use of short acting $beta_2$ agonists FEV_1 or PEF 60 - 80% predicted FEV_1 or PEF variability > 30%
Severe Persistent Symptoms daily Frequent nocturnal symptoms Frequent Exacerbations Limitations of physical activity FEV_1 or PEF < 60 % predicted FEV_1 or PEF variability > 30%

Adapted from [5].

Table 2. Asthma classification by severity before treatment

Characteristic	Controlled (all of the following)	Partly controlled (any measure present in any week)	Uncontrolled
Daytime symptoms	None (twice or less a week)	More than twice a week	Three or more features of partly controlled asthma present in any week
Limitations of activity	None	Any	
Nocturnal symptoms	None	Any	
Need for reliever/ rescue medication	None (twice or less a week)	More than twice a week	
Lung function (FEV_1 or PEF)	Normal	< 80% predicted or personal best	
Exacerbations	None	One or more a year	Once in any week

Adapted from [5].

Table 3. Levels of asthma control

All current international guidelines use asthma control to classify severity and to signal the need for a change in treatment strategy in a step-wise manner. However, many studies of the epidemiology and natural history of asthma still refer to severity in accordance with Table 2.

5. Epidemiology

Studies of asthma epidemiology have been hindered by the lack of an agreed diagnostic standard. There is controversy as to whether symptoms and airway hyper-responsiveness should be assessed separately or jointly, although there is a poor correlation between the presence of symptoms and airway hyper-responsiveness [11,12].

6. Incidence

Incidence rates for asthma vary in accordance with the age of the population under study and the diagnostic criteria used. Global estimates suggest that there are at least 300 million people worldwide with asthma, with a predicted 100 million additional cases by 2025 [5,13]. Asthma incidence rates are highest in early childhood and in male children until puberty [14] and appear to be rising. A study in the USA described childhood asthma incidence rates to be 183 per 100,000 children in 1964 and 284 per 100,000 in 1983 [15]. The incidence of adult-onset asthma is highest in females (3 per 1000 person-years compared with 1.3 per 1000 person-years in males) [16] but these do not appear to be increasing [15].

7. Prevalence

There have been many studies estimating the prevalence of asthma in differing communities. Overall, the global prevalence ranges from 1% to 18% of the population in different countries [17]. Data suggest that there are increases in prevalence of asthma in children and in older adults in developing countries and decreases in the prevalence of asthma in the developed world [18]. Urbanisation appears to be a risk factor for asthma, as its prevalence has consistently been shown to be higher among children living in cities compared with those living outside urban developments [19,20]. Possible explanations for this include atmospheric agents, the hygiene hypothesis where reduced exposure to allergens leads to a less tolerant immune response, a poorer socioeconomic background and differences in healthcare utilization. These remain as yet unproven.

8. Healthcare utilization

The global financial impact of asthma is substantial. Healthcare utilization accounts for the largest proportion of these costs and is increasing annually. In 2000, the estimated annual costs for asthma in the USA was $12.7 billion (8.1 for direct costs, 2.6 related to morbidity, 2.0 related to mortality). In 2007 this figure had risen to an estimated $50.1 billion [21]. On an individual basis, the direct health care costs associated with asthma in the USA are approximately $3,300 per person with asthma each year [21].

Increased hospital admissions account for a significant proportion of the rising costs and have been documented worldwide, including in the UK, New Zealand, USA, and Australia [21-23]. A study comparing asthma hospitalisations in the 1960s and the 1980s reported a 50% increase in cases of children with an exacerbation of asthma and a 200% increase in cases of adults across these decennials [24]. There has also been a significant rise in asthma-related contact with a family physician [25].

9. Morbidity and mortality

Increased utilization of healthcare and monetary spend on asthma has not correlated with vast improvements in mortality or morbidity. The World Health Organisation estimates that 15 million disability-adjusted life years (DALYS) are lost annually due to asthma [13,26]. This represents 1% of the total global disease burden. Annual worldwide deaths from asthma have been estimated at 250,000, but mortality does not correlate well with prevalence. Indeed, the countries that currently suffer the highest prevalence (Northern America, UK, New Zealand) enjoy the lowest mortality rates [26]. In developed countries, death rates appear to be stable. In the USA mortality has remained at approximately 3,500 deaths per year for five years [21], while in the UK annual mortality rates have remained stable at approximately 1300 per annum [27].

10. Demographics and asthma

The epidemiology of asthma is associated with by age-related sex differences. Asthma and wheezing are more prevalent in young boys compared with young girls [14], but this trend disappears during puberty [28]. In a study of 16 countries, it was reported that girls had a lower risk of developing asthma than did boys during childhood, this risk was equal at puberty, and reversed in young adults [29]. Women older than 20 years have both a higher prevalence and higher morbidity rates from asthma, and are more likely to present to hospital and be admitted for treatment [30,31]. They also have more severe disease and higher mortality rates [32] . The reason for this disparity is unclear but genetic and hormonal factors are likely to contribute.

As well as clear gender differences, there are also racial differences in the prevalence of asthma. In the USA, morbidity from asthma has been consistently shown to be greater in children of African American descent (for example, 13.4% of African American children and 9.7% of white children [33]). Furthermore, children of African American descent are reported to have asthma which imposes a greater limitation on activity, with more hospital admissions but fewer family physician visits when compared to white children [34]. Data also suggest that asthma-associated mortality in children of African American and Puerto Rican descent is higher than in any other group [35].

Socioeconomic forces also appear to be important in asthma, and studies suggest that asthma severity is increased in poorer communities [36] . This may reflect environmental factors such as exposure to smoke and occupational hazards, as well as health care utilization.

11. The natural history of asthma

Most models of chronic disease suggest there is a common natural history to all diseases, which begin with a prodromal stage, prior to disease presentation.

This pre-illness period is defined as the period when subjects are free of overt disease but who have the susceptibility for the development of the condition (such as a genetic predisposition towards disease). During this phase, disease development is not inevitable and identifying individuals at risk provides an opportunity to prevent disease emergence. The disease manifests itself only after exposure to necessary environmental triggers (epigenetics). Following disease emergence, the condition can progress unabated (the natural course of the disease), or disease-modifying strategies can be employed to protect or reduce disease presentation, or to affect a cure. See figure 2 for a diagrammatic representation of this.

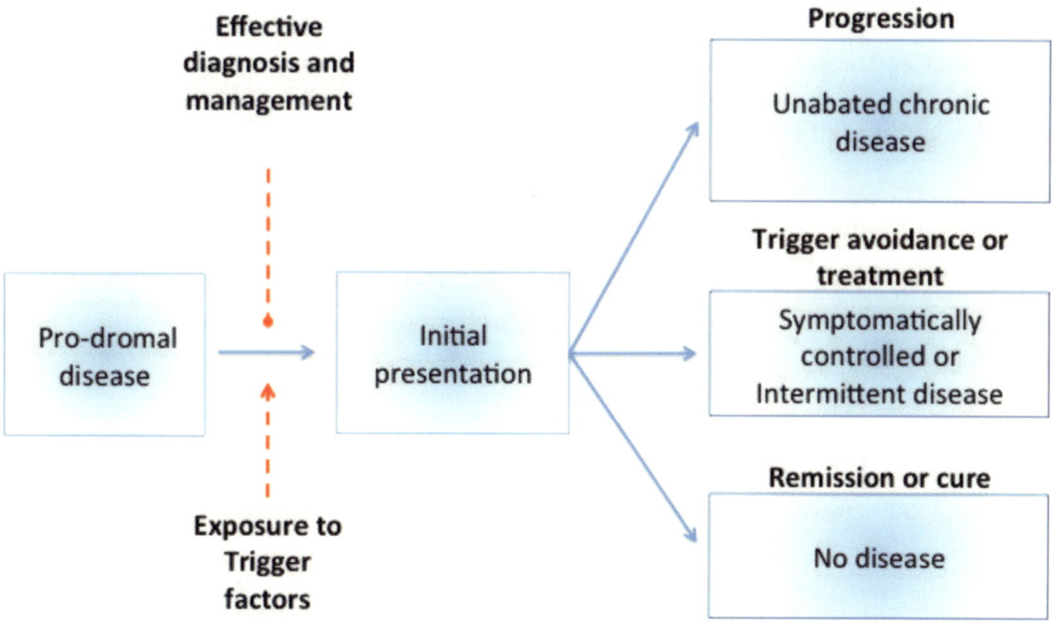

Fig. 2. **A hypothetical representation of the course of a chronic disease** (adapted from [37]).

The prodromal stage equates to disease predisposition before the advent of triggers which cause disease manifestation. Following exposure, the disease presents, but this could theoretically be avoided if disease predisposition were known and exposure avoided. Following presentation, the disease can progress, or could be controlled or cured by appropriate management (treatment or exposure avoidance). Presently asthma is not curable using existing therapeutic strategies and while there is a need to expand treatment regimes, there is also great interest in identifying asthma susceptibility factors, which would allow patients to be diagnosed in the prodromal phase of asthma, before the advent of symptoms. This is likely to involve studies of genetic and environmental factors.

12. The genetics of asthma

There is great interest in understanding the natural course of asthma. Asthma is a heterogenous condition and there remains some controversy as to whether asthma is a single disease entity or whether it represents a common label for a number of disease phenotypes. A disease phenotype represents a set of characteristics that are important in terms of disease progression or prognosis and it is increasingly apparent be that specific cohorts of asthma patients experience different presentations of disease and warrant different treatment strategies. Specific disease phenotypes may also experience different prognoses.

There are now numerous studies of the pattern of inheritance of asthma [38], rhinitis [39], allergic dermatitis [40], and serum IgE levels [41] and these have clearly shown that the familial concordance is partly due to shared genes. There are several loci that may be involved in the pathogenesis of allergy and asthma (see Table 4). In common with other complex diseases, independent investigators have not been able to reproduce many of these results. There are several explanations for this including genetic heterogeneity between populations, differences in phenotype definition, and lack of a consensus over the appropriate significance levels to use in these studies. A number of candidate linked have been repetitively associated with the presence of asthma or asthma severity and have a plausible biological role in the development of the disease.

Candidate Genes

Interleukin 4	B_2 adrenergic receptor
Tumour Necrosis Factor α	Intereukin -4 receptor a
HLA,	N-Acetyltransferase
α_1-antitrypsin	Angiotensin-converting enzyme
Interleukins 5, 9, and 13,	Glucocorticoid receptor,
CD14	Clara cell protein 16,
Transporter antigen peptide 1,	Interleukin 9 receptor,
Immunoglobulin heavy chain genes,	T cell antigen receptor ,
T cell antigen receptor	
β Subunit of the high-affinity IgE receptor	

Table 4. Candidate Genes in Allergy and Asthma

On chromosome 6p21, there is an important region that contains the genes for the major histocompatibility (MHC) molecules as well as the tumor necrosis factor α (TNF-α) and lymphotoxin genes. This area of chromosome 6 has been repeatedly identified in linkage and association studies. Most of the data concerns the association of specific MHC genotypes with sensitization to specific aeroallergens [42]. On chromosome 5q there are many candidate genes for asthma and allergy such as the interleukin 4 and β_2-adrenergic receptor genes both of which have been associated with asthma [43] . Chromosome 11q13 has been linked to a variety of different phenotypes and the β chain of the high-affinity IgE receptor has been proposed as a candidate for this linkage [44]. The region containing the interleukin 4 receptor α chain (16p12) has also been implicated in IgE responsiveness [45].

It is hypothesized that polymorphisms within these candidate gene alter pro-inflammatory protein expression and cellular functions to cause a predisposition towards asthma or alterations in responses to treatment (especially in the case of β2 adrenergic and glucocorticoid receptors). In most cases the functional consequences of genetic variation have not been assessed, and these remain associations only, but there is great interest in characterizing predispositions further in order to modify risk.

13. Asthma phenotypes and progression

There have been longitudinal studies that have addressed how asthma progresses and these have begun to explore the effect of disease phenotype on outcome [46-48].

14. Asthma phenotypes with age

14.1 Early childhood

Longitudinal studies have consistently confirmed that most cases of chronic, persistent asthma start in early childhood, with the initial presentation occurring during the first 5 years of life [15,46,48]. There are some methodological concerns with these studies, as most ask parents to document or recall recurrent symptoms of wheeze or cough. These can represent recurrent viral infections and only a small proportion of these children will go on to develop persistent asthma [49], however the association between childhood symptoms and persistent asthma later in life appears robust.

Further work has tried to understand which children are most at risk of developing asthma. The vast majority of infants who become wheezy during infections do not go on to develop asthma. Most of these infants (representing two thirds of cases of wheeze) have one or two episodes of wheeze before the age of two, but these do not recur after this age and this presentation is termed "Transient wheezing of infancy" [50]. Studies suggest that the most important risk factors for transient wheezing in infancy are exposure to respiratory viruses (especially RSV) [49], maternal smoking in pregnancy and lower lung function values [51,52]. Remission is thought to occur due to growth of the airways and lung parenchyma [53] but currently there is no evidence that any particular active intervention reduces progression to asthma although bronchodilators improve both symptoms and lung function measurements, suggesting disease is related to bronchomotor tone. Sensitisation to aeroallergens is associated with a risk of chronic asthma in later life, but interestingly, symptoms seem to start 2 - 3 years later than in those whose asthma is not associated with atopy [54]. Furthermore, treating this sensitization is associated with a reduction in the development of asthma [55].

14.2 Adolescent to adulthood

Birth cohort studies suggest that over 60% of children who are frequently wheezy or who have a physician diagnosis of asthma go on to experience asthma-like symptoms as an adolescent [56]. Chronic asthma symptoms that persistent into adolescence and early adulthood are associated with both sensitization to allergens and elevated levels of circulating IgE [57]. Different allergens appear important in different geographical regions, for example in desert regions the mould *Alternaria* is associated with asthma [58], while in more temperate and coastal regions, house dust mite is the more likely relevant sensitizing agent [59]. The ability to detect the allergen most closely associated with disease varies according to region, and there are likely to be more unidentified allergens that are associated with disease.

Identifying the exact allergen responsible in each patient may be less important than characterizing the inflammatory reaction present. The key features of asthma including symptoms, disordered airway function, airway inflammation, exacerbations and the decline in lung function, are not closely related to each other within patients and might have different drivers. There is no clear causal link between eosinophilic airway inflammation and airway hyper-responsiveness [60] and infiltration of airway smooth muscle by mast cells may be more relevant [61]. In contrast, asthma exacerbations are more closely related to eosinophilic airway inflammation[60]

15. Asthma remission or progression

Large, long term population based prospective studies have tried to identify factors that predict who will progress and experience persistent, severe asthma, and who will remit [62-64].

In all studies, severity and frequency of symptoms in early childhood predict outcomes in adulthood. Those that experience mild and infrequent symptoms in early life go on to experience no or mild asthma-related symptoms. Those with the most severe symptoms have persistent severe asthma in later life. In one population based study, 52% of children (aged 10) with asthma and 72% of children with severe asthma had frequent or persistent wheeze age 42 [65].

The majority of patients with persistent asthma in later life demonstrated evidence of an allergic predisposition (with allergic rhinitis or eczema in childhood) [47].

Deficits in lung volumes during childhood are also consistently associated with persistent asthma in adulthood [65]. The presence of abnormal lung function in childhood is a predictor of asthma and children who wheeze or who have a diagnosis of asthma, who then go on to have persistent asthma in adulthood have reductions in FEV_1 and FEV_1/ FVC ratio compared with controls throughout life. Interestingly, the slope of decline over time does not alter between wheezers and controls in this group [47], suggesting that developmental factors are important in asthma sustainment in this group, but that these factors do not contribute to accelerated decline in lung function in later life.

In contrast to this, when asthma symptoms occur in later life (aged over 25 years), they are associated both with moderate deficits in FEV_1 and FEV_1/FVC in early adulthood and a faster decline in lung function in subsequent years [53]. This, combined with studies of inflammation [66], suggest that in this group, developmental factors combined with epigenetic influences such as inflammatory polymorphisms or environmental stimuli, lead to progressive disease. Airway hyper-responsiveness appears to be an important component of this, and has been consistently associated with progression to adult asthma in a number of studies [47,56].

Less is known about factors that cause the re-emergence of asthma following a period of remission in early adulthood. There is evidence that remission may be a clinical phenomena rather than a true abatement of disease, as it is not associated with a loss of inflammation or bronchial hyper-responsiveness. Indeed, eosinophil counts, exhaled nitric oxide and concentrations of IL-5 remain higher in asthma patients with no symptoms who are off treatment than sex and age-matched controls [67]. It might be that environmental and genetic factors combine in these patients so that their burden of inflammation crosses a symptomatic threshold, leading to disease re-emergence, but there are no studies that explore this hypothesis.

16. Conclusion

Asthma is a common, chronic inflammatory lung condition associated with variable airflow obstruction and symptoms of breathlessness, cough and wheeze. Age of onset, severity and clinical course varies between patient groups, and these clinical phenotypes are likely to reflect differences in the genetic, developmental and environmental factors which predispose to disease and trigger symptoms. Currently, these factors are not well understood, but they are likely to be vital in determining which patients go on to experience worsening disease outcomes and which patients respond to certain treatment regimes.

The continued presence of inflammation even in quiescent disease suggests that current treatment strategies are not treating the drivers of disease, but instead are modifying disease-related symptoms by transiently reducing inflammation. As effective as current treatments are for the majority of patients, more research is needed to determine the causes of asthma in different patient populations.

Understanding the epigenetics of asthma will allow for new treatment strategies, where specific medications are targeted to specific cohorts of patients based upon their inflammatory make-up and disease presentation.

17. References

[1] Global Strategy for Asthma Management and Prevention. Global Initiative for Asthma (GOLD). *Available from : URL:* http://www.ginaasthma.org (2006).

[2] National Asthma Education and Prevention Program Expert Panel Report 2. Guidelines for the daignosis and management of asthma. *National Institute of Health, National Heart Lung and Blood Institute. NIH Publication*, 97 - 4051 (1997).

[3] Wenzel SE. Asthma: Defining of the persistent adult phenotypes. *Lancet* 368, 804 - 813 (2006).

[4] Jeffery PK. Structural and inflammatory changes in COPD: a comparison with asthma. *Thorax* 53(2), 129-136 (1998).

[5] Global Strategy for Asthma Management and Prevention. Global Initiative for Asthma (GOLD). *Available from :*
URL: http://www.ginaasthma.org, 1 - 119 (2010).

[6] Wenzel Sally e, Szefler Stanley j, Leung Donald yM, Sloan Steven i, Rex Michael d, Martin Richard j. Bronchoscopic Evaluation of Severe Asthma . Persistent Inflammation Associated with High Dose Glucocorticoids. *Am. J. Respir. Crit. Care Med.* 156(3), 737-743 (1997).

[7] Chanez P, Vignola AM, O'shaugnessy T *et al.* Corticosteroid reversibility in COPD is related to features of asthma. *Am J Respir Crit Care Med* 155(5), 1529-1534 (1997).

[8] Taylor DR, Bateman ED, Boulet LP *et al.* A new perspective on concepts of sthma severity and control. *Eur Respir J* 32, 545 - 554 (2008).

[9] Crockcroft DW, Swystun VA. Asthma control versus asthma severity. *J Allergy Clin Immunol* 98, 1016 - 1018 (1996).

[10] Bateman ED, Boushey HA, Bousquet J *et al.* Can guideline-defined asthma control be achieved? The Gaining Optimal Asthma Control study. *Am J Respir Crit Care Med* 170(8), 836 - 844 (2004).

[11] Pekkanen J, Pearce N. Defining asthma in epidemiological studies. *Eur Respir J* 14(4)(1999).

[12] Boushey HA, Holtzman MJ, Sheller JR, Nadel JA. Bronchial hyper-activity. *Am Rev Respir Dis* 121(2), 389 - 413 (1980).

[13] Masoli M, Fabian D, Holt S, Beasley R. The global burden of asthma: Executive summary of GINA Dissemination Committee Report. *Allergy* 59(5), 469 - 478 (2004).

[14] Dodge RR, Burrows B. The prevalence and incidence of asthma and asthma-like symptoms in a general population sample. . *Am Rev Respir Dis* 122(4), 567 - 575 (1980).

[15] Yunginger JW, Reed CE, O'connell EJ, Melton LJ, Iii.,, O'fallon WM, Silverstein MD. A community based study of the epidemiology of asthma. Incidence rates, 1964 - 1983 *Am Rev Respir Dis* 146(4), 888 - 894 (1992).

[16] Toren K, Hermansson BA. Incidence rates of adult onset asthma in relation to age, sex, atopy and smoking. A Swedish population-based study of 15813 adults. *Int J Tuberc Lung Dis* 3(3), 192 - 197 (1999).

[17] Beasley R. The global burden of asthma report, Global Initiative for Asthma (GINA). *Available from* http://www.ginasthma.org (2004).

[18] Ford ES. The Epidemiology of obesity and asthma. *J Allergy Clin Immunol* 115(7), 661 - 666 (2005).

[19] Mannino DM, Homa DM, Pertowski CA, Et Al. Surveillance for asthma - United States 1960 - 1995. *Mor Mortal Wkly Rep CDC Surveill Summ* 47(1), 1 - 27 (1998).

[20] Crain EF, Weiss KB, Bijer PE, Hersh M, Westbrook L, Stein RE. An estimate of the prevalence of asthma and wheezing among inner-city children. *Paediatrics* 94(3), 356 - 362 (1994).

[21] Prevention CFDCA. Asthma in the US: Growing every year. *Available at* http://www.cdc.gov/vitalsigns/asthma (2011).

[22] Mitchell EA. International trends in hospital admission rates for asthma. *Arch Dis Child* 60(4), 376 - 378 (1985).

[23] Wilkins K, Mao Y. Trends in rates of admission to hospital and death from asthma among children and young adults in Canada during the 1980s. *Can Med Assoc J* 148(2), 185 - 190 (1993).

[24] Evans RD, Mullally DI, Wilson RW, Et Al. National trends in the morbidity and mortality of asthma in the US. Prevalence, hospitalization and death from asthma over 2 decades. 1965 - 1984. *Chest* 91(6), 65S - 74S (1987).

[25] Uk. A. Where do we stand? Asthma in the UK today. *Available at* http://www.asthma.org.uk/wheredowestand (2004).

[26] Bousquet J, Bousquet PJ, Godard P, Daures JP. The public health implications of asthma. Public Health Reviews. *Bulletin of the World Health Organization* 83, 548 - 554 (2005).

[27] Asthma Uk. Key facts and statistics about asthma. *Available at* http://www.asthma.org.uk/news (2011).

[28] Venn A, Lewis S, Cooper M, Hill J, Britton J. Questionnaire study of the effect of sex and age on the prevalence of wheeze and asthma in adolescence. *BMJ* 316, 1945 -1946 (1998).

[29] De Marco R, Locatelli F, Sunyer J, Burney P. Differences in incidence of reported asthma related to age in men and women. A retrospective analysis of the data of the European Respiratory Health Survey. *Am J Respir Crit Care Med* 162, 68 - 74 (2000).

[30] Skobeloff EM, Spivey WH, St Clair SS, Schoffstall JM. The influence of age and sex on asthma admissions. *JAMA* 268, 3437 - 3440 (1992).

[31] Baibergenova A, Thabane L, Akhtar-Danesh N, Levine M, Gafni A, Leeb K. Sex differences in hospital admissions from emergancy departments in asthmatic adults. A population based study. *Ann Allergy Asthma Immunol* 96(5), 666 - 672 (2006).

[32] Melgert BN, Ray A, Hylkema MN, Timens W, Postma DS. Are there reasons why adult asthma is more common in females? *Curr Allergy Asthma Rep* 7, 143 - 150 (2007).

[33] Taylor WR, Newacheck PW. Impact of childhood asthma on health. *Pediatrics* 90, 657 - 662 (1992).

[34] Coultras DB, Gong HJ, Grad R, Et Al. Respiratory diseases in minorities of the United States. *Am J Respir Crit Care Med* 149, S93 - S131 (1994).

[35] Weitzman M, Gortmaker SL, Sobal AM, Perrin JM. Recent trends in the prevalence and severity of childhood asthma. *JAMA* 268, 2673 - 2677 (1992).

[36] Mielck A, Reitmeir P, Wjst M. Severity of childhood asthma by socioeconomic stauts. *Int J Epidemiol* 25, 388 - 393 (1996).

[37] Guerra S, Martinez FD. The natural history of asthma and COPD. *In Asthma and COPD. Basic mechanisms and clinical management. Editors P Barnes, JM Drazen, Rennard, S.I., and NC Thomson* Academic Press, 23 - 33 (2009).

[38] The European Community Respiratory Health Survey Group. Genes for asthma? An analysis of the EuropeanCommunity Respiratory Health Survey. *Am J Respir Crit Care Med* 156, 1773 - 1780 (1997).

[39] Dold S, Wjst M, Von Mutius E, Reitmeir P, Stiepel E. Genetic risk factors for asthma, allergic rhinitis and atopic dermatitis. *Arch. Dis. Child* 67, 1018 - 1022 (1992).

[40] Diepgen TL, Blettner M. Analysis of familial aggregation of atopic eczema and other atopic diseases by ODDS RATIO regression models *J Invest Dermatol* 106, 977 - 981 (1996).

[41] Johnson CC, Ownby DR, Peterson EL. Parental history of atopic disease and concentrations of blood IgE. *Clin Exp Allergy* 26, 624 - 629 (1996).

[42] Ansari AA, Shinomiya N, Zwollo P, Marsh DG. HLA-D gene studies in relation to immune responsiveness to a grass allergen LolpIII. *Immunogenetics* 33, 24 - 32 (1991).

[43] Hizawa N., Freidhoff LR, Chiu YF *et al.* Genetic regulation of dermatophagoides pteronyssinus-specific IgE responsiveness - a genome wige multi-point linkage analysis in families recruited through 2 asthmatic sibs. *J Allergy Clin Immunol* 102, 436 - 442 (1998).

[44] Palmer LJ, Daniels SE, Rye PJ *et al.* Linkage of chromosome 5q and 11q gene markers to asthma associated quantitative traits in Austrailian Children. *Am J Respir Crit Care Med* 158, 1825 - 1830 (1998).

[45] Deichmann KA, Heinzmann A, Forster J *et al.* Linkage and allelic association of atopy and markers flanking the IL-4 receptpr gene. *Clin Exp Allergy* 28, 151 - 155 (1998).

[46] Barbee RA, Dodge R, Lebowitz ML, Burrows B. The epidemiology of asthma. *Chest* 87(1), 21S - 25S (1985).

[47] Sears MR, Greene JM, Willan AR, Et Al. A longitudinal population based cohort study of childhood asthma followed into adulthood. *N Engl J Med* 349(15), 1414 - 1422 (2003).

[48] Anderson HR, Pottier AC, Strachan DP. Asthma from birth to age 23: Incidence and relation to prior and concurrent atopic disease. *Thorax* 47(7), 537 - 542 (2004).

[49] Stein RT, Holberg CJ, Morgan WJ, Et Al. Peak flow variability, methacholine responsiveness and atopy as markers for detecting different wheezing phenotypes in childhood. *Thorax* 52(11), 946 - 952 (1997).

[50] Martinez FD, Helms PJ. Types of asthma and wheezing. *Eur Respir J* 27, 3s - 8s (1998).

[51] Tager IB, Ngo L, Hanrahan JP. Maternal smoking during pregnancy. Effects on lung function during the first 18 months of life. *Am J Respir Crit Care Med* 152(3), 977 - 983 (1995).

[52] Martinez FD, Morgan WJ, Wright AL, Holberg CJ, Taussig LM. Diminished lung function as a predisposing factor for wheezing respiratory illness in infants *N Engl J Med* 319, 1112 - 1117 (1988).

[53] Martinez FD. Sudden infant death syndrome and small airways occulsion. Facts and a hypothesis. *Pediatrics* 87(2), 190 - 198 (1991).

[54] Halonen M, Stern DA, Lohman C, Wright AL, Brown MA, Martinez FD. Two subphenotypes of childhood asthma that differ in maternal and paternal influences on asthma risk. *Am J Respir Crit Care Med* 160(2), 564 - 570 (1999).

[55] Moller C, Dreborg S, Ferdousi HA *et al.* Pollen immunotherapy reduces the development of asthma in children with seasonal rhinoconjunctivitis (the PAT study). *J Allergy Clin Immunol* 109, 251 - 256 (2002).

[56] Guerra S, Wright AL, Morgan WJ, Sherrill DL, Holberg CJ, Martinez FD. Persistence of asthma symptoms during adolsecent. Role of obesity and age at onset of puberty. *Am J Respir Crit Care Med* 170(1), 78 - 85 (2004).

[57] Burrows B, Martinez FD, Halonen M, Barbee RA, Cline MG. Associations with asthma with serum IgE levels and skin test reactivity to allergens. *N Engl J Med* 320, 271 - 277 (1989).

[58] Halonen M, Stern DA, Wright AL, Taussig LM, Martinez FD. Alternaria as a major allergen for asthma in children raised in a desert environment. *Am J Respir Crit Care Med* 155(4), 1356 - 1361 (1997).

[59] Peat JK, Tovey E, Toelle BG, Et Al. House dust mite allergens. A major risk factor for childhood asthma in Australia. *Am J Respir Crit Care Med* 153(1), 141 - 146 (1996).

[60] Green RH, Brightling CE, Mckenna S, Et Al. Asthma exacerbations and sputum eosinophil counts, a randomised controlled trial. *Lancet* 360, 1715 - 1721 (2002).

[61] Brightling CE, Bradding P, Symon FA, Et Al. Mast cell infiltration of airway smooth muscle in asthma. *N Engl J Med* 346, 1699 - 1705 (2002).

[62] Strachan DP, Butland BK, Anderson HR. Incidence and prognosis of asthma and wheezing illness from early chilhood to age 33 in a national British cohort. *BMJ* 312(7040), 1195 - 1199 (1996).

[63] Jenkins MA, Hopper JL, Bowes G, Carlin JB, Flander LB, Giles GG. Factors in childhood as predictors of asthma in early adult life. *BMJ* 309, 90 - 93 (1994).

[64] Williams H, Mcnicol KN. Prevalence, natural history and relationship of wheezy bronchitis and asthma in children. An epidemiological study. *BMJ* 4(5679), 321 - 325 (1969).

[65] Phelan PD. Asthma in children and adolescents: An overview. *London: Balliere Tindall* (1995).

[66] Fabbri LM, Romagnoli M, Corbetta L, Et Al. Differences in airway inflammation in patients with fixed airflow obstruction due to asthma or chronic obstructive pulmonary disease. *Am J Respir Crit Care Med* 167(3), 418 - 424 (2003).

[67] Van Den Toorn LM, Overbeek SE, De Jongste JC, Leman K, Hoogsteden HC, Prins JB. Airway inflammation is present during clinical remission of atopic astma. *Am J Respir Crit Care Med* 164, 2107 - 2113 (2001).

2

Bronchial Challenge Testing

Lutz Beckert and Kate Jones
University of Otago, Christchurch
New Zealand

1. Introduction

Airways hyper-responsiveness (AHR) is found in almost every patient with asthma. The degree of AHR is variable between individuals with asthma and can correlate to the severity of the underlying asthma. Equally treatment of asthma can modify the degree of underlying AHR. Measures of Airway hyper-responsiveness or bronchial challenge testing are therefore important in both the assessment and management of asthma.

The appraisal and assessment of the currently available bronchial challenge testing is hampered by the lack of a 'gold standard' for the diagnosis of asthma. In addition to basing this overview on published evidence, we are also integrating some our own research and clinical experience as clinicians and director of a respiratory physiology laboratory.

Some tests including the **direct challenge tests** with methacholine or histamine are highly sensitive; this makes them particularly useful to exclude a diagnosis of asthma. The disadvantage of these tests is a general lack of specificity. Although one is unlikely to miss asthma using these highly sensitive tests, the clinical importance of a positive test is not always clear. In addition, the methacholine challenge test may be positive in physiological scenarios which cause airways reactivity.

At times it is clinically more meaningful to choose a less sensitive but more specific test, which reflects the physiological airway response such as one of the **indirect challenge tests** for example; exercise challenge, hypertonic saline, adenosine or mannitol testing. These tests are particularly helpful if one wishes to assess the response to treatment. If asthma is well controlled these tests are often negative and are not useful in excluding asthma.

The performance of bronchial challenge testing requires adherence to international quality guidelines for the performance of spirometry and well trained staff. Most tests use a change in the FEV_1 by 200mls as the minimum cut-off, which reflects the historic belief that spirometry, (in particular FEV_1) is only reversible within 200mls; i.e. 200mls is thought to be the minimum standard of a coefficient variation of these tests. However, new equipment and the latest ERS / ATS guidelines suggest a variability of 150ml or even 100mls could be achieved. This becomes particularly important if one were to comment on trends within a series of tests.

Finally, as in any other clinical tests the risk benefit ratio needs to be considered. Although it may be interesting to know whether a patient with advanced COPD still has significant reversibility, a possible positive response to methacholine may cause distressing respiratory compromise. Challenge testing should not be performed if the baseline FEV_1 is less than 1.5 L or less than 60% of the predicted FEV_1. The expected response should also be taken into account when performing tests, particularly the methacholine challenge and eucapnic voluntary hyperventilation test can potentially cause significant changes in a susceptible airway. Many laboratories will only perform a eucapnic voluntary hyperventilation (EVH) test when other tests like hypertonic saline are negative, and a clinical suspicion of asthma persists.

2. History of challenge testing

Much of this chapter, actually much of this book, is devoted to preventing the smooth muscle cells contracting or maybe turning the process of altogether. Considering the mental energy spent controlling contraction of the airway smooth muscle cells and witnessing the, at times devastating clinical outcome may lead the clinician to relate to this metaphore of the airway smooth muscle cell described by Seow and Fredberg " … we might think of the airway smooth muscle as the Hell's Angels of cells, sitting on a Harley-Davidson, unshaven, a cigarette in one hand, a can of beer in the other, and a tattoo on its arm reading 'Born to Lose'" (Seow & Fredberg, 2001).

The same authors argue the airway smooth muscle cell, although first described in 1804, may not have a specific physiological function. It seems plausible that there is no explanation for the utility of airway smooth muscle. It is probably that during the ontological development of the lung from the foregut, some of the vestigial gut smooth muscle may have become displaced into the airway as an 'accident of nature' not fulfilling any useful function in the lung.

It was during the 1940's that Curry first reported a greater degree of bronchoconstriction to inhalation of histamine and methacholine in patients with asthma compared to those without asthma (Curry, 1947). In the same decade Tiffenaeu described the change in the airway using either histamine or methacholine by describing the provoking concentration (PC) to induce a 20% reduction in the FEV_1 (PC_{20}). (Tiffeaneu & Pinelli, 1947). From then onwards bronchial challenge testing started to make its way from a research tool into the clinical arena.

In 1987 Pauwels and colleagues proposed that bronchoprovocation tests could be divided into direct and indirect stimuli. Direct stimuli like methacholine, histamine, leukotrienes and prostaglandins act directly on the smooth muscle receptors. Indirect stimuli act through one or more intermediate pathways which cause a release of mediators from inflammatory cells and cause bronchial constriction. Many naturally occurring stimuli in asthma cause symptoms through indirect mechanisms and these tests may correlate better with clinical features of asthma. Indirect tests include exercise, hypertonic saline, adenosine monophosphate, eucapnic voluntary ventilation and mannitol.

The current Global Initiative for Asthma Guidelines (GINA) include these indirect challenges as a diagnostic and management tool because the response to these challenges is modified or even completely inhibited by inhaled steroids. The availability of dry powder mannitol capsules has the potential to bring challenge testing from the specialist laboratory to the patient bedside or more relevant the ambulatory setting.

3. Reversibility testing

Bronchodilator reversibility testing is clinically easier to perform and generally safer than bronchial challenge testing. Although the sensitivity is only approximately 50% to detect asthma, the specificity is approaching 90%. We have included a short description on reversibility testing in this chapter because depending on the clinical question, a positive bronchodilator response may make a bronchial challenge test redundant.

The bronchodilator response is complex and dependent on the interaction between airway epithelium, nerves and smooth muscle. The relationship between bronchoconstriction and bronchodilator response is not straightforward as the presence of one cannot guarantee the presence of the other. In general when performing reversibility testing the referrer is looking to answer one of the following questions:

1. Is there evidence of reversible airflow limitation?
2. Can the subjects' lung function be improved by the addition of a bronchodilator?

3.1 Methods

The ERS/ATS consensus guidelines (Pellegrino 2005) suggest that prior to giving a bronchodilator, baseline spirometric measurements are taken including FEV_1, FVC and PEFR. After baseline measurement, 400mcg salbutamol or 160mcg ipatropium is given via a spacer in four divided doses at 30 second intervals. Spirometry is then repeated after 10-15 minutes if using a short acting beta agonist or 30 minutes if using a short acting anticholinergic drug.

When testing is being performed to assess for the presence of a possible therapeutic benefit, then it is suggested that the subjects' usual drug, dose and mode of delivery is used. The class of drug, dose and mode of delivery vary widely. The repeat testing should be performed according to the time of the reported drugs onset of activity.

Nebulised bronchodilators are sometimes used in reversibility testing however there are a number of issues surrounding their use. The administered dose can vary widely depending on rate and output, particle size, distribution and concentration, respiratory rate, and inspiratory to expiratory ratio. The administration of bronchodilators without nebuliser or spacer is not recommended as in general the respirable fraction is low and heavily technique dependent (Pellegrino 2005). Spacers are preferred because of the reduced risk of aerosol generation of infected particles.

3.2 What defines a positive response?

Current ATS/ERS guidelines use an increase in FEV_1 and/or FVC (not due to an increased expiratory time) of 12% **and** 200ml as being suggestive of significant bronchodilatation.

The definitions of significant reversibility vary surprisingly widely in standard consensus guidelines. For example the British NICE COPD guidelines suggest that significant reversibility suggestive of asthma is achieved with a change in the FEV_1 of 400ml (NICE COPD guidelines 2010) Many studies have investigated the appropriate cut-off for significant reversibility. The choice of cut-points needs to balance the chance of an event occurring by random variation; the co-efficient of variant of the measurement has its upper limits approaching 8% or 150ml. Even if bronchodilator testing is positive it may not infer a symptomatic improvement or proof of a diagnosis of asthma as increasingly it is recognised that other pathological processes including COPD can result in significant bronchodilator reversibility.

Our own research suggests that the ATS / ERS definition is sensitive, meaning that significant bronchodilation is unlikely to be missed. It does however come at the cost of reduced specificity. If one were to use mid-flow parameters like the FEF_{25-75} or even the volume based standard FEV_{25-75}, the co-efficient of variation is significantly reduced and this improves the positive predictive value (Swanney 2003). Most of these parameters are measured routinely by the software of modern electronic spirometers, therefore making them easy to measure and apply. However, clinical experience with these new parameters is lacking.

The lack of a bronchodilator response should not be used to withhold the use of this class of agent in clinical practice as they may still produce a clinical response including improved symptoms and performance. If it is clinically important to accurately determine the response then referral for bronchial challenge testing should be considered.

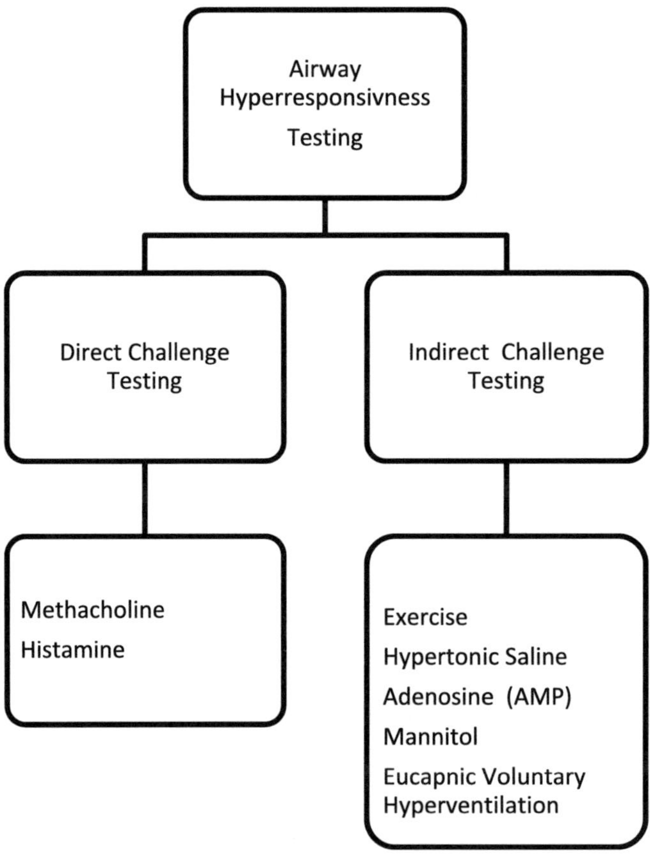

Fig. 1. Diagram of direct and indirect challenge testing

4. Direct bronchial challenge testing

In 1987, Pauwels distinguished bronchial challenges for AHR into direct and indirect testing (Pauwels et al., 1988). Direct stimuli act on the airways smooth muscle causing contraction. Indirect stimuli act via the inflammatory cells within the airway.The two main components of AHR are persistent and variable (O'Byrne et al., 2009). The persistent component consists of the anatomical and structural changes including airway remodelling and smooth muscle hypertrophy. The variable component is thought to be related to external or environmental influences and the subsequent inflammatory process involving mast cells and eosinophils. These processes are not independent. We know that over time, persisting airways inflammation contributes to structural changes within the airway (Grainge et al., 2011).

4.1 Use in the diagnosis of asthma?

In our experience, the main clinical utility of direct challenge testing is to exclude asthma. The direct challenge tests stimulate the airway smooth muscle cell directly and have significant negative predictive power for the diagnosis of asthma; i.e. almost all patients who are asthmatic will have a positive test. The most commonly used direct stimuli are histamine and methacholine. As they act directly on the smooth muscle it is thought that their effects are predominantly via the persistent or structural changes associated with AHR.

In contrast, indirect challenge tests exert their effect through inflammatory cells, epithelial cells and bronchial nerves, which release mediators like leukotrienes or interleukins subsequently resulting in bronchial smooth muscle constriction. Indirect challenges may therefore reflect the degree of bronchial hyper responsiveness and the effect of treatment more accurately (Jooes et al., 2003).

4.2 Methacholine challenge testing

Methacholine challenge testing (MCT) is a type of direct bronchial challenge testing. Methacholine is a muscarinic agonist. In our experience, the MCT is a sensitive test with high negative predictive value, better for ruling asthma out rather than ruling it in. The MCT has its maximal diagnostic content in those patients with a pre-test probability of asthma i.e. between 48-70%. (Perpina, 1993). One of the difficulties with the MCT is its poor positive predictive value. It is difficult to determine the false negative response rate as there is a wide variability in the literature of the definition of "current asthma symptoms". This necessitates the need to remain open to idea of repeating the test or escalation to other forms of bronchial challenge testing if the clinical suspicion remains high.

Methacholine powder with Food and Drug Administration (FDA) certification validating it for human use and purity should be used. The two most common methods published by Crapo et al (Crapo et al., 2000) and Cockcroft (Cockcroft, 1977) which involves tidal breathing and inhalation of an aerosol from a nebuliser at an output of 0.13 mL/min. The other method is the dosimeter method (Chai, 1975) which involves inhalation of an aerosol with 5 breaths to TLC with a 5 second breath hold for each. Otherwise the methods are the same with saline as control and doubling of concentrations from 0.03mg/mL to 16mg/mL and 5 minutes between each inhalation. The FEV_1 is measured at 30 and 90 seconds after completed inhalation. The percentage decline in FEV_1 is calculated and the test is stopped when a drop of 20% in FEV_1 occurs, or the highest concentration is administered. The PC20 can be calculated from a log concentration vs. dose response curve.

The two methods were previously believed to give similar results based on a single study with small numbers using histamine. More recently it has been shown that the tidal breathing method can produce a lower PC20. The reasons for this are thought to be a combination of a greater dose with the tidal breathing method and the potential for the 5 breath hold method to produce bronchodilatation in subjects with mild AHR to methacholine (Allen, 2005).

A number of contraindications to methacholine challenge test exist. According to the ATS guidelines the following are considered to be absolute contraindications; severe airflow obstruction with FEV_1 <50% or 1L (this is controversial and varies within the literature from 60% to 80% predicted), myocardial infarction or stroke within 3 months of testing, uncontrolled hypertension or aortic aneurysm. Relative contraindications include an FEV_1 <60% or <1.5L, the inability to perform adequate spirometry, pregnancy or current breastfeeding and the current use of cholinesterase inhibitor for myasthenia gravis.

Methacholine testing should only be performed by trained staff in an appropiately equipped Bronchial Challenge Laboratory. Serious side-effects of MCT are rare. Transient symptoms such as wheeze, cough, and dyspnoea are reported. Very rarely death after Methacholine exposure has been reported. (Becker, 2001)

There are a number of other factors which can lead to an increase in AHR and therefore false positive MCT. These factors include exposure to environmental antigens, occupational or environmental sensitizers, respiratory tract infection, allergic rhinitis and smoking related lung disease. In general the MCT has a poor positive predictive value.

Conversely, there are other agents which can reduce airways hyper reactivity, therefore potentially giving a false negative result. On the whole this is not as great an issue as that of false positives. The negative predictive value exceeds 90% when the pre-test probability of asthma is 30-70%. If the patient has current symptoms present over the previous 2 weeks and the MCT is negative, one can be fairly confident in ruling out asthma as the diagnosis. Agents which can modify the result of the MCT include oral or inhaled bronchodilators such as cromolyn sodium, necrodomil, hydralazine, cetirizine and leuktriene modifiers. In addition some foods can reduce bronchial hyper reactivity including coffee, tea, cola and chocolate. Inhaled or systemic corticosteroids can modify the effect of MCT, however in general it is not necessary to stop them prior to MCT. (Crapo 2000).

The MCT does have a number of other limitations which should be considered when interpreting the result. As it is a direct challenge test, it is predominantly testing the smooth muscle contraction and fixed component related to airways remodelling. This is highly likely to relate to the chronicity of the problem and may therefore be absent in those with recent onset of their disease or alternatively in those with chronic asthma and fixed airflow obstruction with airways remodelling. AHR can also have significant variability within a subject. This is important to acknowledge, particularly in children where the presence of a negative direct bronchial challenge may be heavily dependent on recent exposures.

There are other factors that need to be taken into consideration when interpreting the MCT; firstly the pre-test probability, the interpretation of the results may be different depending on whether you are screening an asymptomatic population or testing on the basis of symptoms. Other important issues include the presence or absence of any post-test symptoms and the degree of recovery in symptoms and lung function after bronchodilator is given.

The cut-points for a positive test have been chosen to produce the highest sensitivity. Initially the cut point was set at 8mg/mL (Cockcroft et al., 1985 & Cockcroft, 1977). This produces a very high sensitivity, however the specificity was lower with a large number of positives in patients with rhinitis and up to 5% of asymptomatic individuals. This has now been modified to include the 4-16mg/mL as a borderline positive result. At a level of 16mg/mL up to 20% of asymptomatic people from a random population will have a positive test (Cockcroft, 1992). The best PC20 cut point to give highest positive and negative predictive values based on ROC curve analysis is 8-16mg/ml.

The ATS guidelines suggest that in the presence of no baseline airways obstruction a PC20 greater than 16mg/ml should be considered normal, values between 4-16 indicate a borderline response and should be interpreted in the light of the clinical history and pre-test probability as above, between 1-4mg/ml indicates mild AHR and PC20 of less than 1mg/ml demonstrates moderate to severe AHR.

For example, if the PC20 is less than 1mg/ml and the pre-test probability is high then you can be relatively confident of a diagnosis of asthma. However if there is a low pre test probability and PC20 is between 1-16mg/ml then the interpretation is less clear. Options would include poor perception of symptoms, other causes of AHR, a subject who has never previously been exposed to triggers, or a number of individuals with subclinical disease who may go on to develop asthma in the future.

It is difficult to interpret a positive MCT when the baseline spirometry is abnormal or demonstrates significant airflow obstruction and in the presence of a positive bronchodilator challenge. In these situations MCT may be inappropriate and unnecessary.

Many patients with COPD and fixed airflow obstruction will have a positive MCT but no asthma symptoms and no bronchodilator response. These two diseases are best differentiated on the basis of the clinical history including patient age, smoking history, allergies and triggers.

4.3 Histamine challenge

In the 1940's it was first observed that histamine had the potential to induce bronchoconstriction; it has been used in laboratories since the 1960s. It was the use of histamine by Tiffeneau in 1947, who introduced the concept of incrementally increasing the provoking dose in order to induce a 20% reduction in the FEV_1. As discussed, one of the main limitations of direct tests is that a positive response is not necessarily specific for identifying asthma and can occur in healthy people with no symptoms, smokers and in the presence of a number of other lung diseases. A recent article in the NEJM suggests that we need to keep an open mind regarding the role of airways remodelling rather than airways inflammation as a cause of asthma symptoms (Grainge 2011). The authors used the direct challenge agent, Methacholine, to induce bronchoconstriction because it doesn't cause airway inflammation or eosinophilia. They even went to the lengths of taking bronchial biopsies to show the absence of inflammation but there is still evidence of airway remodelling and increased mucus production. The clinical implications are wide; it raised the possibility of airway remodelling secondary to airway injury after a chronic cough and the importance of addressing bronchial constriction in addition to inflammation. It may ultimately lead to new therapeutic approaches, bearing in mind that anti-inflammatory treatment has not been shown to modify the natural history of lung function changes in prospective studies (Guilbert 2006).

Practically, methacholine and histamine have a very similar action on the airway smooth muscle. By chance they can even be used in equivalent doses to cause an effect on the airway. Histamine acts not only on airway smooth muscle, but also on sensory fibres in the airway. So although it is classified as a direct stimulus it may actually have some of its effects via an indirect pathway. Histamine is associated with more flushing and systemic side effects.

Many laboratories prefer the use of methacholine over histamine for the lack of these systemic reactions, if they wish to perform a direct bronchial challenge test. Others continue to use histamine as they are familiar with its use. Histamine is not licensed as a medical product in all countries, in particular the United States.

5. Indirect challenge testing

5.1 Overview of indirect challenge testing

A number of indirect stimuli are also used to detect airways hyper-responsiveness including exercise challenge, hypertonic saline, adenosine monophosphate (AMP), mannitol, and eucapnic voluntary hyperventilation. Exercise testing was the first standardized indirect bronchial challenge test. Following this, there has been an increase in the use of osmotic agents such as hypertonic saline and mannitol, stemming from the theory that exercise induced bronchoconstriction (EIB) is induced by an increase in airways osmolarity.

These agents act indirectly on smooth muscle via the existing inflammatory cells in the airway causing release of inflammatory mediators such as histamine, leukotrienes and prostaglandins. AMP also acts by direct stimulation of mast cells in an IgE independent fashion. They result in smooth muscle contraction and consequently reduction in airway calibre.

Indirect tests are felt to be more physiological and clinically relevant than direct testing as they stimulate both neural and inflammatory pathways. Most asthma stimuli in 'real life' are more likely to be indirect than direct stimuli; the bronchoconstricting effect of endogenous mediators like prostaglandins or leukotrienes display a stronger effect on the smooth muscle than methacholine or histamine. The presence of a positive indirect test infers the presence of inflammation, and an airway which is responsive to inflammatory mediators. AHR to indirect tests tends to improve or resolve with the use of inhaled corticosteroids (ICS). This implies that an improvement in airways inflammation leads to subsequent benefits in the variable component of AHR. Although a positive indirect challenge test infers the presence of airways inflammation and a positive response to ICS, this is not always due to eosinophilic inflammation as mast cells are often also important in the pathogenesis. Many indirect tests are dose limited, meaning the dose cannot be increased any further due to the inherent limits of the test such as the solubility of AMP or the physiological limits of an individual for exercise.

Other uses of indirect stimuli are in those individuals who present with diagnostic uncertainty and have ongoing symptoms whilst taking ICS. If the indirect test is positive it confirms the presence of ongoing active inflammation with asthma. In contrast a negative test may indicate that either their asthma is not currently active at the time, or an alternative diagnosis should be considered.

5.1.1 Guide to therapy?

We know that AHR in response to indirect testing decreases and can resolve after the use of inhaled corticosteroids (ICS), in contrast to direct testing. EIB also improves after use of ICS (Koh 2007). The degree of AHR to indirect stimuli correlates with the degree of airways inflammation. For example, the numbers of eosinophils and mast cells present in the airway. These markers of airways inflammation are in turn known to reduce in number with the use of ICS. Therefore indirect bronchial challenge testing can be used as a meaningful measure to assess control of airways inflammation and could potentially be used as a tool in clinical decision making regarding ICS dose. Tests including fraction of exhaled nitric oxide (fENO) and sputum eosinophils have been used as measures of ongoing airways inflammation in eosinophilic asthma. Indirect tests of AHR have the advantage that they can be used in all phenotypes of asthma as AHR to indirect stimuli has been shown to be present in non-eosinophilic asthma when fENO may be normal. This observation suggests the involvement of mast cells amongst others in non-eosinophilic asthma.

5.2 Exercise challenge testing

Exercise challenge testing is one of the oldest forms of challenge testing, with the intention of reproducing the physiological response of the airways during exercise. Exercise causes airway narrowing in the majority of patients with asthma. It is generally believed that exercise related hyperventilation causes a drying of airway mucosa, thereby creating a hypertonic environment which in turn leads to airways bronchoconstriction (Crapo 1999) . Clinically this is of particular relevance to people who have to perform demanding or even life saving work in adverse conditions like police persons, military personal, CUBA divers or fire fighters. This is also of concern in athletes, and tends to be aggravated in people exercising in cold environments, particularly cross country skiing or ice-skating.

5.2.1 Indications

Exercise testing is particularly useful in patients with a history of exercise induced symptoms. In our experience exercise testing is more useful in people who perform recreational exercise rather than high performance athletes. These tests are intuitive for the patient, and don't need expensive equipment or administration of medication.

5.2.2 Methods

Whilst several protocols exist, the most widely accepted protocol is based on the Guidelines for Methacholine and Exercise Challenge Testing, produced by the ATS in 1999. The guiding principle is to create a degree of hyperventilation by pushing the participants quickly to perform high cardiac output exercise. This is classically done on a treadmill or exercise bike with the aim of achieving 80 - 90% of the maximal heart rate in 4 - 6 minutes (Crapo 2000).

The heart rate is normally monitored through an ECG or pulse oximetry and the test is stopped when the patient has achieved 80 - 90% of the maximal cardiac output. However although the end of test criteria is dependent on heart rate, the respiratory rate is also very important. Some protocols suggest measuring the respiratory rate aiming for 40 - 50% of the maximal calculated respiratory rate. It is equally feasible to allow the athlete to perform his or her usual exercise, like swimming, canoeing or track running. Since the aim of the asthma exercise testing is to create hyperventilation, protocols designed for cardiac testing, like the Bruce protocol, are not meaningful in this setting.

The principle outcome variable of exercise testing is the FEV_1. Baseline spirometry should be performed prior to exercise, not during testing and then at 5, 10, 15, 20 and 30 minutes post exercise. This is important as a significant percentage of patients have a late reaction to exercise with a significant fall in their FEV_1. The criteria for a positive response has been extensively discussed. While most laboratories have now adopted greater than 10 % from baseline to be abnormal, a fall of 15% appears to be more diagnostic of exercise induced bronchospasm (Crapo 2000).

The contraindications to exercise testing are similar to those for other forms of challenge testing, in particular a low baseline FEV_1 of less than 60% and less than 1.5L. In addition patients with unstable cardiac ischemia or malignant arrhythmias should not be tested. Patients with orthopaedic limitation are not likely to achieve exercise ventilation high enough to elicit airway narrowing. Bronchodilator medication should be withheld up to 48 hours prior to testing.

High performance athletes often find it difficult to reach a high degree of cardiac output and hyperventilation under laboratory conditions, particularly when an exercise bike is used. In our experience with elite athletes, although the clinical utility of this test is meaningful when the test is positive, the sensitivity is not high. False negative exercise tests have been reported in patients who are in a stable phase, patients who are on treatment and also athletes who clearly do have airway related problems at high performance but don't reach a state of hyperventilation under laboratory conditions.

5.3 Hypertonic saline testing

Hypertonic saline testing (HTS) was developed to establish whether EIB was caused by an increase in osmolarity of the airway surface liquid when humidifying large volumes of dry air during a period of exercise.

5.3.1 Methods

A high-output ultrasonic nebuliser of hypertonic saline is delivered for progressively longer intervals from 0.5 up to 8 minutes. The ultrasonic nebuliser integrates analog devices to control ultrasonic nebulisation. An oscillator develops electrical power, which is transmitted to a transducer in the nebuliser chamber. When energised by the high frequency electrical signals (approximately 1.63 MHZ), the transducer changes its thickness, oscillating at the frequency of the applied voltage. This results in an energy transfer between the transducer and the liquid in the chamber, causing the liquid to be nebulised into minute droplets.

The patient is asked to inhale the fine hypertonic saline mist through a mouth piece (a towel is provided) for 30 seconds. You must ensure the output setting and airflow of the nebuliser is set to maximum. Nebulisation is stopped and two spirometry manoeuvres are performed. If no significant fall in the FEV_1 has been detected further hypertonic saline is nebulised. The exposure time doubles at each level: 30secs, 1min, 2mins, 4mins, 8mins.

The test is positive when the patient demonstrates a 15% reduction in FEV_1. The test should be stopped when the patient has had a total exposure time of 15.5 minutes and >20 g saline has been delivered.

The major indications for using hypertonic aerosols are to identify bronchial hyper-responsiveness consistent with active asthma or exercise-induced asthma and to evaluate bronchial responsiveness that will respond to treatment with anti-inflammatory drugs. In a study by Riedler (1994), children with a history of current wheeze were seven times more likely to have a positive response to hypertonic saline than asymptomatic children. In an occupational study in people responding positively to the question "have you ever had an attack of asthma" the mean percentage fall in FEV_1 was 17.6% compared with 5.8% for those who responded negatively. From the evidence to date, it would appear that bronchial responsiveness to a hypertonic aerosol is consistent with an asthma diagnosis.

A challenge with a hypertonic aerosol can be used in the assessment of a patient with a past history of asthma that wishes to join the armed forces. The hypertonic saline test has become the test of choice in some states in Australia. A positive test confirms the suspicion of asthma. If the test becomes negative with appropriate anti-inflammatory treatment it also confirms that the airways disease can be controlled and applicants are not discriminated against.

An interesting variant highlighted by the ERS task force report is that the hypertonic saline challenge may play a particular role in assessing people with chronic cough. Hypertonic saline may prove the presence of asthma by causing a fall in the FEV_1. It may also provoke excessive cough in the absence of airway narrowing and indicate that the cough is not due to asthma but a different airway mechanism (Joos et al., 2003).

The benefit of HTS when compared to exercise testing is the ability to also collect sputum for analysis. The PD20 to HTS after 6 weeks of ICS reflects the percentage of airways mast cells and sputum eosinophilia. (Gibson, et al., 2000).

Finally, testing with hypertonic saline may by the agent of choice if a bronchial challenge is indicated during pregnancy.

5.4 Adenosine (AMP) challenge testing

Unlike the previous indirect challenges mentioned, the mode of action for the inhaled AMP challenge is not osmotic. When inhaled, AMP quickly dephosphorylates into adenosine causing mast cells to degranulate and release histamine and leukotrienes, which have a potent effect on bronchoconstriction.

AMP is prepared for inhalation by mixing AMP with a phosphate-buffered solution. It is administered by doubling concentration doses within the range of 0.09 to 800 mg/mL. The doubling concentrations of AMP are delivered to the participant via nebulizer for 2 minutes with spirometric measurement every two minutes until a 20% fall in FEV_1 is recorded.

AMP may provide a good demonstration of airway inflammation based on sputum eosinophils. AMP is cheap and may be a good way to monitor inflammation. It can also cause sputum eosinophilia within 1 hour of the challenge. An inflammatory response after the AMP challenge could present a problem and needs to be considered before using the AMP challenge as a diagnostic tool. AMP is not widely licensed around the world. (Mohsenin &Blackburn, 2006)

It has been shown that mannitol produces results similar to those from the AMP challenge in terms of airway hyper-responsiveness and recovery time without airway eosinophilia and may potentially replace adenosine testing in the future.

5.5 Mannitol testing

The Mannitol challenge test was developed in an attempt to imitate the physiological response to exercise by creating a hypertonic airway environment but avoiding the inherent limitations of exercise testing and allowing testing to leave the specialised laboratory to become a point of care test. Mannitol is a natural sugar which is not normally absorbed in the airways and slowly causes an increasingly hypertonic environment. In susceptible subjects, it induces bronchoconstriction. (Anderson et al., 1997)

Mannitol testing has been well researched, has excellent data available and is a commercially available product. Mannitol testing is leaving the research environment and lung function laboratories and entering the clinical arena. Laboratories that work with mannitol have found it easy to use and in general patients report finding it acceptable. Some patients are not able to tolerate testing with mannitol due to significant coughing (Anderson 2010).

5.5.1 Methods

As in other challenge test, mannitol challenge should also not be performed if the FEV_1 is less than 60% of the predicted value. Using the dry powder capsule and the inhaler device which is part of the Bronchial Challenge Test Kit (aridol™, Pharmaxis Ltd, Frechs Forest, Australia) the participant is asked to inhale an escalating dose of Mannitol. The typical regime is an inhalation of 5mg, 10mg, 20mg, 40mg, 80mg, 160mg, 160mg and 160mg of mannitol leading to a total cumulative dose of 635mg. The FEV_1 is measured 60 seconds after inhalation.

A test is positive if the FEV_1 falls more than 15% from baseline or the FEV_1 falls more than 10% between two incremental does of mannitol. The test is negative when no significant fall, i.e. a fall of less than 15% from baseline, has been observed after 635mg of mannitol has been administered.

The limitations of the mannitol test are related to the availability of the medications, and also the response from the patients. Since mannitol testing is a form of indirect testing by monitoring a physiological response, it can be negative in patients with well-controlled asthma. This feature can be used clinically, as a mannitol challenge test, similar to an exercise, and hypertonic saline challenge test can be negative in patients whose asthma is very well controlled. If a clinical suspicion of exercise induced asthma persists then performance of the Eucapnic Hyperventilation Test should be considered.

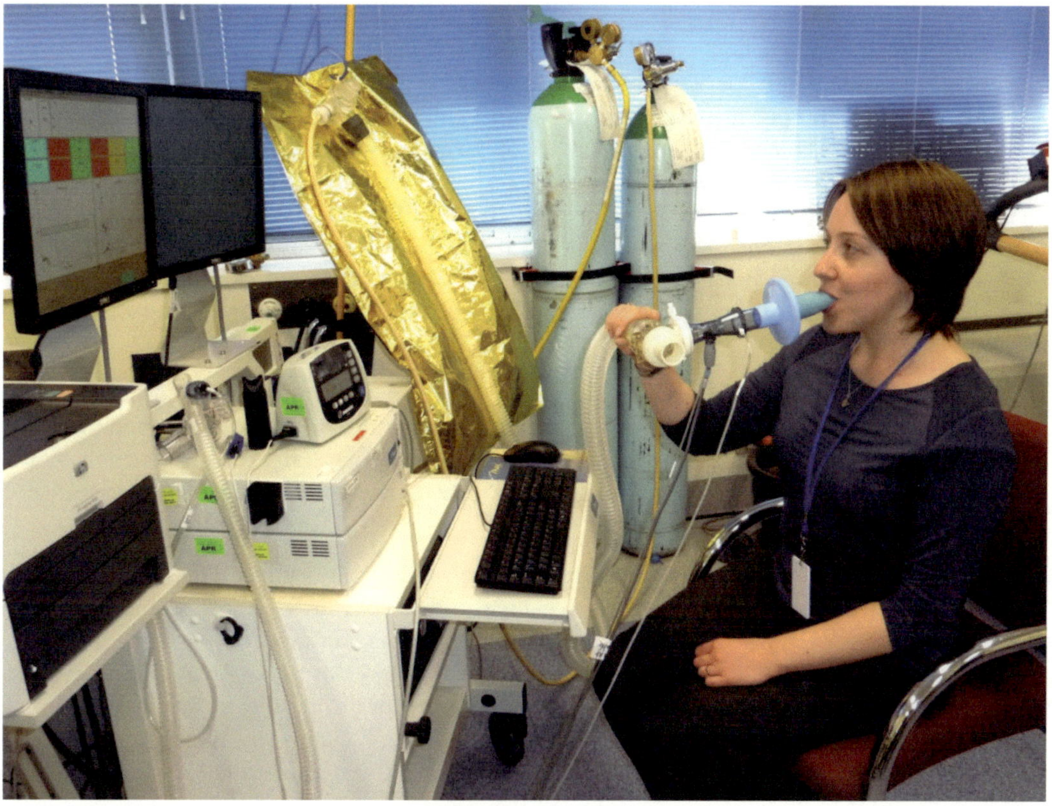

Picture 1. Eucapnic Voluntary Hyperventilation testing

Picture showing the setup for Eucapnic Voluntary Hyperventilation. In the background is a gas cylinder with 5% CO2 and 21 % O2 balanced with N2, a large, (golden), non-diffusing gas bag and a two way non-rebreathing valve. The patient is instructed to actively hyperventilate through the mouthpiece inhaling the balanced gas mixture for six minutes.

5.6 Eucapnic Voluntary Hyperventilation

This test has been developed as a physiological test to assess the airways response to exercise. During episodes of hyperventilation the airways mucosa can dry out, creating a hypertonic environment. In exercise challenge testing this is often limited by the inability to reach an appropriate level of hyperventilation, as exercise is usually cardiac limited, however we are looking for the respiratory stimulus. We have previously discussed the role of hypertonic saline testing and mannitol testing which use different methods to mimic this response. Normal hyperventilation is limited by the development of hypocapnoea which can cause significant dizziness, neurological symptoms and syncope. Bronchial provocation testing using eucapnic voluntary hyperventilation came into favour when it was realised that exercise is not needed to achieve high respiratory rates. The possible side effects of hyperventilation were counteracted with the addition of 4.9% Carbon dioxide (Philllips, et al., 1985).

5.6.1 Method

The eucapnic voluntary hyperventilation test allows significant hyperventilation at a rate of approximately 30 - 60 per minute. The rate to be achieved can be calculated assessing 30 x FEV_1 or .85 x MVV, whichever is greater. Using a large, non-diffusing gas bag filled with 5% CO2 and 21 % O2 balanced with N2, and a two way non-rebreathing valve the patient is instructed to actively hyperventilate through the mouthpiece inhaling the balanced gas mixture. The patient is encouraged to maintain this hyperventilation for six minutes. The FEV_1 is measured immediately after the end of test (two manoeuvres within 150ml), and then at 5, 10, 15 and 20 minutes. The test is positive if the FEV_1 falls more than 10% from the baseline.

Although the test is relatively easy to set up, responses can be very profound with reductions in FEV_1 in excess of 50% after only a minute of hyperventilation. Cardio-respiratory emergencies have been described. Given the potentially strong reaction to the EVH, it is common to only perform an EVH test, if the participant has a negative hypertonic saline or methacholine challenge test.

This test has been shown to be particularly useful if a high clinical suspicion of EIB persists despite negative simple challenge tests like hypertonic saline or methacholine challenge. In the setting where asthma needs to be excluded, for example amongst commercial divers or where asthma persists and patients wish to continue taking asthma medication, for example in elite athletes during competition, the eucapnic voluntary hyperventilation may be a simple, elegant and useful tool. After careful consent has been obtained, the patient is instructed to hyperventilate whilst carbon dioxide is added and removed in order to maintain a eucapnic environment.

The eucapnic voluntary hyperventilation test is usually restricted to tertiary laboratories given the need for balanced gas mixture and resuscitation equipment. One limitation of EVH is that it can be modified by the use of certain agents used in asthma management. Athletes therefore may need to stop their asthma medication prior to performance of a eucapnic hyperventilation test which may interfere with their training schedule. Because EVH has demonstrated high sensitivity it is currently the IOC Medical Commission-recommended challenge to identify EIB among Olympic athletes (Rundell & Slee, 2008).

6. Summary and clinical vignettes

The choice of bronchial challenge test will be determined by a number of factors including the physicians experience, the skill set in the local laboratory and also by emerging evidence. Evidence on the best use of bronchial challenge testing is still emerging, highlighted by some more recent publications (Grainge 2011). A very important aspect when choosing a challenge test is the patients medical background and the specific clinical question being asked.

In this last section we outline some clinical vignettes which focus on the choice and interpretation of bronchial challenge testing. These are based as much on our clinical experience as on evidence and certainly remain open for interpretation. If these clinical vignettes inspire discussion and debate we would be delighted and we will endeavour to engage in correspondence. We also accept that our approach may change as new evidence comes to light.

Chest tightness in a runner

A 24 year-old female presents to respiratory outpatients with 9 months of paroxysmal exertional dyspnoea and chest tightness. She is a competitive marathon runner and her symptoms are only present after running over 10km. She has been given a clinical diagnosis of asthma and prescribed inhaled corticosteroids and sodium chromoglycate with little effect. How would you further investigate her?

The assessment of exercise induced asthma in elite athletes can pose some difficulties and it is known that symptoms often correlate poorly with the results of challenge testing. The use of clinical exercise testing is of high specificity but only moderate sensitivity due to the frequent inability of available testing protocols to achieve adequate workload to induce symptoms. The current test of choice by the international Olympic committee's medical commission (IOC-MC) is eucapnic voluntary hyperventilation (EVH) (Fitch et al 2008). The advantage of EVH is the increased ability to achieve minute ventilation of a magnitude equivalent or in excess of that obtained at extreme levels of exercise. Other options in centres where EVH may not be available would include the use of a "field exercise challenge" or an indirect challenge tests such as hypertonic saline or mannitol. In the event of these tests being negative with ongoing symptoms, supervised withdrawal of her current inhaled medications could be considered prior to repeating the testing.

Shortness of breath after treated sleep apnoea

A 45 year old man is referred from the sleep unit. After successful treatment for sleep apnoea he increased his activity levels and noticed wheezing and shortness of breath on exercise. His current body mass index is 45; he is planning on losing weight and wonders if he can improve his exercise tolerance with asthma treatment.

Shortness of breath in an obese person is a common problem. The additional load on the upper airway, which already has the highest resistance, can cause airway narrowing and exertional wheeze. However fat tissue itself also releases pro-inflammatory cytokines which can cause airways inflammation in susceptible subjects. Spirometry can be helpful as it may show a restrictive pattern. In that case measurement of the total lung capacity is frequently reduced, with a marginally reduced DLCO but well maintained and often high kCO. If spirometry shows an obstructive pattern the test of choice here would be a direct test, like methacholine challenge test. If no other clinical features are suggestive of asthma besides wheeze on exercise, a negative methacholine test would exclude asthma and the patient could be reassured to continue exercising and attempting to lose weight, which will ultimately improve his respiratory function.

Chronic cough in a never smoker

A 55 year-old female who has never smoked, presents with a 3 year history of chronic cough, worse at night.. There are no symptoms of breathlessness, wheeze, gastro-oesophageal reflux or nasal drip. She is worried about the possibility of underlying asthma.

In the first instance baseline spirometry with reversibility testing may be useful if positive due its high specificity. If the reversibility testing was negative, given the intermediate pre-test probability of asthma a direct challenge test could be considered. If a methacholine challenge test was negative this could be helpful in ruling out asthma as the cause of her cough. Many excellent guidelines are available to help the physician to investigate chronic cough. The evidence based Australian cough guidelines suggest that the most remediable causes which respond well to specific treatment include protracted bacterial bronchitis, angiotensin-converting enzyme inhibitor use, asthma, GORD, obstructive sleep apnoea and eosinophilic bronchitis (Gibson 2010).

Asthma in a police recruit

A 21 year old man comes to see you after applying for the police force. In the screening questionnaire he answered that he'd had mild asthma since early childhood. He has always taken a small dose of inhaled corticosteroids and his asthma has never caused him to miss any school, wake him at night, or have any unscheduled visits to medical facilities. He has been successful in competitive sports.

This is a frequent question in a respiratory laboratory and the choice of test may be influenced by the regulatory authorities. From a patient advocate point of view a direct challenge test with methacholine for example would only confirm that he indeed has asthma. Several medical examiners within the armed forces request indirect testing either with mannitol or hypertonic saline. If he did have asthma and it was poorly controlled, he would demonstrate a fall in his FEV1 indicating a positive test. However even if he did have underlying asthma and it was well controlled, no fall in the FEV1 would be shown. This is seen by medical examiners as reassuring that his asthma would be well controlled (or absent) and he will not be discriminated against during the selection process.

7. Conflict of interest

The authors have no conflict of interest to declare.

8. References

Allen, N.D, Davis, B.E, Hurst, T., Cockcroft, D.W. (2005) Difference between Dosimeter and Tidal Breathing Methacholine Challenge. Contributions of dose and Deep Inspiration Bronchoprotection. *Chest* 128 (6): 4018-4023

Anderson, S.D., Brannan, J., Spring, J., Spalding, N., Rodwell, L.T., Chan K., Gonda, I., Walsh, A., Clark, A.R. (1997). A new method for bronchial provocation testing in asthmatic subjects using a dry powder of mannitol. *Am J Respir Crit Care Med* 156 (3Pt 1):758-765)

Anderson, S. D. (2010). Indirect Challenge Tests: Airway Hyperresponsiveness in asthma: Its measurement and clinical significance. *Chest* 138 (2)(Suppl):25S-30S

Becker , L.C. (2001). Report of internal investigation into the death of a volunteer research subject, www.hopkinsmedicine.org/press/2001/july/report_of_internal_investigation.htm. (accessed 5 August 2011.)

Chai, H., Farr, R.S., Froehlich, L.A., Mathison, D.A., McLean, J.A., Rosenthal, R.R., Sheffer, A.L., Spector, S.L., Townley, R.G. (1975) Standardization of bronchial inhalation challenge procedures. *J Allergy Clin Immunol.* 56 (4); 323-327

Cockcroft, D.W., Killian, D.N., Mellon, J.J., Hargreave, F.E. (1977) Bronchial reactivity to inhaled histamine: a method and clinical survey. *Clin Allergy* (3); 235-243).

Cockcroft DW. (1985) Bronchial inhalation tests. I. Measurement of non-allergic bronchial responsiveness. *Review Ann Allergy. 55(4):527-34..*

Cockcroft, D.W., Murdock, K.Y., Berschied, B.A., Gore, B.P. (1992) Sensitivity and specificity of histamine PC20 determination in a random selection of young college students. *J Allergy Clin Immunol* 89: 23-30).

Crapo, R.O., Casaburi, R., Coates, A.L., Enright, P.L., Hankinson, J.L. Irvin, C.G., MacIntyre, N.R., McKay, R.T., Wanger, J.S., Anderson, S.J., Cockcroft, D.W., Fish, J.E., Sterk, P.J. (2000) Guidelines for methacholine and exercise challenge testing - 1999. The official statement of the American Thoracic Society was adopted by the ATS Board of Directors, July 1999. *Am J Respir Crit Care Med* 161 (1): 309-329)

Curry, J.J. (1947) Comparative action of acetyl-B-methy choline and histamine on the respiratory tract in normals, patients with hay fever, and subjects with bronchial asthma. *J Clin Invest.* 26(3):430-438.

Fitch, KD, Sue-Chu, M, Anderson, SD, Boulet, L-P, Hancox, RJ, Mckenzie, DC, Backer, V, Rundell KW, Alonso, JM, Kippelen, P, Cummiskey, JM, Garnier, A, Ljungqvist, A. Asthma and the elite athlete: Summary of the International Olympic Committee's Consensus Conference, Lausann, Switzerland, Jan 22-24, 2008. J. Allergy. Clin Immunol 122: 254-260

Gibson, P.G., Saltos, N., Borgas, T. (2000) Airway mast cells and eosinophils correlate with clinical severity and airway hyperresponsiveness in corticosteroid-treated asthma. *J Allergy Clin Immunol.* 105(4):752-759

Gibson PG, Chang AB , Glasgow NJ , Holmes PW, Katelaris P, Kemp AS, Landau LI, Mazzone S, Newcombe P, Van Asperen P and Vertigan AE (2010). CICADA: Cough in Children and Adults: Diagnosis and Assessment. Australian Cough Guidelines summary statement. MJA 192 (5): 265-271

Guilbert TW, Morgan WJ, Zeiger RS TM David, Boehmer SJ , Szefler SJ,. Bacharier LB, Lemanske RF, Strunk RC, Allen DB,. Bloomberg GR, Heldt G, Krawiec M, Larsen G, Liu AH Chinchilli VM, Sorkness CA, Taussig LM, . Martinez FD, (2006) Long-Term Inhaled Corticosteroids in Preschool Children at High Risk for Asthma. N Engl J Med; 354:1985-1997

Global Strategy for asthma management and prevention. Global Initiate for Asthma (GINA) 2006. http://www.ginasthma.org.1-110 Accessed 12 August 2011

Grainge, C.L., Lau, L.C., Ward, J.A., Dulay, V., Lahiff, G., Wilson, S., Holgate, S., Davies, D.E., Howarth, P.H. (2011) Effect of Bronchoconstriction on airway remodelling in asthma. *N Engl J Med* 364 (21):2006-2015.

Joos, G.F. (Chairman), O'Connor, B. (Co-Chairman), Anderson, S.D., Chung, F., Cockcroft, D.W., Dahle´n, B., DiMaria, G., Foresi, A., Hargreave, F.E., Holgate, S.T., Inman, M.,

Lötvall, J., Magnussen, H., Polosa, R., Postma, D.S., Riedler, J. (ERS Task Force) (2003) Indirect airway challenges. *Eur Respir J* 21: 1050–1068

Koh MS, Tee A, Lasserson TJ, Irving LB. (2007) Inhaled corticosteroids compared to placebo for prevention of exercise induced bronchoconstriction. Cochrane Database Syst Rev. 18;(3):CD002739.

Mohsenin, A. & Blackburn, M.R. (2006) Adenosine signaling in asthma and chronic obstructive pulmonary disease *Curr Opin Pulm Med* 12:54-9

National Institute for Health and Clinical Excellence (2010) Chronic obstructive pulmonary disease (updated) http://www.nice.org.uk/guidance/CG101 accessed 15 August 2011

O'Byrne, P.M., Gauvreau, G.M., Brannan, J.D. (2009) Provoked models of asthma: what have we learnt? *Clin Exp Allergy* 39 (2): 181-192).

Pauwels, R., Joos, G., Van der Straetem, M. (1988) Bronchial hyper-responsiveness is not bronchial hyperresponsiveness is not bronchial asthma. *Clin Allergy* 18;(4): 317-321

Pellegrino R, Viegi G, Brusasco V, Crapo RO et al. (2005) Interpretative strategies for lung function tests. Eur Respir J. 26(5):948-68.

Perpina, M, Pellicer, C., de Diego, A., Compte, L., Macian, V. (1993) Diagnostic value of the bronchial provocation test with methacholine in asthma. A Bayesian analysis approach. *Chest* 104 (1): 149-54

Philllips, Y.Y., Jaeger, J.J. , Labue, B.L., Rosenthal, R.R. (1985) Eucapnic voluntary hyperventilation of compressed air mixture. A simple system for bronchial challenge by respiratory heat loss. *Am Rev Respir Dis* 131(1):31-135)

Riedler J, Reade T, Dalton M, Holst D, et al. (1994) Hypertonic saline challenge in an epidemiologic survey of asthma in children. Am J Respir Crit Care Med. 150:1632-9.

Rundell, K.W., Slee, J. (2008) Exercise and other indirect challenges to demonstrate asthma or exercise-induced bronchoconstriction in athletes . *J Allergy Clin Immunol* 122:238-46

Ryan G., et al. (1981) Standardization of inhalation provocation tests: two techniques of aerosol generation and inhalation compared. *Am Rev Respir Dis* 123(2): 195-199.

Seow, C.Y. & Fredberg, J.J. (2001) Historical perspective on airway smooth muscle: the saga of a frustrated cell. *J Appl Physiol* 91(2):938 – 52

Swanney, MP., Sallaway, K.A., Beckert, L.E. (2003) Comparison of FEV1 and mid-flow parameters as markers of bronchial hyperresponsiveness to methacholine. *Proceedings of ANZSRS ASM Adelaide Meeting,* Australia 2003.

Tiffeaneu, R. & Pinelli, A. (1947) Air circulent et air captive dans l'exploration de la function ventilatrice pulmonaire, *Paris Med* . 133:624-628.

3

Determination of Biomarkers in Exhaled Breath Condensate: A Perspective Way in Bronchial Asthma Diagnostics

Kamila Syslová[1], Petr Kačer[1], Marek Kuzma[2], Petr Novotný[3] and Daniela Pelclová[4]
[1]*Institute of Chemical Technology, Prague,*
[2]*Institute of Microbiology, Prague,*
[3]*ESSENCE LINE, Prague,*
[4]*1st Medical Faculty, Charles University, Prague,*
Czech Republic

1. Introduction

The nowadays commonly used term asthma comes from Greek language and means "panting". Currently, asthma is defined as a chronic inflammatory disorder of the airways where many cells and cellular elements play significant roles. In susceptible individuals, this inflammation causes recurrent episodes of wheezing, breathlessness and chest tightness accompanied by coughing, occurring very often during the night or early morning. These episodes are widely associated with a variable airflow obstruction that is either spontaneously reversible, or controllable by a suitable treatment. Asthma can be controlled by recognizing its alarming signs and by avoiding stimuli triggering the attack. During an asthma episode, the airways become extremely narrow due to a muscle constriction, swelling of the inner lining and a mucus production. Fig. 1 compares the airway bronchi of a healthy subject and a patient with an ongoing asthmatic bronchoconstriction. These repetitive episodes can cause a very limited airflow and may lead to unexpected fatalities. Factors, playing role in bronchial asthma can be divided into three groups. Among the first, internal factors are such as genetic predisposition and the state of immune system. The second factors are classified as external triggers and include for example allergens like pollen, mold spores, dust mites or animal dander. However, indoor and outdoor pollutants and irritants such as smoke, perfumes, cleaning agents, etc., can also belong to this group. The third group consists of physical factors, especially exercise and cold air, and physiological factors like stress, gastroesophageal reflux disease (GERD) or viral and bacterial upper respiratory infection. Severity of asthma is traditionally classified as mild, moderate and severe depending on its symptoms, rescue inhaler use and function parameters of lungs. While on controller therapy, each of these groups is further classified as well controlled, not well controlled or poorly controlled, based on the presence and frequency of symptoms, and lung function (GINA 2010).

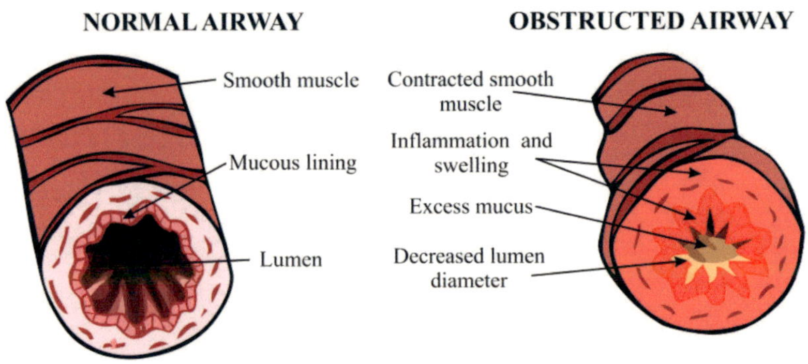

Fig. 1. Airways of healthy (left) and asthma (right) subjects

Bronchial asthma is one of the top public health problems affecting both children and adults globally. According to WHO, asthma is currently underdiagnosed and it is more than obvious it often unnecessarily reduces the quality of life, restricting individuals' activities for a lifetime. It is the most common chronic illness in children, while currently, 300 million people are suffering from it and 250,000 annual deaths are attributed to this disease. It is therefore a significant burden to the public health (GINA 2010). Workplace conditions, such as exposure to fumes, gases or organic and/or inorganic dust, are responsible for 11 % of asthma cases worldwide (occupational bronchial asthma), while about 70 % of asthmatics also suffer from various allergies. The prevalence of asthma increased by 95 % from 1995 to 2010 and the asthma rates in children under the age of five increased by more than 190 % from 1995 to 2010. It is estimated that the number of people with asthma will grow by more than 100 million by 2025. Without a proper management, asthma exacerbations often require frequent treatment and monitoring at emergency departments (ED), hospitalizations, and may lead to premature deaths. In the United States, almost 2.2 million people visited an ED in 2010 because of asthma and almost half a million of those were hospitalized. It generally affects people of all races and ages but some populations are burdened by the disease disproportionately more than others. Although asthma most often starts in the childhood, affecting more boys than girls, it affects more women than men in the adulthood (WHO, 2011).

However, asthma diagnosis can be rather difficult. Currently, there is no precise physiological, immunological, or histological test for diagnosing asthma. Early diagnosis of this potentially life-threatening disease is essential to allow a physician initiating an effective therapy and minimize the harm to the patient. The diagnosis is usually made based on the pattern of symptoms (airways obstruction and hyper-responsiveness) and/or response to the therapy (partial or complete reversibility) over a period of time. Signs and symptoms can range from mild to severe and are often similar to those of other conditions, including chronic obstructive pulmonary disease (COPD), early congestive heart failure or vocal cord problems. Children often develop temporary breathing conditions that have symptoms similar to asthma. For example, it can be hard to distinguish asthma from wheezy bronchitis, pneumonia or reactive airway disease. In order to rule out other possible conditions, lung function is generally tested first in an asthma diagnosis process. Tests to measure the lung functions include: (1) Spirometry Pulmonary Function Tests (PFT), which measures the narrowing of bronchial tubes by measuring how much air is exhaled after a deep breath and how fast it is breathed out. (2) Peak

Expiratory Flow Rate method (PEFR) measures the degree of obstruction in the airways. PEFR is a simple method that measures the level by which the peak flow readings are lower than usual. This is a sign that the airways may have deteriorated their functioning and that asthma could be exacerbating. Lung function tests are often done before and after taking a bronchodilator such as salbutamol to open the airways. If the lung function improves with the use of a bronchodilator, it is likely to be asthma. (3) Methacholine or histamine challenge tests consist in provoking bronchoconstriction or narrowing of the airways by a methacholine or histamine stimulus. Histamine causes nasal and bronchial mucus secretion and bronchoconstriction *via* the H1 receptor, whereas methacholine utilizes the M3 receptor for bronchoconstriction. The degree of narrowing can then be quantified by spirometry. Subjects with pre-existing airway hyperreactivity, such as asthmatics, will react to lower doses of bronchoconstriction drug. This test may be used if the initial lung function test is normal. (4) Fractional exhaled nitric oxide (FeNO) test appears useful to diagnose and monitor asthma, where the amount of nitric oxide present in patient breath is measured. If airways are inflamed - a sign of asthma - the nitric oxide levels are higher than normal. However, this test is not widely available.

At present, quantification of inflammation in the lungs is based on invasive (open lung biopsy (Chuang et al., 1987; Jarjour et al. 1998; Jeffery et al., 2000), bronchoalveolar lavage (Jarjour et al., 1998; Reynolds, 2000)) or *semi*-invasive (for example, induced sputum (Dworski et al., 2004; Green et al., 2002; Holz et al., 2000)) methods and the measurement of inflammatory markers in plasma and urine, which are likely to reflect systemic rather than lung inflammation. The analysis of exhaled breath condensate (EBC) is a relatively novel method with a good potential to become the preferred and completely non-invasive alternative to the currently practiced invasive and *semi*-invasive diagnostic methods for bronchial asthma. New approaches are based on attempting to identify robust biomarkers which could be utilized in establishing the diagnosis of asthma. The former studies investigated the predictive value of EBC pH for asthma, the latter chose to research hydrogen peroxide, nitrogen oxides, arachidonic acid derivatives, cytokines and others. Besides arachidonic acid derivatives, especially cysteinyl leukotrienes (cys LTs) have shown the most consistent results for the diagnosis of asthma (Hatipoglu & Rubinstein, 2004).

Thus, in the current clinical practice, spirometry and symptom scores are used to assist in the diagnosis of the disease severity and control in individual patients. EBC analysis and determination of concentration levels of the bronchial asthma biomarkers is an exciting new approach to monitoring lung inflammation. Many studies have attempted to associate changes in the EBC biomarkers - pH, hydrogen peroxide, arachidonic acid derivatives, especially cys LTs with diagnostic parameters, stratification of asthma severity, therapy effectiveness, etc. Because the technique is relatively inexpensive, it might be useful in large clinical studies and in clinical practice. In the near future, it might be possible to detect multiple asthma biomarkers in EBC (multimarker screening) to aid diagnosis, to predict the most effective therapy, and monitor the response to a treatment. The detection of elevated inflammatory mediators in EBC of subjects with relatively asymptomatic asthma and normal pulmonary function tests could offer a novel way monitoring the lung inflammation and perhaps initiating treatment in an earlier stage. They could also be helpful for the diagnosis of occupational asthma (Klusáčková et al., 2008) and monitoring work-related asthma control at the condition of either elimination from the workplace or reducing exposure, as the clinical benefit from workplace interventions is not sufficiently proven.

2. Exhaled Breath Condensate – A matrix for diagnostics

Every person breathes out 15 to 25 m^3 of air *per* day. In addition to gas exchange, lungs are involved in many metabolic processes (defence against pathogens, airway clearance, arachidonic acid metabolism etc.). They contain different cell types responsible for various functions (respiratory regulation, defence reactions and surfactant production). The surface of lungs and airways is abundant with a number of substances (e.g. enzymes, tumour markers, antibodies, proteins, metabolites etc.) whose presence and concentration level reflects the physiological/pathological conditions of an organism. Metabolites generated in the lungs can be examined by invasive or semi-invasive methods - bronchoalveolar lavage (BAL), methods of induced sputum and open lung biopsy. These diagnostic methods impose a considerable strain on the patients and cannot be repeated as often as the efficient health monitoring would require. By contrast, the measurements of metabolite products in the EBC are non-invasive and conspicuously reflect the composition of the extracellular lung fluid (Piotrowski et al., 2007).

During the collection of an EBC, it is often assumed that the monitored biomolecules are merely contained in the gas phase of the exhaled air. This assumption neglects the fact that the exhaled air also contains a liquid fraction, i.e. aerosol which inevitably carries important biochemical information as well (Fig. 2). In addition to gases as nitrogen, oxygen, carbon dioxide or carbon monoxide contained in the gaseous phase, there are substances with a sufficient vapour pressure at the body temperature and the atmospheric pressure such as water, hydrogen peroxide, hydrocarbons and other volatile organic compounds. In parallel, there are substances insoluble in water which form binary systems with water in the epithels of lungs and airways. In this case, the vapour pressure of water and hardly volatile biomolecules add up, greatly facilitating the evaporation of biomolecules. As a consequence, these can be present in the vapour phase of the exhaled air. Eicosanoids (leukotrienes and prostaglandins) are the example of substances entering the exhaled air by this described mechanism. Molecules of water-soluble substances, for example vasoactive peptides, enzymes, DNA and proteins flow within the exhaled air as aerosol particles. They are released from the mucous surface due to a turbulent airflow throughout bronchi and bronchioles (Effros et al., 2004). EBC is a water-based matrix. The collection of an EBC sample is a simple, non-invasive procedure that can be beneficially applied especially to children (older than 3 years), seniors as well as patients with different disease-impaired health conditions.

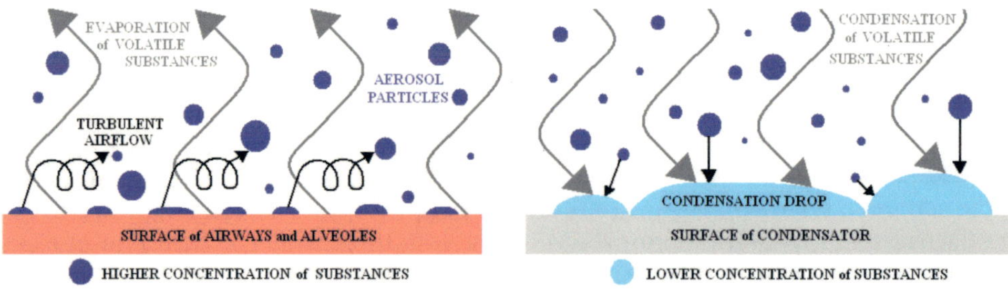

Fig. 2. Generation of exhaled breath condensate. Occurring on the airways surface and in alveoli: (1) evaporation of volatile substances and substances insoluble in water forming a binary system with water on the airways surface and (2) aerosol particles carried away by the turbulent airflow. Aerosol droplets are collected in the exhaled air condenser, where condensation of the water vapour and other volatile substances occurs.

Furthermore, its repeated usage in short time intervals is another advantage compared to invasive methods, enabling monitoring of an ongoing disease as well as an effective pharmacotherapy. The equipment for the collection of EBC generally consists of a mouthpiece with a one-way valve connected to a collecting system (Fig. 3).

The subjects wear a noseclip and breathe tidally *via* the mouthpiece and the one-way valve, in which expiratory and inspiratory air is separated. The valve block is connected to the collecting system which is composed of a lamellar condenser and a polypropylene tube (a sample collection container) that is inserted into a cooling cuff maintained at a stable cold temperature by a refrigerator.

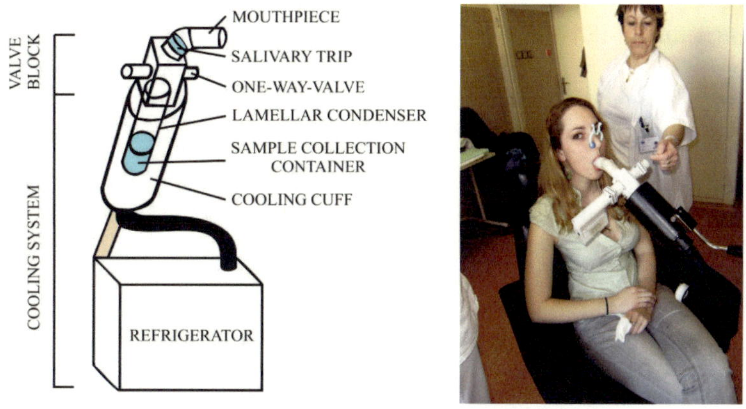

Fig. 3. Scheme of an exhaled breath condenser (left) and clinical EBC collection (right)

During the collection of EBC, the following parameters must be monitored: (1) the condenser temperature, (2) the nasal contamination, (3) the contamination by saliva, (4) humidity and (5) the time of EBC collection. The condenser temperature plays a crucial role in monitoring biomarkers contained in the gas phase (e.g. aldehydes, eicosanoids) and the amount of the condensed water (affecting the dilution rate of the EBC sample). In condensers utilizing cooling water at the temperature of 10 °C, about 81 % of water vapour condenses from exhaled air, whereas using ice, 89 % is captured on the condenser surface. The condensers using a counter flow cooling system reach temperatures of -10 °C achieving 93 % of the water condensed (Horváth et al., 2005). This low temperature is important for the preservation of heat-labile substances, i.e. a number of biomarkers including leukotrienes, aldehydes, etc. Inflammatory mediators such as leukotrienes and prostaglandins are also formed in the nose and paranasal sinuses (Howarth, 2000). Using simple experiments, the nasal contamination (alternatively the determination of whether the monitored biomarkers occur in the mucosa of the nose and nasopharynx and influence the quantity of substances detected in EBC) can be determined. In particular, the level of monitored substances in EBC is determined with/without using a nasal clip during the collection of EBC. Since leukotrienes are contained in high concentrations in saliva (McKinney et al., 2000; Tufvesson et al., 2010; Zakrzewski et al., 1987), it is important to exclude the contamination of EBC by saliva. This can be achieved by measuring amylase concentrations in the samples (the limit of detection for amylase activity in saliva is 0.078 $U.mL^{-1}$, it is approximetly the contamination of 0.2 μL of saliva in 1 mL of EBC (Gaber et al., 2006)). When collecting EBC using devices equipped with a saliva trap, the contamination by saliva has not been evidenced (Montuschi et al., 2000; Syslová et al., 2011). The often neglected factor is the humidity, affected either by the environment (air humidity) in which the collection is carried out or in which the individual was present just prior to the collection and the amount of water that entered into the lungs from the body (dependent on the hydration/dehydration of the organism). Experiments carried out with the constant exhaled air volume of 120 L and the equal humidity demonstrated that a significant difference in monitored biomarkers could be determined in one subject owing to different bodily hydration (the first situation - hydration: drinking about 1 L of fluid before the collection of EBC *versus* the second situation - dehydration: drinking absence for 12 hours before the collection). With the fluid intake, the concentration of biomarkers was reduced by 33.8 ± 5.22 % for LTC_4, 36.8 ± 4.27% for LTD_4 and 36.3 ± 6.99 % for LTE_4. The absence of the fluid intake caused a concentrating of the monitored analytes to 162.7 ± 15.63 % for LTC_4, 161.3 ± 7.23 % for LTD_4 and 155.7 ± 14.50 % for LTE_4. Further to the humidity factor, the timing of the collection of EBC can affect the final detected concentration. The level of substances can be increased by 15 % during 18-20 hours without sleeping (valid for the sum of cys LTs) (Syslová et al., 2011).

EBC has been determined to have its pH in the range of 7.8 - 8.1 immediately after the collection; however it rapidly decreased (pH 6.0 - 6.5) due to the absorption of CO_2 from the ambient air, which could have been one of the causes for the consecutive changes occurring in this matrix after its collection (Effros et al., 2004). It was demonstrated that storing EBC under an inert atmosphere (argon) did not cause any change in pH; however this did not appear to be the main parameter with regards to the determination of some biomarkers concentration levels (e.g. leukotrienes, prostaglandins). The storage and the manipulation with the samples after the collection of EBC were the parameters capable of affecting the levels of the substances detected in EBC. The main risk factor was primarily the thermal and light instability of certain substances, in particular leukotrienes, prostaglandins, aldehydes and protein substances. For this reason, samples are required to be stored frozen at the temperature of -80 °C (or at -20 °C for up to one month). At this temperature, it was proven that the decomposition had been preserved and possible *in vitro* changes in the composition of the most important EBC asthmatic biomarkers had been prevented. Otherwise, the deteriorating changes started already at room temperature and took place in a short time interval (see section 4) (Syslová et al., 2008, 2011). A repeated freezing/thawing of the sample (freeze-thaw cycle was performed between -80 °C and laboratory temperature) had a negative impact on the stability of substances. Apparently, the critical point for the stability of the substances was the transformation of the sample from their solid to their liquid state (temperature of 0 °C). With regards to the lability of the biomarkers to a number of factors (described above), it is critical to respect them and prevent the circumstances that would otherwise had a negative effect on their precise determination. It is essential that an isotope-labelled internal standard (known amounts of deuterium labelled analytes to 1 mL of EBC) be added to the sample immediately after the collection. Performing the so-called "stable-isotope-dilution assay" allows a highly precise quantification as well as monitoring of changes in the sample composition, occurring during its processing.

3. Biomarkers of bronchial asthma present in exhaled breath condensate

Asthma is a chronic inflammatory disease of the airways characterized by reversible airways obstruction. Clinically, the severity of asthma is determined by evaluation of the expiratory flow rate and the symptoms. Smouldering inflammation is present even in patients with mild to moderate asthma. Long-term presence of inflammation and repeated episodes of acute inflammation result in structural changes in the airways (airways remodelling), which might cause chronic airflow obstruction. It is apparent that molecular diagnostics based on the detection of inflammatory biomarkers facilitate the diagnosis earlier than clinical symptoms develop, and in parallel, the start of a therapy decreasing a potential harm to the patient. It also allows optimal monitoring of the inflammation and the disease activity. All the facts head to an improved asthma management beneficial to the patient as well as to the health system owing a predictable enhanced cost-effectiveness of the medical treatment.

In medicine, a biomarker is a term often used to refer to a substance (small/large size molecule), gene, cell, etc. measured in a biological matrix whose concentration reflects the severity or even presence of a certain disease state. More generally, a biomarker is anything that can be used as an indicator of a particular disease state or another physiological state of an organism. They may indicate either normal or diseased processes in the body. Although the term biomarker is relatively new, biomarkers have been used in pre-clinical research and clinical diagnosis for a considerable period of time (e.g. acetone present in breath as a sign of ketoacidosis, which may occur in diabetes, cholesterol as a biomarker and a risk indicator for coronary and vascular diseases, C-reactive protein (CRP) as a marker of inflammation, etc.). A biomarker is a parameter that can be used to measure the progress of a disease or the effects of its treatment. In molecular terms, biomarker is "the subset of markers that might be discovered using metabolomics, proteomics, genomics and other "-omics" or imaging technologies. Biomarkers also play a major role in medicinal biology. Biomarkers probably represent the future paradigmatic approach allowing us an early diagnosis, a more efficient disease prevention and monitoring of a drug response, a faster drug target identification etc.

Compound/Factor	**pH**
	H_2O_2
	Eicosanoids
	1) LTs: a) cys LTs = (LTC_4, LTD_4, LTE_4), b) LTB_4
	2) 8-isoprostane
	Nitrate/Nitrite, Nitrotyrosine
	Aldehydes (Malondialdehyde)
	Thiobarbituric acid reactive products (TBAR)
	Glutathione
	Adenosine
	Cytokines (IL-4, IL-6, TFN-α)
	Interferon-γ (IFN-γ)

Table 1. Inflammatory mediators detected in EBC in bronchial asthma

Collection and analysis of substances present in EBC procures a simple, non-invasive, real-time, point-of-care clinical and research tool for evaluating lung pathophysiology based on a molecular diagnostics approach. In the case of asthma, a chronic inflammatory disease of the airways, a row of biomarkers/factors present in EBC have been referenced (Table 1). Various inflammatory markers present in EBC have been investigated as possible asthma biomarkers.

The pH value of the airway lining fluid reflects the underlying homeostatic balance between acid and the base production of inflammatory cells and the buffering capacity of resident airways cells. EBC pH has been proved to be one of the robust biomarkers of asthma associated inflammation and resulting acid stress. In general, EBC pH values are lower in asthmatics and well correlate with sputum eosinophililia, which is the hallmark of asthmatic airway inflammation, and resulting oxidative stress (Murugan et al., 2009). EBC pH is unstable at room temperature because CO_2 diffuses in and out of solution readily. Determination of EBC pH obtained after de-aeration with an inert gas (usually argon or nitrogen) has provided the most reproducible pH values to date (Kullmann et al., 2007). EBC pH measurement and its application to non-invasive assessment of asthmatic airway inflammation had first been received with optimism, but there have later been published several negative studies as well (Zhao et al., 2008; Ojoo et al., 2005). This fact may be explained by the proposition that EBC pH reflects asthma control more than it reflects asthma severity, and hence is unable to distinguish healthy subjects from asymptomatic quiescent asthmatics. In spite of these drawbacks, pH values of EBC posses established reference values in healthy subjects (normal median pH is 8.0 with interquartile 25 – 75 % range of 7.8 – 8.1) (Paget-Brown et al., 2006) and also shows a good reproducibility in asthmatics (the intra-class correlation ICC = 0.97) over a one-year period with minimal seasonal variation (Accordino et al., 2008). Asthma subjects demonstrate values with the median 7.4. Endogenous airway acidification has been assessed in asthma in many studies (Rozy et al., 2006; Ojoo et al., 2005; Hunt et al., 2000; Niimi et al., 2004). Regarding EBC pH values in non-deaerated samples, the mean values ranged from 6.0 to 7.4 (Brooks et al., 2006; Gessner et al., 2003). Nevertheless, EBC pH value after deaeration has been extensively validated and it has been found to represent a simple, robust and reproducible biomarker. Continuous EBC pH measurement may provide an option for monitoring of airways inflammation.

Hydrogen peroxide (H_2O_2) is one of the best asthma biomarkers ever studied. The activation of inflammatory cells in the airways leads to the production of superoxide anion (O_2^-), which undergoes spontaneous or enzyme-catalyzed dismutation to the less reactive H_2O_2. It has strong oxidizing properties which lead to further cellular injury. Thus, elevated values of exhaled H_2O_2 indicate airway oxidative damage. As hydrogen peroxide is unstable, it must be manipulated carefully. It has been determined spectrophotometrically (colorimetric assay) (Dekhuijzen et al., 1996), spectrofluorimetrically (fluorimetric assay) (Hyslop & Sklar, 1984; Ruch et al., 1983; Nowak et al., 2001), by a flow injection analysis with flurescence detection (Svensson et al., 2004), by a chemiluminescent method (Zappacosta et al., 2001) and with an amperometric biosensor (Ecocheck, Jaeger, Germany) (Gerritsen et al., 2005; Thanachasai et al., 2002). Besides pH, EBC H_2O_2 is the only other biomarker with established reference values in healthy subjects. The mean normal value is reported to be 0.13 μM, with a 2.5 – 97.5 % reference range of < 0.01 – 0.48 μM. In asthma subjects, they have been found to be elevated when compared to the healthy controls (Koutsokera et al., 2008). Elevated exhaled H_2O_2 levels enable distinction of asthmatics from controls and correlate with the disease severity and the lung function deterioration (Emelyanov et al., 2001). In parallel to H_2O_2 concentration, a reduction has been found in patients treated with inhaled corticosteroids (monitoring of pharmacotherapy). A series of studies have also shown correlations between airway senzibilization and H_2O_2 concentration levels. These findings suggested that exhaled H_2O_2 might be more useful than the FeNO test in monitoring asthmatic patients. However, poor reproducibility due to the high variability in values (including variability due to changes in flow) and poorer correlations in corticosteroid-naive asthma patients (Horváth et al., 1998) have been reported and thus the optimism with use of this marker has been moderated.

As mentioned, exhaled nitric oxide (NO) is an established marker of airway inflammation and is increased in patients with asthma. NO is a free radical due to its unpaired electron and it may react with oxygen to yield nitrogen oxides (NO_x) or with superoxide anion to yield peroxynitrite, a highly reactive substance that may lead to the production of NO-derived products (Ricciardolo et al., 2006). NO-related products (nitrite, nitrate, nitrotyrosine and nitrosothiols) form some other groups of substances elevated in asthma patients compared to healthy controls (Kharitonov & Barnes, 2001). NO synthesis and release in the respiratory system has been determined indirectly by quantifying nitrite/nitrate, nitrotyrosine and *S*-nitrothiols in EBC. Nitrite/nitrate detection in EBC has been performed by the following methods: colorimetric assay (Griess reaction), fluorimetric assay (DAN reaction) (Marzinzig et al., 1997), chemiluminescence (Nguyen et al., 2005) and ion chromatography/conductivity detection (Tate et al., 2002). The normal values of nitrite/nitrate exhibited a significant discrepancy in the literature (Koutsokera et al., 2008) which is attributed to different assays used, efficiency of the method utilized for the reduction of nitrite to nitrate and NO_x present in the environment as a pollutant. Nitrite and/or nitrate elevated levels in asthma patients were determined (68 μM) and compared to healthy controls (9.6 μM) (Koutsokera et al., 2008). In contrast, a subsequent report showed no difference between concentration levels of nitrite/nitrate in asthmatic and healthy subjects (Kazani & Israel, 2010).

Several independent studies (Csoma et al., 2002; Montuschi & Barnes, 2002a; Koutsokera et al., 2008; Kazani & Israel, 2010) have indicated the presence of elevated levels of arachidonic acid derivatives (Cys LTs, leukotriene B_4 (LTB_4), 8-isoprostane) in EBC of asthma patients (Fig. 4). Therefore, measurements of these mediators are considered as potentially effective in the establishment of the diagnosis of asthma in a large cohort.

Inflammatory molecules called leukotrienes belong to the group of several substances released by mast cells during an asthma attack, and it is leukotrienes which are primarily responsible for bronchoconstriction. In chronic, more severe cases of asthma, general bronchial hyperreactivity (or smooth muscle twitchiness) is largely caused by eosinophils, which are attracted into the bronchioles by leukotrienes (and other chemoattractants) and which themselves also produce leukotrienes. Thus leukotrienes seem to be critical both in triggering acute asthma attacks and in causing a longer term hypersensitivity of the airways in chronic asthma. Leukotrienes are derived from arachidonic acid, the precursor of prostaglandins. There are two families of leukotrienes (LTB_4 and cys LTs - LTC_4, LTD_4 and LTE_4). The first group acts primarily in conditions in which the inflammation is dependent on neutrophils, such as cystic fibrosis, inflammatory bowel disease, and psoriasis. The second group (cys LTs) is concerned primarily with eosinophil and mast cell induced bronchoconstriction in asthma. They bind to highly selective receptors on bronchial smooth muscle and other airway tissue. Drugs have now been designed which can interfere with the activity of leukotrienes. Both leukotriene synthesis inhibitors and cysteinyl-leukotriene receptor antagonists have recently been shown to protect asthmatic patients against asthma attacks, but they are not useful as "rescue remedies" once an attack has already started. They act by preventing the relevant leukotriene release from mast cells and eosinophils or by blocking the specific leukotriene receptors on bronchial tissues, thus preventing bronchoconstriction, mucus secretion, and oedema. These drugs also reduce the influx of eosinophils and this way limit the inflammatory damage in the airway. For patients with moderate to severe asthma symptoms despite corticosteroid treatment, concomitant treatment with LT modifiers significantly improves asthma control.

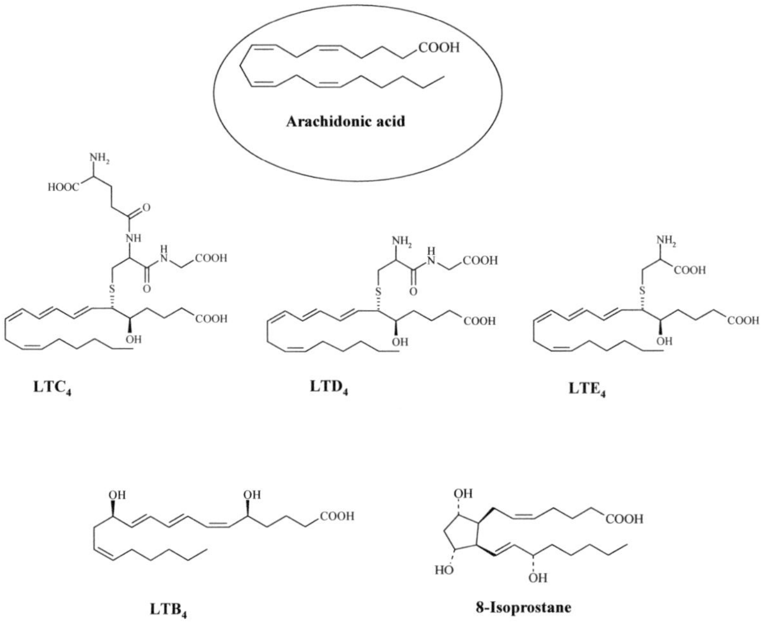

Fig. 4. Arachidonic acid derivatives - potential biomarkers of bronchial asthma

Leukotrienes, in particular cys LTs (LTC_4, LTD_4, LTE_4) have a potentially important role in asthma biomarker based diagnostics (Kazani & Israel, 2010). Concentrations of cys LTs in EBC are elevated in patients with asthma when compared to healthy controls. Their levels often decrease after LT directed anti-inflammatory therapy. The values of cys LTs in asthmatics and also controls are rather contradictory. On the other hand, the majority of works have found reasonably different values in asthma patients and healthy controls. The levels of LTB_4 and its relation to asthma are rather conflicting. Elevated levels in asthmatics were reported (97.5 pg/mL) when compared to the control (32.3 pg/mL) (Kostikas et al., 2005) and also by other authors (Csoma et al., 2002; Montuschi & Barnes, 2002a). On the other hand, no difference in the levels between well-controlled asthmatics (4.6 pg/mL) and controls (4.3 pg/mL) were referenced either (Carraro et al., 2005).

Isoprostanes are formed by the free-radical lipid peroxidation of arachidonic acid, representing *in-vivo* markers of oxidative stress (Janssen, 2001). The most studied is 8-isoprostane (8-iso prostaglandin $F_{2\alpha}$). Elevated levels of 8-isoprostane in asthmatics (42.4 pg/mL) when compared with controls (32.3 pg/mL) were observed by several authors (Montuschi, 2009; Zhao et al., 2008).

Several other biomarkers have been assessed in EBC, including adenosine (Csoma et al., 2005), aldehydes (Corradi et al., 2004), glutathione (Csoma et al., 2005), thiobarbituric acid reactive substances (TBARs) (Nowak et al., 1999), ammonia (Gessner et al., 2003), several cytokines, such as interleukin-4 (IL-4), interleukin-6 (IL-6), tumour necrosis factor-α (TNF-α), interferon-γ (IFN-γ) (Koutsokera et al., 2008) etc. However, it is believed that the pursuit of normal/pathological (asthma) concentration values for these biomarkers is not yet feasible and further studies focusing on standardization of measurement are needed in that direction.

4. Cysteinyl leukotrienes – The most prominent biomarkers of bronchial asthma

Leukotrienes (LTs) are a family of inflammatory lipid mediators synthesized from arachidonic acid ((5Z,8Z,11Z,14Z)-5,8,11,14-eicosatetraenoic acid) by a variety of cells (eosinophils, mast cells, basophils and macrophages). The name leukotriene is derived from their main producer, leukocytes, and from the specific structure of these substances, i.e. three conjugated double bonds. An overproduction of LTs is a major cause of inflammation in bronchial asthma. The biosynthetic pathway can be triggered in the organism by a variety of stimuli, including antigens, microbes, cytokines, immune complexes, and toxins. These stimuli activate signal transduction cascades that in turn activate LTs, forming enzymes, i.e. phospholipase and lipooxygenase (Peters-Golden & Brock, 2003).

Arachidonic acid is a twenty-carbon polyunsaturated ω-6 fatty acid bound in the cell membrane phospholipids, mostly in phosphatidylinositol in the C_2 position. Arachidonic acid is released into the organism by the enzyme phospholipase (Fig. 5 and Fig. 6). The phospholipase pathway is active in leukocytes, including mast cells, eosinophils, neutrophils, monocytes, and basophiles. The split of arachidonic acid from phospholipids may occur in three ways (Fig. 6). The first direct pathway, producing arachidonic acid and lysophospholipid, is catalyzed by phospholipase A_2.

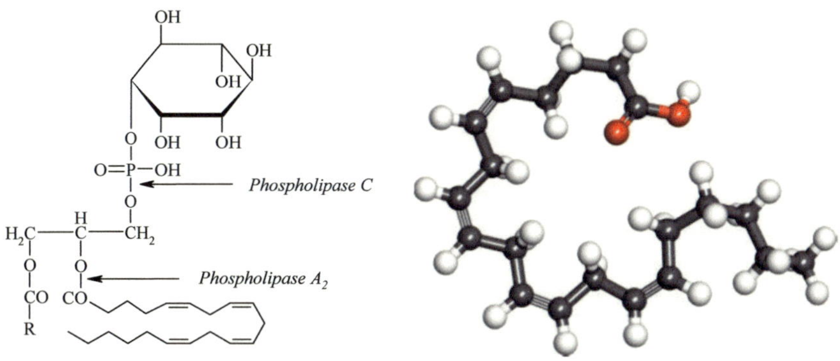

Fig. 5. Phosphatidylinositol with arachidonic acid in the most common position (C_2) with arrows pointing at hydrolyzes sites for phospholipase enzymes (left); arachidonic acid structure (right)

The other two metabolic processes lead to an intermediate, 1,2-diacylglycerole, which is produced by the action of phospholipase C enzyme. 1,2-diacylglycerol can be split into arachidonic acid and monoacylglycerols by diacylglycerollipase. In addition, diacylglycerolkinase can also convert it to phosphatidic acid which is further split by phospholipase A_2 to arachidonic acid and lysophosphatidic acid. In the organism, arachidonic acid is metabolized by three reaction ways: (1) it is transformed to leukotrienes by 5-lipoxygenase enzyme (5-LO); (2) it is converted to prostaglandins by cycloxygenase and (3) it is nonenzymatically converted to isoprostane (arachidonic acid is attacked by reactive oxygen species). Leukotrienes are synthesized in the cells from free arachidonic acid by the action of 5-lipoxygenase enzyme. The catalytic mechanism involves the insertion of an oxygen species at the C-5 position of the carbon skeleton of arachidonic acid to form an intermediate 5-HPETE (5-hydroxyperoxy-6,8,11,14-eicosatetraenoic acid) which is spontaneously reduced to 5-HETE (5-hydroxy eicosatetraenoic acid). The enzyme 5-LO participates in the next step of the transformation of 5-HETE to the reactive epoxide leukotriene A_4 (LTA_4). The efficient utilization of endogenous arachidonate by 5-LO requires activation of a protein termed "5-lipoxygenase activating protein" (FLAP).

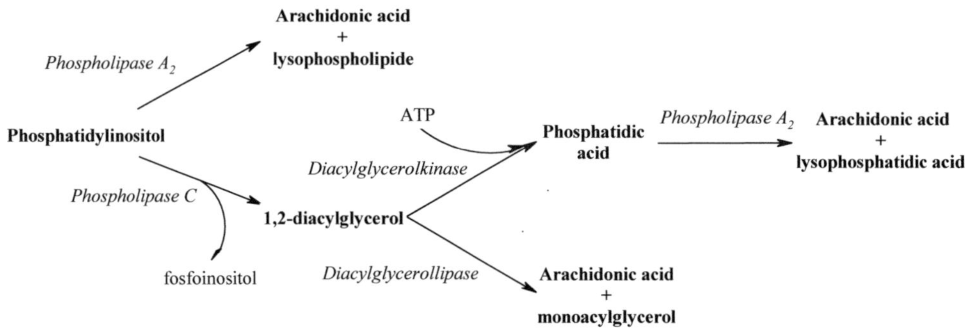

Fig. 6. Different pathways of generation of arachidonic acid from membrane phospholipids

LTA_4 can be further transformed by one of two possible enzymatic pathways. During inflammation, the levels of LTB_4 are elevated by the action of LTA_4 hydrolase, while the second pathway is dominant during allergic reactions and produces cys LTs. The first member of the family of cys LTs, LTC_4, is produced by coupling of LTA_4 and reducing glutathione. This transformation is catalysed by LTC_4 synthetase. The next members of the cys LT series (LTD_4 and LTE_4) are produced by a gradual transformation occurring sequentially ($LTC_4 \rightarrow LTD_4 \rightarrow LTE_4$) by a consecutive action of γ-glutamyl transpeptidase enzyme ($LTC_4 \rightarrow LTD_4$) and dipeptidase ($LTD_4 \rightarrow LTE_4$) (Montuschi, 2004) (Fig. 7). The biological effect of cys LTs is mediated *via* specific receptors classified as Cys-LT receptors. Their two subtypes, Cys-LT_1 and Cys-LT_2 receptors, are mainly located on smooth muscle cells, eosinophils and other cells throughout the body. Binding of leukotrienes to Cys-LT_1 receptors located in the lungs and the airways leads to the constriction of bronchi and bronchioles. It can also cause mucosal oedema and an increased secretion of viscous mucus, which leads to narrowing of the airway lumen and repetitive episodic states of dyspnoea expiratory wheezing. The Cys-LT_2 receptor is responsible for the constriction of blood vessels in the lungs (Barnes & Smith, 1999; Izumi et al., 2002). These effects can even be caused by very low concentrations of cys LTs with values around 10 mol/L. In excess, cys LTs can induce anaphylactic shock. (Brocklehurst, 1960). For this reason, cys LTs are known as "slow reacting substances of anaphylaxis (SRS-A)"

In order to properly handle and monitor cys LTs in body fluids, the knowledge of their physico-chemical properties is of vital importance. The temperature and light stability in different environments (e.g. EBC, solvents) is a crucial point for an analytical/diagnostic method development. Although the effect of daylight on the stability of cys LTs was experimentally tested, none was actually found. On the contrary, temperature was found to be the parameter with the most significant effect on the stability of cys LTs. It was demonstrated that the composition of EBC with regard to cys LTs was rapidly changed at ambient temperature (25 °C) as a result of (1) their enzymatic inter-conversion and (2) their limited temperature stability. Fig. 8 depicts the behaviour of cys LTs in EBC and in organic solvents (mixture of acetonitrile and water 70 : 30 – v/v was used as the mobile phase in LC-MS) where the negative effect of temperature (25 °C) on the composition of individual cys LTs was demonstrated. In the matrix of EBC, besides the degradation of individual substances (very apparent in the mobile phase), inter-conversion of individual cys LTs was observed in the series of $LTC_4 \rightarrow LTD_4 \rightarrow LTE_4$, evidently catalyzed by the present enzymatic systems. At the temperature of -80 °C, EBC samples could be stored without any detectable change in the cys LTs content for a period of 3 months (similarly, the temperature of -20 °C seemed to be acceptable) (Ohanian et al., 2010). On the other hand, the temperature of 4 °C was not sufficient for the storage of the EBC sample. Although the inter-conversions as well as the degradations were slowed at this temperature (in comparison to 25 °C), the degradations of all the studied biomarkers still occurred in a period of hours in both experimentally studied matrices (EBC, organic solvent). Effects of sample handling, time and storage conditions on cys LTs in EBC have also been studied by other authors (Ohanian et al., 2010; Beyer, 1987).

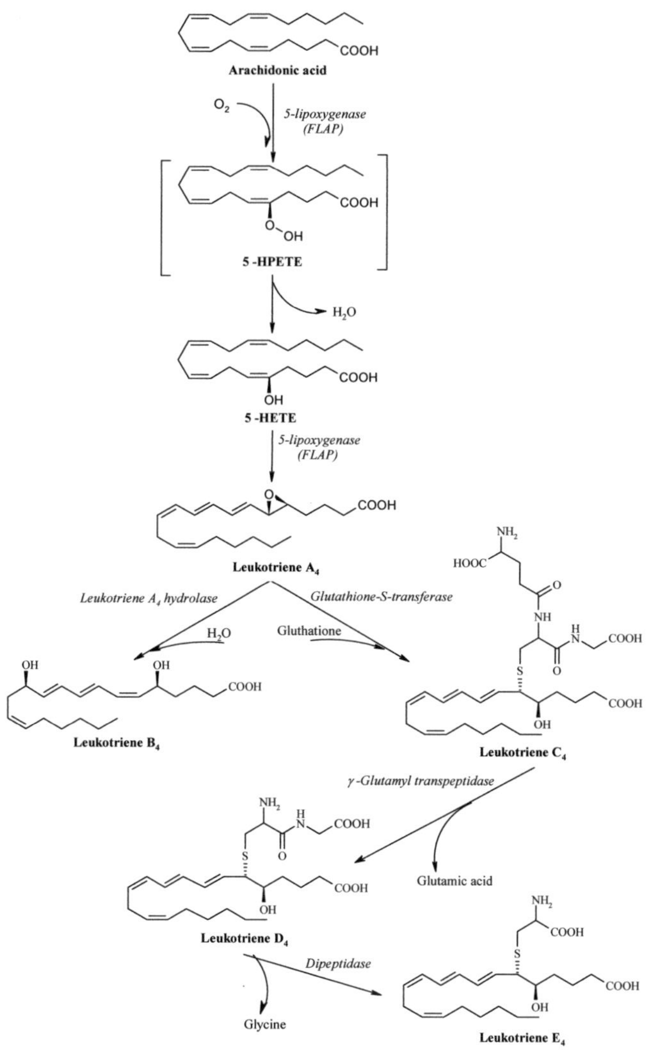

Fig. 7. Synthesis of leukotrienes

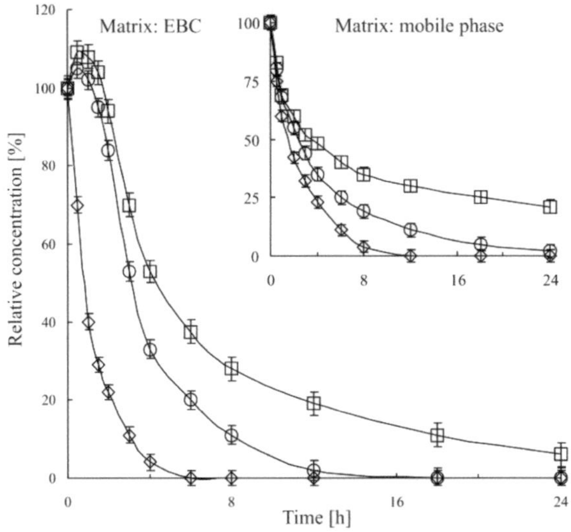

Fig. 8. Stability of cys LTs in EBC matrix and in organic solvent; LTC_4 (◇), LTD_4 (○) and LTE_4 (□)

It was also essential to map the behaviour of the biological system with respect to the production of cys LTs during the circadian biorhythm. The intra-day physiological variations were determined by analyzing EBC samples collected from volunteers (age 18 ± 1, non-smokers, without the diagnosis of bronchial asthma). EBC samples were obtained at different times throughout the day (6, 12, 18 and 24 h). An identical trend was demonstrated in the concentration profiles of cys LTs in all subjects, increasing during the day and returning to its original level during the night. The level of cys LTs increased by an average of 15.4 %. The inter-day physiological variations of the method were assessed by analyzing samples of healthy volunteers obtained from each subject in one week period. Regarding the inter-day physiological variations in a group of 10 healthy people, the total level of cys LTs did not differ by more than 6.6 % for each individual over a period of 5 consecutive days. The clinical studies should respect the circadian biorhythm and collect EBC clinical samples in a similar day-time (e.g. all samples should be collected between 8 and 12 a.m.).

5. Methods for determination of cysteinyl leukotrienes

Since the discovery and elucidation of the structures of leukotrienes and other eicosanoids (prostaglandin and thromboxane) and their metabolites, numerous analytical techniques have been developed for their analysis in complex biological matrices. Various publications have described the determination of leukotrienes in the blood plasma (Shindo et al., 1997; Henden et al., 1993) urine (Armstrong et al., 2009; Misso et al., 2004; Higashi et al., 2004), EBC (Syslova et al., 2011; Brussino et al., 2010; Biko et al., 2010) and saliva (McKinney et al., 2000; Tufvesson et al., 2010). At present, immunochemical methods are used for the quantitative determination of leukotrienes formed *in vivo*, namely Enzyme Linked Immunosorbent Assay (ELISA, sometimes also denoted as Enzyme Immunoassay – EIA) (Samitas et al., 2009; Csoma et al., 2002; Baraldi et al., 2003; Antczak et al., 2002; Chappell et al., 2011) or instrumental analytical methods based on gas or liquid chromatography (GC, LC) coupled to a variety of detectors, preferentially mass spectrometer (MS), (Sanak et al., 2010; Čáp et al., 2004; Montuschi & Barnes, 2002b; Syslová et al., 2011) but also ultra-violet detector (UVD), fluorescence detector (FLD), or electrochemical detector (ECD).

Immunochemical methods offer simple, rapid, robust yet sensitive, and easily automated methods for routine analyses in clinical laboratories. Immunoassays are based on highly specific binding between an antigen and an antibody. An epitope (immunodeterminant region) on the antigen surface is recognized by the antibody's binding site. The type of antibody and its affinity and avidity for the antigen determines the sensitivity and specificity of the assay. Depending on their format, immunoassays can be qualitative or quantitative. They are able to measure low levels of disease biomarkers and therapeutic or illicit drugs in a patient's blood, serum, plasma, urine, or saliva.

Antigen is a substance of natural or synthetic (artificial) origin. When exposed to antigens, the immune system reacts by synthesis of antibodies in plasmatic cells (lymphocytes). The antibodies then bond to the antigen molecules through weak interactions (hydrogen bonds, non-polar hydrophobic interactions, van der Waals forces, Coulomb forces, London dispersion attractive forces and steric repulsive forces) and block the antigen effects. In the organism, antibodies are represented by glycoproteins denoted as immunoglobulins (Ig). The Y-shaped immunoglobulin molecule consists of two identical heavy H-chains and two light L-chains (Fig. 9). The heavy chain is connected to the light chain by one disulfide bridge, while the heavy bridges are interconnected by multiple disulfide bridges. Apart from these, each chain has its own intrachain disulfide bonds (Daussant & Desvaux, 2007).

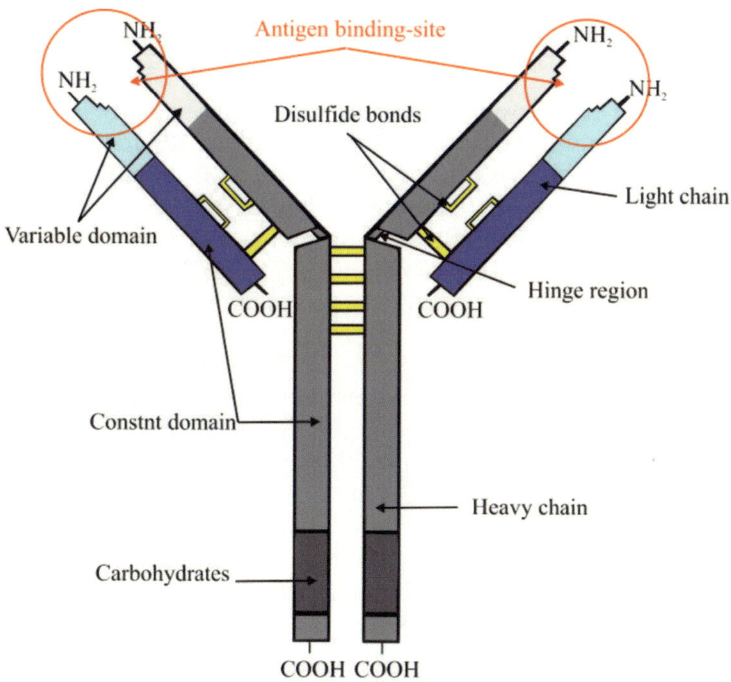

Fig. 9. Structure of an immunoglobulin monomer.

According to the types of H-chains, immunoglobulins can be divided into five main groups: IgA, IgD, IgE, IgG a IgM. The most abundant in the blood serum are IgG, representing about 75 % of the total Ig amount. Both heavy and light chains can be subdivided into their functional domains: while the part closer to the amino-end is termed variable (V), the fragment containing a carboxyl group is said to be constant (C). The variable (heterogeneous) moiety forms a unique part of immunoglobulin which is complementary to antigen *via* a highly specific key-lock mechanism between the antigen and antibody. The immunoglobulin molecules can be cleaved into so-called hinge regions by the action of papain (a plant enzyme) and it is thus possible to split the antibody molecule into three parts: two Fab-fragments containing arms (i.e. the entire light chain and a part of the heavy chain) and one crystalline Fc-fragment. The latter contains the remaining parts of both H-chains interconnected by disulfide bridges. The Fab-fragments allow the bonding of antigens and the Fc-fragments bond to receptors on the surface of leukocytes or can be employed in antibody immobilization upon various surfaces without losing the functionality of the antigen binding place (immunochemical methods) (Daussant & Desvaux, 2007).

ELISA (Enzyme Linked Immunosorbent Assay), also called EIA (Enzyme ImmunoAssay), belongs to the most frequently used methods applicable in the quantitative analysis of antigens. This method comes in a range of modifications which are all based on a highly specific interaction of antigen and antibody. One of these binding partners is covalently bound to an enzyme (usually peroxidase, acetylcholinesterase or alkaline phosphatase) whose role is the catalytic conversion of the added substrate to a coloured product. The colour intensity, determined spectrophotometrically or fluorimetrically, directly or indirectly reflects the amount of antigen present in the sample. A common attribute of all ELISA methods is the immobilization (*via* adsorption or a covalent bonding) of the antibody (when the antigen is determined) on a solid support such as microtiter plate, which facilitates the separation of immunochemically bond molecules. Either direct or direct sandwich ELISA can be utilised for the antigen detection (Fig. 10). In direct ELISA methods, antigens (e.g. cys LTs as biomarkers of bronchial asthma) from biological matrices (EBC, blood plasma, urine) bind to the immobilized antibodies (mouse monoclonal anti cys LTs IgG). Direct ELISA relies upon competitive binding of cys LTs from the biological sample and cys LTs bound to an enzyme (acetylcholinesterase). After the incubation period (usually overnight), during which the antigen-antibody complex is formed, sample removal and washing of the complex, a mixture of substrates (acetylcholine and 5,5′-dithio-bis(2-nitrobenzoic acid) is added. Acetylcholine is cleaved by an enzyme to thiocholine, further reacting with 5,5′-dithio-bis(2-nitrobenzoic acid) and yielding yellow 5-thio-2-nitrobenzoic acid, which can be determined spectrophotometrically. In sandwich ELISA, only cys LTs contained in the biological sample bind to the anchored antibodies. Colour assignment is allowed as a result of the substrate conversion by the enzyme linked to free antibodies against cys LTs added to the solution. The antibodies with enzyme form a sandwich complex with anchored cys LTs (the antibody captured with an enzyme uses other interaction with the antigen than the immobilized antibody). As in the direct method, enzyme cleaves the substrate into a detectable coloured product.

Radioimmunoassay (RIA) works on a similar principle as the direct competitive ELISA where the main difference lies in the use of a labelled antigen. The enzyme on antigen is replaced by a tyrosine moiety containing a γ-radioactive iodine isotope. The γ-radiation is then monitored for the non-bonded labelled antigen present in the sample. However, operating with radioactive species can only be carried out at specialized facilities with appropriate equipment which represents a relevant disadvantage and explains the less frequent utilization of RIA in practice. At present, this method is not used for the determination of cys LTs (Lindgren et al., 1983).

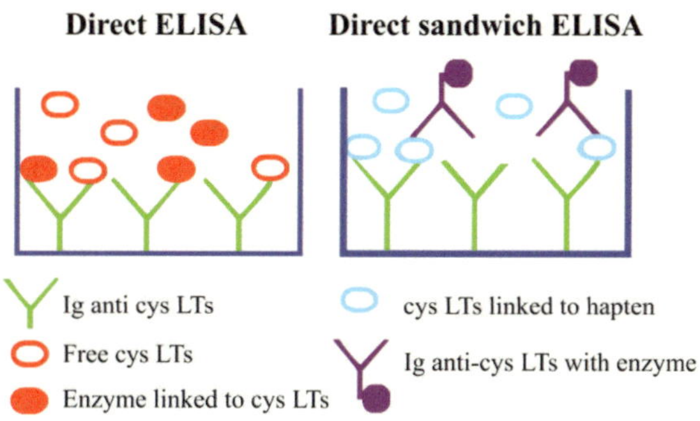

Fig. 10. The principles of direct ELISA and direct sandwich ELISA

Gas chromatography coupled with mass spectrometry (GC-MS) can be used for the analysis of leukotrienes giving information both about their structures and quantities. This analytical method takes advantage of its (1) high separation selectivity determined by the type of capillary columns used and (2) high specificity and sensitivity enabled by the integration of a mass spectrometric detector. Therefore, GC-MS method allows the quantification of substances in biological matrices on ng/mL-level. The most significant disadvantage is the need of a sufficient volatility and thermal stability of analytes in the sample, which is not the case of leukotrienes. To resolve it, pre-treatment procedures (extraction and derivatization) are necessary to be included in this particular case prior to quantitative and qualitative analysis. Derivatization is a chemical reaction of an analyte with a suitable derivatization reagent which changes its physical and chemical properties (in this case mainly volatility and thermal stability). Additionally, derivatization prior to a GC-MS analysis is carried out to improve the sensitivity of MS detection by enabling a better fragmentation in the detector. Leukotrienes contain several functional groups which can be employed in the derivatization reaction. The following are among the most popular: esterification of the carboxyl group, etherification of the hydroxyl group or hydrogenation of the double bonds. However, when cys LTs are hydrogenated on a rhodium catalyst (reaction time 20 min, temperature 0 °C), the cysteinyl moiety is cleaved off by a parallel desulfuration and thus only a sum of cys LTs can be determined by a GC-MS analysis. (Fauler et al., 1991; Balazy & Murphy, 1986). When other reactions are utilized, such as esterification by ethyl chloroformate (Čáp et al., 2004), pentafluorobenzyl ester-trimethyl silyl ether (PFB-TMS) (Awad et al., 1993; Ferretti et al., 1992), pentalfuorophenyl diazoalkanes (Hofmann et al., 1990), or etherification by *N,O*-bis(trimethylsilyl) trifluoroacetamide (BSTFA), followed by suitable extraction steps, individual cys LTs can be quantified by this method. Although there are only few different derivatization reactions used together with the analysis of leukotrienes by GC–MS, many variations of these reactions have been reported with regards to the type of a solvent, amount (excess) of derivatizing agent, temperature, reaction time and the storage of the samples to be injected into the GC–MS.

High Performance Liquid Chromatography (HPLC) in combination with mass spectrometry is generally used for the analysis of low volatile and thermally labile substances and thus it is highly suitable for the analysis of leukotrienes. The high selectivity of separation is achieved by a suitable choice of chromatographic phase systems, i.e. the liquid and stationary phase. Reversed-phase HPLC is the most commonly used with the stationary phase consisting of silica gel modifiable by non-polar octadecyl groups and the polar liquid phase usually consisting of water, acetonitrile or methanol, optionally with addition of buffers. For the detection, usually UV, fluorescence, electrochemical or MS methods are used. Nowadays, the combination of HPLC and MS allows facile separation and parallel detection of even very low analyte concentrations present in complex matrices. Since the remaining detectors mentioned above do not allow the quantification of analytes and lack the high specific structural information, HPLC-MS is becoming the first choice method for the analysis of substances in biological matrices. Therefore, the analysis of complex body fluids on a picogram scale is viable using HPLC-MS and also suitable for the future routine practice. In order to increase the detector precision and sensitivity, the following is advisable prior to the HPLC-MS analysis: (1) addition of an isotopically labelled internal standard and (2) use of a pre-treatment method (immunoextraction, solid phase extraction and lyophilisation) to remove undesired species and concentrate the sample.

When an MS detection is utilized, the analytes need to be evaporated and ionized. As this can be carried out at atmospheric pressure (API - atmospheric pressure ionization), it is also feasible with thermally labile substances (leukotrienes). Electrospray ionization (ESI) is one of the most frequently used API techniques. It belongs to the soft ionization techniques characterized by the preservation of a molecular ion peak with minimal fragmentation of the analyzed molecule. Depending on the molecule charge of a measured analyte, two measurement modes can be distinguished, i.e. positive electrospray ionization (ESI^+) in which protonated molecular ion $[M+H]^+$ is produced and negative electrospray ionization (ESI^-), where the molecule is deprotonated $[M-H]^-$. Ionization of cys LTs is possible in both modes but the $[M-H]^-$ ion is preferred especially because of a higher response in the detector. The combination of ESI ionization and a triple-stage quadruple analyzer (TSQ) is a suitable detection technique for the quantification of the given analytes. The first and the third quadruples (Q1 and Q3) are identical and capable of using the same scan modes. On the contrary, the second quadruple (Q2) is different both in its construction and function, allowing fragmentation of the analyte upon elastic collision with an inert gas (argon). Therefore, it is often referred to as the collision cell. A mass spectrometer equipped with a triple quadruple uses a highly selective single reaction monitoring mode (SRM) for the quantification and structural identification of substances. In the case of cys LTs, Q1 isolates the deprotonated $[M-H]^-$ molecular ions (LTC_4 m/z = 624 Da, LTD_4 m/z = 495 Da and LTE_4 m/z = 438 Da, see Fig. 11 - MS/MS spectra of cys LTs), which are further used as precursor ions for the subsequent collision-induced dissociation (CID) in Q2. In the collision cell, the molecule selectively degrades and yields product ions which are analyzed on quadrupole Q3, giving MS/MS spectra. For the quantification of cys LTs, the following SRM transitions are used: LTC_4 - 624.1 $\rightarrow$ 351.2 (collision energy 27eV); LTD_4 - 495.2 $\rightarrow$ 477.3 (21 eV) and LTE_4- 438.2 $\rightarrow$ 333.1 (19 eV).

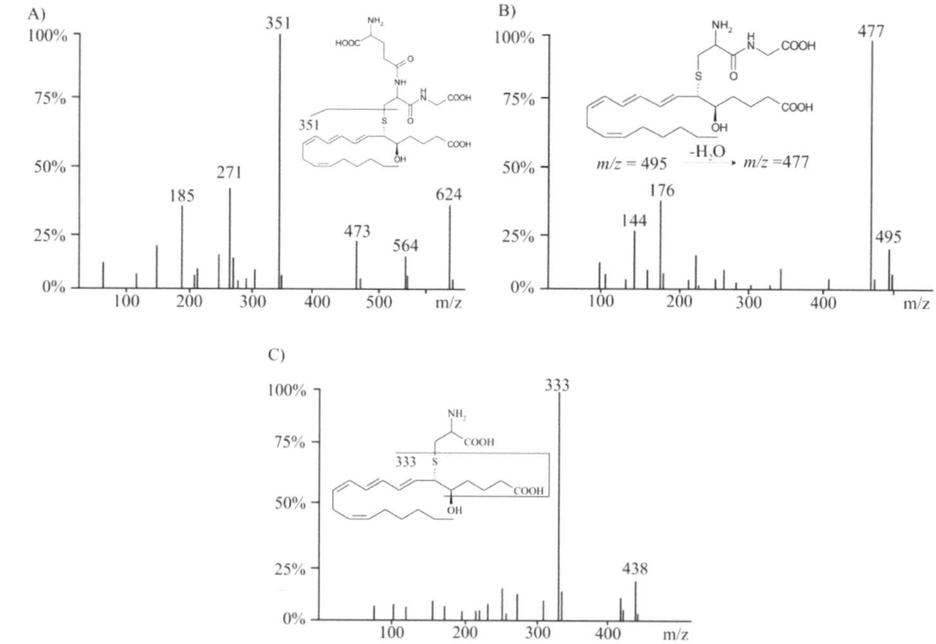

Fig. 11. ESI^- collision spectra of cys LTs (A -LTC_4, B-LTD_4, C-LTE_4)

Metabolomic techniques ("breathomics"), based on nuclear magnetic resonance (NMR), have also been applied in the EBC analysis, leading to the characterization of the biochemical fingerprints of airways (Carraro et al., 2007). Selected signals from NMR spectra offered a slightly better discrimination (linear discriminant analysis (LDA) of approximately 86 %) for asthmatics *versus* healthy children, as compared to the success rate of approximately 81 % for the combination of exhaled nitrogen oxide (ENO) and the forced expiratory volume at one second (FEV_1). The selected NMR variables were derived from the region of 3.2 – 3.4 ppm, indicative of oxidized compounds, and from the region of 1.7 - 2.2 ppm, indicative of acetylated compounds.

Introduction of internal standards may increase the precision of a quantification analysis. To achieve this, it is desirable to select a substance with physical and chemical properties identical to the observed endogenous cys LTs. It should act in the same manner not only during the detection but also in all preceding pre-treatment steps (extraction, derivatization). With some methods (ELISA, RIA), inner standards cannot be used as they are not separable from the endogenously present substance. Other methods (LC with UV, fluorescence or electrochemical detection) require using substituted analogues of cys LTs such as derivatized cys LTs. However, the use of these substances only partially resolves the drawbacks of separation and quantification methods. A successful MS detection requires the usage of ideal internal standards meeting the condition of identical physical and chemical properties and differing only in their molecular weight by the substitution of ^{1}H, ^{12}C or ^{16}O by corresponding stable isotopes ^{2}H, ^{13}C or ^{18}O. The minimal difference in the molecular weight between an endogenous cys LT and an isotopically labelled cys LT is 3 Da. Cys LTs labelled with ^{2}H and ^{13}C are nowadays commercially available and easily used in the quantification of cys LTs (Syslová et al., 2011; Montuschi, 2009).

6. Pre-treatment methods used for isolation and concentration of biomarkers

With only minor exceptions, the first step of analytical methods (including LC-MS, ELISA) in analysis cys LTs is their extraction from a biological matrix (EBC, urine, plasma, cerebrospinal fluid etc.). In principle, only few extraction techniques have been reported for the separation of cys LTs from EBC samples. These methods include immunoaffinity extraction (IAE) (Syslová et al., 2011), solid phase extraction (SPE) (Mizugaki et al., 1999; Ohanian et al., 2010; Chappell et al., 2011; Yang et al., 2009; Debley et al., 2007; Syslová et al., 2011), lyophilization (LYO) (Debley et al., 2007; Syslová et al., 2011) and solvent extraction (Huwyler & Gut, 1990). The applied methods varied primarily in their selectivity related to the given analytes. IAE showed the highest selectivity for cys LTs, which was determined by the highly specific reaction between the antigen (cys LTs) and the antibody (mouse monoclonal antibody against leukotriene C_4, D_4 and E_4 covalently bound to Sepharose 4B). This highly specific interaction not only enabled the separation of organic metabolites from salts contained in EBC, which was similar to SPE, but also cys LTs from other compounds present in EBC and especially from arachidonic acid derivatives. Identical specificity was achieved when immunoaffinity columns with antibodies immobilized to cys LTs were utilized. When SPE was used, the salts were eliminated together with potentially present other substances with a markedly different retention factor at the applied stationary phase of the SPE column (i.e. the eliminated substance was not retained within the stationary phase or it could have remained sorbed on it during the elution of cys LTs). The substances with a similar retention index (e.g. LTB_4, isoprostanes, thromboxanes) were contained in the solution together with cys LTs even after the SPE. For the separation of cys LTs, various stationary phases have been described in a number of papers including octadecyl (C18) (Syslová et al., 2011; Mizugaki et al., 1999) and various other kinds of copolymers (Ohanian et al., 2010; Chappell et al., 2011; Yang et al., 2009; Debley et al., 2007). SPE method enabled to supplement a less precise method of separation, i.e. the liquid–liquid extraction using the following solvents: water/propan-2-ol/dichloromethane (Huwyler & Gut, 1990; Clancy & Hugli, 1983). The liquid-liquid extractions are time-consuming since multi-step extractions may be needed in some cases or large volumes of organic solvents may be necessary for an efficient extraction. In addition, liquid-liquid extraction has not yet been demonstrated to be efficient for leukotrienes (Salari & Steffenrud, 1986). LYO is a useful method for concentrating non-volatile (or slightly volatile) substances dissolved in water. Cys LTs contained in EBC fall into this category. During the freeze-drying of the sample, no temperature stress of labile cys LTs occurred, which could have led to preferring freeze vacuum drying over IAS, SPE and solvent extraction (in this case, samples, when stored, had to be defrosted and processed at laboratory temperature). However, in contrast to this temperature-related advantage, there was no selectivity at all for the given analytes resulting in a deteriorated ionization during the mass-spectrometric determination even with the preceding liquid chromatography step. Apparently, this was caused by the presence of large quantities of substances including salts (Debley et al., 2007; Syslová et al., 2011). The methods of SPE, solvent extraction and LYO cannot eliminate possible analyte isomers potentially affecting the detectable level of cys LTs and thus there are higher requirements on the analysis, especially on the chromatographic part of the method.

Using the pre-separation methods based on antigen immunoextractionis connected with only minor errors and more accurate substance quantification is achieved (Table 2). Commercially available immunoaffinity sorbents and columns are burdened with a number of drawbacks, such as (1) time consumption (processing one sample takes approx. two hours), making the integration of non-compliance with the stability of cys LTs at room temperature more difficult, (2) the method labour input (in sorbents, it is especially difficult to separate EBC from an immunoaffinity sorbent and it is necessary to perform a series of mechanical operations, i.e. vortexing and centrifugation) and (3) limited repetitive use (the binding capacity in immunoaffinity columns is rapidly deteriorated by regeneration as a consequence of washing of antibodies from the support, while immunoaffinity sorbents exhibit a poor mechanical separation from an aqueous environment since boundless layers of water–sorbent are produced).

Analyte	Precision RSD (%)	Accuracy RE (%)
IAS		
LTC_4	9.7	-9.6
LTD_4	8.7	-8.0
LTE_4	8.1	-7.0
SPE-C18		
LTC_4	10.1	-10.4
LTD_4	9.2	-8.5
LTE_4	8.7	-8.2
LYO		
LTC_4	11.2	-14.2
LTD_4	9.9	-11.5
LTE_4	9.7	-9.3

Table 2. Validation parameters (precision and accuracy) for various pre-treatment methods (IAS, SPE and LYO) combined with LC-MS (n = 5)

Efforts to immobilize antibodies on more suitable supports by producing magnetic immunoparticles or encapsulating antibodies to polymeric matrices (e.g. polyvinyl alcohol) strive to minimize the above mentioned drawbacks. The very basic element of every magnetic immunoparticle (Fig. 12) is the magnetic core (1) composed of a magnetic material (e.g. magnetite, maghemite, cobalt, nickel, etc.). The magnetic core is ensphered in a functionalized outer coating (2), which usually stabilizes it (e.g., chitosan, carbon, polyethylene glycol, polyvinyl alcohol, etc.). On the surface, a cross-linker (3) is commonly bound (glutaraldehyde, carbodiimide, hydroxymethyl phosphine, etc.), which allows anchoring of an antibody. Such a prepared immunoparticle can be used for the separation of biomarkers from complex matrices. The produced antigen-antibody complex is separated from the solution using an external magnetic field (Fig. 12). The covalent bond between a magnetic particle and an antibody allows carrying out the regeneration of immunoparticles without any significant loss of the binding capacity.

By encapsulating antibodies to polyvinylalcohol (PVA) hydrogel (consisting of a mixture of two polymers: PVA with the function of a supporting matrix and polyethylene glycol (PEG) as a plasticizer) and producing porous immunolenses (Fig. 13), a rapid, accurate and very easy-to-handle tool is achieved for the separation of biomarkers from EBC. It was found experimentally that even after a repeated regeneration, no reduction occurred in the binding capacity of the immunolenses.

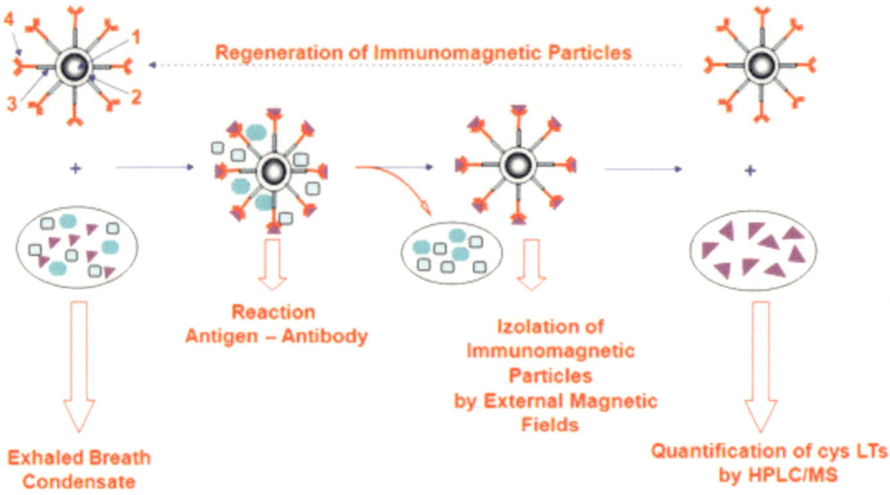

Fig. 12. Scheme of magnetic immunoparticles and their utilization for separation of biomarkers from EBC

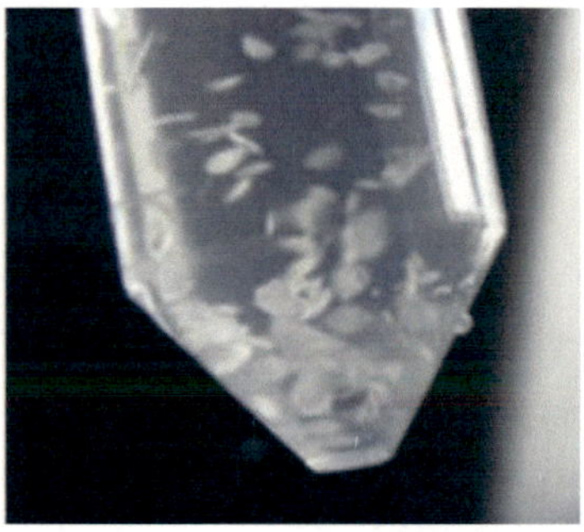

Fig. 13. Polymeric immunoparticles with encapsulated antibodies

7. Detection based on mass spectrometric methods and comparison with others

The following analytical methods are currently used for the quantitative determination of cys LTs in EBC: EIA (ELISA), HPLC-MS and GC-MS. These individual methods can be optimally compared on the basis of method validation parameters (including pre-treatment methods and derivatization), i.e. precision, accuracy, limit of detection (LOD) and limit of quantification (LOQ), which are listed in the table 3. The least utilized method is the derivatization of cys LTs with a consecutive GC-MS detection (Čáp et al., 2004). The method is accompanied by several shortcomings: (1) the choice of derivatization reagent (ethylchloroformate) which causes the degradation of LTC_4, while the referenced authors provide that LTC_4 is not quantified in clinical studies, even though its presence in EBC has been demonstrated using LC-MS method; (2) unsuitable use of an internal standard, i.e. arachidonic acid, which is endogenously present in EBC and its physico-chemical properties are significantly different from cys LTs for both its derivatization step and the very GC-MS analysis; (3) GC-MS analysis using thermal transfer of substances to the gas phase, which is not an appropriate method for the thermally labile cys LTs. In the literature, we have encountered different LOQs for immunochemical methods, while other validation parameters have not been provided (owing to the manufacturer's validation of an EIA/ELISA kit being applicable only to a urine matrix). Using immunochemical methods with a monoclonal antibody for cys LTs, only Σ cys LTs can be determined (contrary to LC-MS methods permitting precise quantifications of individual leukotriene levels). Furthermore, with this method, one can encounter a false positive or negative effect on the results owing to a cross-reaction with other substances contained in EBC. The specificity of antibodies against cys LTs are different and vary with each EIA and ELISA kit. We have encountered, for instance, the following values in immunoglobulin specificity: 1) LTC_4 - 100 %, LTD_4 - 100 %, LTE_4 - 79 %, LTD_5 - 61 %, LTC_5 - 54 %, LTE_5 - 41 %, N-acetyl LTE_4 = 10.5 % (Cysteinyl Leukotriene EIA kit, Cayman Chemical Company, Ann Arbor), 2) LTC_4 - 100 %, LTD_4 - 100 %, LTE_4 - 65 %, N-methyl LTC_4 - 124 %, LTB_4 - < 0.01 % (Cysteinyl Leukotriene Express EIA kit, Cayman Chemical Company, Ann Arbor). Such variable values of specificity may be the source of inconsistent results reported in the literature projected in the values for clinical studies. Due to antibody's low specificity, acquired structural (qualitative) information cannot be selectively attributed to the detected cys LTs using EIA. The determined concentration of cys LTs in EBC are significantly lower using immunochemical methods than using LC-MS. This may be due to disrespecting the thermal stability of the analyte, because the reaction between antigen and antibody are incubated for about 12 hours at room temperature or at 4 °C. At these temperatures, a relatively rapid decomposition of cys LTs occurs (see section 4). Most of the shortcomings of GC-MS and EIA (ELISA) methods are resolves by the unification of liquid chromatography with mass spectrometry. LC-MS method in a highly selective and accurate SRM mode (see section 5) affords both quantitative and qualitative information about the monitored biomarkers. Liquid chromatography can be used in both HPLC mode (high performance liquid chromatography) and UHPLC mode (ultra-high performance liquid chromatography). In UHPLC, the separation of substances is carried out at higher flow rates of the mobile phase (1 mL/min) on LC columns with a smaller average particle size of the stationary phase (diameter of particles 2 μm), shortening the time of LC-MS analysis.

When using the so-called "stable-isotope-dilution assay", the accuracy and precision of the LC-MS method can be increased by suitable deuterated internal standards ((19,19,20,20,20-$^2H_5$) LTC_4, (19,19,20,20,20-$^2H_5$) LTD_4, (19,19,20,20,20-$^2H_5$) LTE_4). Immediately after the collection, a known amount of isotopically labelled internal standard is added to 1 mL of EBC sample (in order to monitor the substance amount from the very beginning and eliminate the error of cys LTs disintegration during the sample handling), which has the identical physico-chemical properties as the endogenously present biomarkers with the only exception of a different molecular weight. This is beneficially utilized in MS detection and both substance resolution (deuterium-labelled cys LTs are characterized by identical retention times in the LC separation, such as the unlabelled cys LTs, but they can be well separated in the mass spectrometer). The disadvantage of the LC-MS analysis of cys LTs still remains the inclusion of the pre-treatment step (SPE, immunoaffinity extraction), during which EBC sample is exposed to room temperature. This problem is resolved using 2D technology for liquid chromatography. In the first dimension, it is possible to carry out an on-line SPE using the SPE column Hypersil GOLD (20x 2.1 mm, particle size 12 μm, Thermo Scientific, USA) and the subsequent dimension using the LC chromatography.

Methods	LOQ	References	Note
EIA	78.1 pg/mL	Hoffmeyer et al, 2009	determined as cys LTs
EIA	13 pg/mL	Debley et al., 2007	determined as cys LTs
EIA	13 pg/mL	Piotrowski et al., 2007	determined as cys LTs
EIA	13 pg/mL	Antczak et al., 2002	determined as cys LTs
EIA	7.8 pg/mL	Goldbart, et al., 2006	determined as cys LTs
EIA	5 pg/mL	Leung et al., 2006	determined as cys LTs
ELISA	14 pg/mL	Soyer et al., 2006	determined as cys LTs
GC-MS	1pg/mL	Čáp et. al., 2004	only LTD4, LTE4; determined separately for each LT
LC -MS	<10 pg/mL	Syslová et al., 2011	determined separately for each LT

Table 3. Limit of quantification (LOQ) for detection methods for cys LTs

8. Clinical experience in biomarker-based diagnostics of occupational bronchial asthma

Occupational asthma is an occupational condition defined as: "A disease characterized by variable airflow limitation and/or airway hyper-responsiveness due to causes and conditions attributable to a particular occupational environment and not stimuli encountered outside the workplace". The proper diagnosis of occupational asthma is important for the prognosis of the disease and can be based on several tests. Out of these, controlled exposure to suspected occupational allergens in the laboratory is considered to be the gold standard. Occupational allergens are either applied with a special bronchoprovocation device or the patients are exposed to allergens in the challenge chamber under conditions reproducing the workplace exposure. An integral part of the specific bronchoprovocation tests is the monitoring of subjective complaints, objective findings and the repeated lung function measurement over 24 h. Exposure to allergens can also be performed directly in the workplace. Nevertheless, it is not always possible to make an unequivocal diagnosis of occupational asthma. It may pose difficulty especially in the case of a borderline decrease in ventilatory parameters, or, on the other hand, in patients with advanced or persisting obstructive ventilatory defect, in whom the specific bronchoprovocation tests cannot be performed. If the specific test is not feasible, other tests (and their combinations) like non-specific bronchoprovocation tests, skin prick tests, serum-specific imunoglobuline E (IgE) can be helpful in the determination of final diagnosis (each with various specificity and sensitivity compared to the specific bronchoprovocation test) (Klusáčková et al., 2008). Patients on permanent antiasthmatic treatment whose reaction to allergens is partially mitigated by the treatment represent another diagnostic problem. Therefore, a need arises to look for other markers (in addition to the ventilatory parameters), which would enable the verification of the reaction to the occupational allergen. Induced sputum analysis is one of the procedures previously reported to be helpful in occupational asthma diagnosis. However, it has the disadvantage that, despite the induction of sputum by hypertonic saline, some people do not produce a satisfactory sample of sputum for analysis. Multiple studies reported eosinophils increase after a bronchoprovocation test

(Lemiere, 2007). Exhaled nitric oxide could be another helpful marker in occupational asthma diagnosis. A definite advantage is that its collection is non-invasive but the sticking point is the lack of unambigouos data after the alergen testing. Exhaled breath condensate (EBC) contains many substances reflecting changes in the airways and it offers further possibilities for the diagnosis and monitoring of occupational asthma and other respiratory diseases. Collection of the EBC enables to study the concentration of leukotrienes directly in the airways and to detect individual cys LTs - LTC_4, LTD_4, LTE_4. The other parameters of interest for the monitoring during the bronchoprovocation are leukotriene B_4 and 8-isoprostane, known to be elevated in asthmatics (Hatipoglu & Rubinstein, 2004).

The aim of our study was to monitor changes in EBC concentrations of cys LTs in patients with occupational asthma diagnosis (without any lung pharmacotherapy) and healthy subjects. The pilot clinical study was performed in a group of 20 subjects with a given diagnosis (56–64 years old, male, nonsmokers) and with the equal number in the control group (52–66 years old, male, non-smokers). EBC samples collected during the clinical study were worked up by the IAS (pre-treatment method used for LC-MS determination) (Syslová et al., 2011) and the results were statistically evaluated. A significant difference was found between the control group and the group with the diagnosis in the values of concentration of LTC_4 (57.4 ± 8.6 pg/mL of EBC in the control group and 80.1 ± 6.2 pg/mL of EBC in those diagnosed with bronchial asthma) and LTE_4 (25.3 ± 5.1 pg/mL in the control group *versus* 35.7 ± 4.8 pg/mL in the bronchial asthma group). The difference in the levels was highlighted in the sum values of cys LTs, where the control group reached values of 77.8 ± 13.8 pg/mL of EBC and the asthmatic group reached 133.2 ± 20.1 pg/mL of EBC. Although a difference in the levels of LTD_4 was observed in its average value as well, differing from 19.9 ± 4.3 pg/mL of EBC in positively diagnosed subjects to 13.8 ± 5.2 pg/mL of EBC in the healthy subjects, the significance of this biomarker for the differential diagnostics of bronchial asthma was not entirely proven as the difference in the confidence intervals was statistically insignificant (Fig. 14).

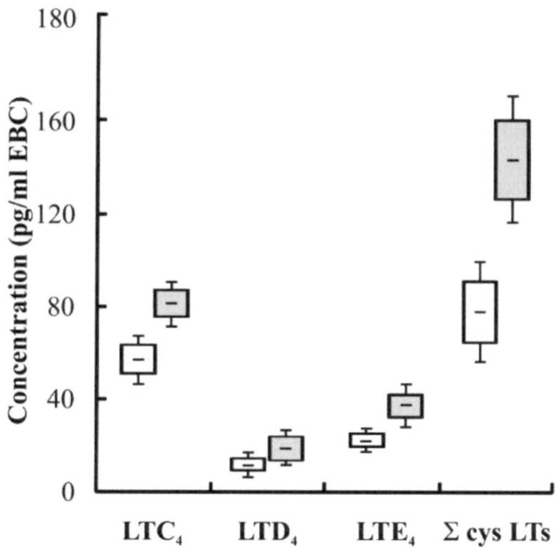

Fig. 14. Clinical study - concentration of cys LTs in EBC; bronchial asthma (grey), healthy subjects (white)

9. Bronchial asthma multimarker screening in exhaled breath condensate

Increased concentration levels of cys LTs in EBC do not always signify a proven diagnosis of bronchial asthma. High levels of cys LTs in EBC could also point to other lung diseases such as cystic fibrosis (Lammers, 2008), COPD (chronic obstructive pulmonary disease) (Usery et al., 2008) or a mere interindividual variation can be involved, where the increased concentration of cys LTs may represent the physiological level compared to other healthy individuals. For this reason, it is even convenient to monitor other substances that have been detected in EBC. Besides cys LTs, other low-molecular substances, considered as relevant biomarkers of other diseases, were monitored in EBC: 8-isoprostane (damage of phospholipids membrane, biomarker of oxidative stress, potential biomarker of bronchial asthma), leukotriene B_4 (damage of phospholipids membrane, biomarker of inflammation, potential biomarker of bronchial asthma), *o*-tyrosine (damage of amino acids, biomarker of oxidative stress), nitrotyrosine (damage of amino acids, biomarker of oxidative stress), 8-hydroxyguanosine (damage of RNA, biomarker of oxidative stress), 8-hydroxy-2′-deoxy-guanosine (damage of DNA, biomarker of oxidative stress), 5-hydroxymethyluracil (damage of DNA, biomarker of oxidative stress), malondialdehyde (damage of phospholipids membrane, potential biomarker of bronchial asthma, biomarker of oxidative stress) and 4-hydroxy-*trans*-nonenale (damage of phospholipids membrane, biomarker of oxidative stress). For their detection, 2D LC-MS method was developed. In the first dimension, on-line SPE (Hypersil GOLD column; 20 x 2.1 mm, particle size 12 μm, Thermo Scientific, USA) was carried out. Water was employed as the mobile phase for the column activation and a mixture of water : acetonitrile (30 : 70) was used for its regeneration. The separation of eluted components from the SPE column was performed on an analytical column (Hypercarb 100 x 2.1 mm column, particle size 5 μm, Thermo Scientific, USA) utilizing gradient elution (0:00 – 70 % A → 10.00 – 70 % A → 25:00 – 5 % A → 55: 00 to 5 % A → 60:00 – 70 % A). Here, solvent A consisted of water with pH adjusted to 10.5 with ammonia and solvent B was composed of methanol and acetonitrile in the ratio 60 : 40 (v/v) with an addition of ammonia (0.1 %). Using an MS detector, the developed method allows to separate and subsequently quantify not only the substances mentioned above but also diastereomers and several other prostaglandins (prostaglandin D_2 and E_2), as shown in the sample chromatogram. Fig. 15 shows the resulting chromatographic record. Using this method, a pilot study was carried out monitoring the levels of substances in healthy individuals (n = 10, age = 66 ± 1.5) and in people with occupational asthma (n = 11, age = 67 ± 2.7). Fig. 16 shows the clinical study results where a statistically significant difference was determined in addition to Σ cys LTs for LTB_4, malondialdehyde, 4-hydroxy-*trans*-nonenal and 8-isoprostane.

EBC analyses in healthy subjects and patients with a diagnosis of occupational asthma using high-resolution mass spectrometry (HRMS; LTQ Orbitrap Velos, Thermo, USA) or nuclear magnetic resonance (NMR) and processing of the obtained data by the so-called principal component analysis (PCA) can reveal and determine differences in individual samples and thus identify substances statistically significant for the given disease (Wan et al., 2008). In the context of PCA, the data can be regarded as a multivariate statistical problem where the metabolite or protein concentrations represent the true variables. Spectra are divided into "bins" of discrete spectral width (ppm in the case of NMR, m/z in the case of MS) and the areas under the curve (AUC) in these "bins" are integrated and serve as *pseudo*-variables. PCA therefore reduces a large number of (usually correlated) "true" variables into a smaller number of (uncorrelated) variables, the so-called principal components (PC). PCA results in the decomposition of raw data into "scores", which reveal the relationship among samples and into "loadings" that show the relationships among the variables. The first PC interprets the greatest variability in data, the second PC (independent of/orthogonal from the first) interprets the second best and so on. If one assumes the data space can be reduced to a cube, PCA resembles turning the cube in different angles and identifying planes in the data space, separating the investigated and compared groups (typically control and case).

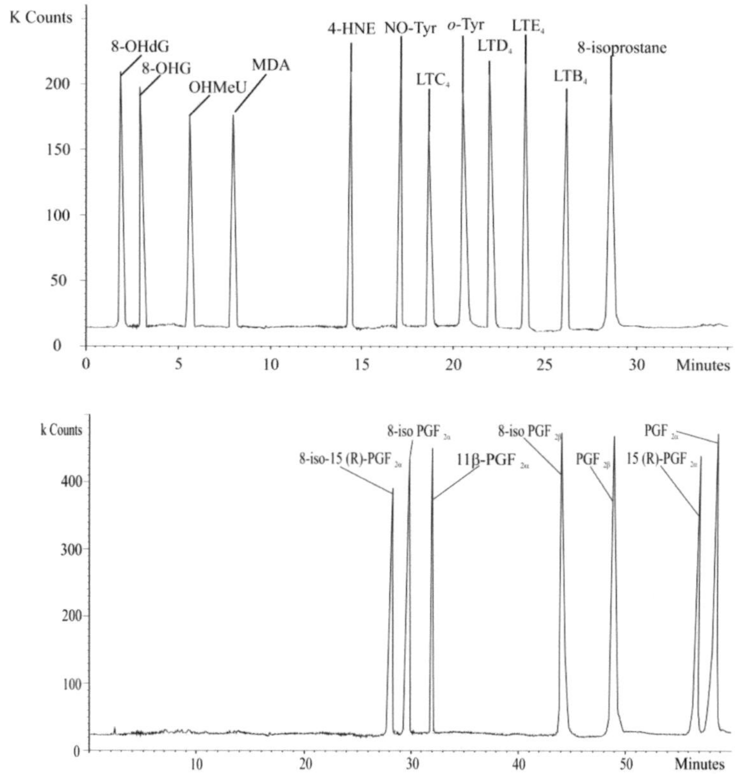

Fig. 15. Chromatogram of detected biomarkers (above) and chromatogram of diastereomers of 8-isoprostane (below)

The above-mentioned approach will be combined with a recent significant advance in chemometric modelling, which uses full-resolution data sets that represent each data point in the spectrum rather than binned data that represent summed segments of a spectrum. The use of full-resolution (all computer points in spectrum) data allows the spectral structure to be retained, and this together with models of orthogonal partial least squares discriminant analysis (O-PLS-DA) incorporate the correlation weight of the variables, enabling plotting of the loadings that are colour-coded and easily interpretable. O-PLS-DA modelling together with a back-scaling step can be successfully applied to determine the metabolic and variable allergenic consequences in multiple bio-fluid compartments.

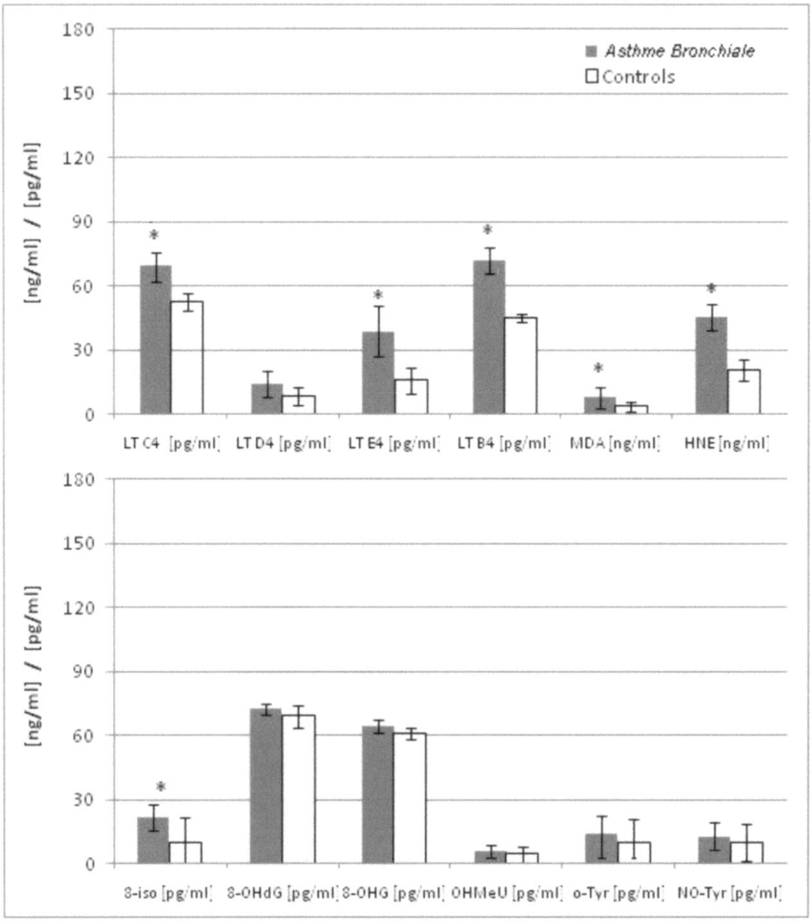

Fig. 16. Concentration of biomarkers in EBC; bronchial asthma (grey), healthy subjects (white)

Alternative approach to the multimarker analysis of both leukotrienes and other biomarkers including cytokines, chemokines as well as genetic profiling is based on a relatively novel technology, i.e. microarrays, or very recently, nanoarrays. Microarrays are two-dimensional platforms, typically based on a glass microscope slide, upon which specific biological probes are anchored, using either deposition or *in-situ* synthesis, in a high-density (tens of thousands to millions of probes) matrix in a predetermined spatial order. The analytical principle is based on a selective hybridization of the immobilized probes with targets contained in the biological sample, in this case EBC, using most commonly fluorescence or color detection. In the case of leukotrienes, antibody microarrays with specific probes to cys LTs are commercially available. Nevertheless, commercially available antibody as much as protein microarrays, have exhibited a rather low or very variable sensivity for each probe and thus further development was required to increase the sensitivity for clinical and research applications (Kricka et. al, 2002). The very novel platform though, nanoarrays, produced by nanolitographic methods (Bearingers et al., 2009; Rosa & Liang, 2009), e.g. the patented dip pen nanolithography (Lee et al., 2006) is exhibiting a principally much better and consistent sensitivity. This technology has already been verified by several applications exhibiting high sensitivity in analyses of e.g. interleukins and THF-α markers. More applications are yet to be developed and validated, while it can be predicted that this platform may well function and be validated for cys LTs in the near future. I.e. nanoarrays thus can be anticipated to eventually create a solid multimarker alternative suitable for a routine screening, providing to have accomplished necessary validations.

10. Conclusions: Future perspective of biomarkers in exhaled breath condensate

Measurements of asthma biomarkers in EBC offer a novel way of monitoring lung inflammation and provide insight into the pathophysiology of the disease. The diagnostics based on determination of biomarkers present in EBC is completely non-invasive, well accepted by the patients, applicable to children, suitable for longitudinal studies, patient follow-up and potentially useful for monitoring drug therapy. From the medicinal point of view, biomarkers present in EBC reflect lungs information, rather than they give systemic information. Characterisation of selective profiles of exhaled biomarkers (cys LTs, LTB_4, 8-isoprostane, etc.) might be relevant to the differential asthma diagnosis. However, EBC analysis requires standardisation and validation of the whole diagnostic process including sample collection, sample pre-analysis handling (e.g. storing, internal standardisation, pre-treatment method application) and uniform analytical technique application.

Future research should be oriented on the identification of reference values for the different asthma biomarkers in healthy subjects (children and adults), on large longitudinal studies to ascertain if sequential measurements in the individual patient reflect asthma severity and the degree of lung inflammation, studies on relationship between the concentrations of asthma biomarkers and its symptoms, lung function, and other indices and results from other diagnostic methods. Unavoidable will also be to conduct controlled studies in order to establish the usefulness of EBC analysis for guiding pharmacological treatment in asthma and the effect of drugs on asthma markers present in EBC. Studies to determine the usefulness of EBC analysis for predicting treatment response and assessment of new therapies should also be carried out. Last but not least is also the knowledge on the feasibility of gene expression analysis in EBC. From the point of complex approach to EBC analysis it will also be important to determine the biomarker concentrations and profiles in regard to different lung diseases as well as to identify other inflammation mediators. This represents a great deal of work remaining. The truth is that EBC analysis is currently used in various clinical trials and studies. On the other hand, it is important to proclaim that the fact whether and when EBC analysis will be applicable to the clinical settings is still difficult to predict.

11. Acknowledgements

The authors wish to acknowledge with gratitude the financial support from the Ministry of Health of the Czech Republic (Grant NS 10298-3/2009), Ministry of Education of the Czech Republic (Grant CEZ: MSM 604 613 301 and EUREKA E!4091/OE09009) the Grant Agency of the Czech Republic (Grant GA CR 203/08/H032).

12. References

Accordino, R.; Visentin, A.; Bordin, A.; Ferrazzoni, S.; Marian, E.; Rizzato, F.; Canova, C.; Venturini, R. & Maestrelli, P. (2008). Long-term repeatability of exhaled breath condensate pH in asthma. *Respiratory Medicine*, Vol. 102, No. 3, (March 2008), pp. 377-381, ISSN 0954-6111

Antczak, A.; Montuschi, P.; Kharitonov, S.; Gorski, P. & Barnes, P.J. (2002). Increased Exhaled Cysteinyl-Leukotrienes and 8-Isoprostane in Aspirin-induced Asthma. *American Journal of Respiratory and Critiacal Care Medicine*, Vol. 166, No. 3, (August 2002), pp. 301 - 306, ISSN 1535-4970

Armstrong, M.; Liu, A. H.; Harbeck, R.; Reisdorph, R.; Rabinovitch, N. & Reisdorph, N. (2009). Leukotriene-E_4 in human urine: Comparison of on-line purification and liquid chromatography-tandem mass spectrometry to affinity purification followed by enzyme immunoassay. *Journal of Chromatograph, B*, Vol. 877, No. 27, (October 2009), pp. 3169-3174, ISSN 1570-0232

Awad, J.A.; Morrow, J.D. & Roberts, L.J.II. (1993). Simplification of the mass spectrometric assay for the major urinary metabolite of prostaglandin D2. *Journal of Chromatography, Biomedical Applications*, Vol. 617, No. 1, (1993), pp. 124-128, ISSN 1572-6495

Balazy, M. & Murphy, R.C. (1986). Determination of sulfidopeptide leukotrienes in biological fluids by gas chromatography mass spectrometry. *Analytical Chemistry*, Vol. 58, No. 5, (May 1986), pp. 1098-1101, ISSN 0003-2700

Baraldi, E.; Carraro, S.; Alinovi, R.; Pesci, A.; Ghiro, L.; Bodini, A.; Piacentini, G.; Zacchello, F. & Zanconato, S. (2003). Cysteinyl leukotrienes and 8-isoprostane in exhaled breath condensate of children with asthma exacerbations. *Thorax*, Vol. 58, No. 6, (June 2003), pp. 505–509, ISSN 1468-3296

Barnes, N.C. & Smith, L.J. (2002). Biochemistry and physiology of the leukotrienes. *Clinical Reviews in Allergy and Immunology*, Vol. 17, No. 1-2, (March 1999), pp. 27-42, ISSN 1559-0267

Bearinger, J. P.; Stone, G.; Dugan, L.C.; El Dasher, B.; Stockton, Ch.; Conway, J.W.; Kuenzler, T. & Hubbell J. A. (2009). Porphyrin-based Photocatalytic Nanolithography. *Molecular & Cellular Proteomics*, Vol. 8, No. 8, (August 2009), pp. 1823–1831, ISSN 1553-9484

Beyer, G.; Meese, C.O. & Klotz, U. (1987). Stability of leukotrienes C4 and D4 in human urine. *Prostaglandins, Leukotrienes and Medicine*, Vol. 29, No. 2-3, (October 1987), pp. 229-235, ISSN 0262-1746

Bikov, A.; Gajdocsi, R.; Huszar, E.; Szili, B.; Lazar, Z.; Antus, B.; Losonczy, G. & Horvath, I. (2010). Exercise increases exhaled breath condensate cysteinyl leukotriene concentration in asthmatic patients. *Journal of Asthma*, Vol. 47, No. 9, (September 2010), pp. 1057-1062, ISSN 1532-4303

Brocklehurst, W.E. (1960). The release of histamine and formation of a slow-reacting substance (SRS-A) during anaphylactic shock. *The Journal of Physiology*, Vol. 151, No. 3, (June 1960), pp. 416–435, ISSN 1469-7793

Brooks, S.M.; Haight, R.R. & Gordon, R.L. (2006). Age Does Not Affect Airway pH and Ammonia as Determined by Exhaled Breath Measurements. *Lung*, Vol. 184, No. 4, (August 2006), pp. 195-200, ISSN 1432-1750

Brussino, L.; Badiu, I.; Sciascia, S.; Bugiani, M.; Heffler, E.; Guida, G.; Malinovschi, A.; Bucca, C. & Rolla, G. (2010). Oxidative stress and airway inflammation after allergen challenge evaluated by exhaled breath condensate analysis, *Clinical & Experimental Allergy*, Vol. 40, No. 11, (November 2010), pp. 1642-1647, ISSN 1365-2222

Carraro, S.; Corradi, M.; Zanconato, S.; Alinovi,R.; Pasquale, M. F.; Zacchello, F. & Baraldi, E. (2005). Exhaled breath condemsate cysteinyl leukotrienes are increased in children with exercise-induced bronchoconstriction. *Journal of Allergy and Clinical Immunology*, Vol. 115, No. 4, (April 2005), pp. 764-770, ISSN 0091-6749

Carraro, S.; Rezzi, S.; Reniero, F.; Héberger, K.; Giordano, G.; Zanconato, S.; Guillou, C. & Baraldi, E. (2007). Metabolomics applied to exhaled breath condensatein childhood asthma. *American Journal of Respiratory and Critiacal Care Medicine,* Vol. 175, No. 10, (May 2007), pp. 986-990, ISSN 0002-9378

Chappell, G.P.; Xiao, X.; Pica-Mendez, A.; Varnell, T.; Green, S.; Tanaka, W.K. & Laterza, O. (2011). Quantitative measurement of cysteinyl leukotrienes and leukotriene B4 in human sputum using ultra high pressure liquid chromatography–tandem mass spectrometry. *Journal of Chromatography B*, Vol. 879, No. 3-4, (Febuary 2011), pp. 277–284, ISSN 1570-0232

Chuang, M.T.; Raskin, J.; Krellenstein, D.J. & Teirstein, A.S. (1987). Bronchoscopy in diffuse lung disease: evaluation by open lung biopsy in nondiagnostic transbronchial lung biops. *The Annals of otology, rhinology, and laryngology*, Vol. 96, No. 6, (December 1987), pp. 654-657, ISSN 0003-4894

Clancy, R.M. & Hugli, T.E. (1983).The extraction of leukotrienes (LTC4, LTD4, and LTE4) from tissue fluids: The metabolism of these mediators during IgE-dependent hypersensitivity reactions in lung. *Analytical Biochemistry: Methods in the Biological Sciences*, Vol. 133, No. 1, (August 1983), pp. 30-39, ISSN 0003-2697

Corradi, M.; Pignatti, P.; Manini, P.; Andreoli, R.; Goldoni, M.; Poppa, M.; Moscato, G.; Balbi, B. & Mutti, A. (2004). Comparison between exhaled and sputum oxidative stress biomarkers in chronic airway inflammation. *European Respiratory Journal*, Vol. 24, No. 6, (December 2004), pp. 1011-1017, ISSN 0903-1936

Csoma, Z.; Kharitonov, S.A.; Balint, B.; Busch, A.; Wilson, N.M. & Barnes, P.J. (2002). Increased Leukotrienes in Exhaled Breath Condensate in Childhood Asthma. *American Journal of Respiratory and Critiacal Care Medicine*, Vol. 166, No. 10, (November 2002), pp. 1345 -1349, ISSN 1535-4970

Čáp, P.; Chládek, J.; Pehal, F.; Malý, M.; Petrů, V.; Barnes, P.J. & Montuschi, P. (2004). Gas chromatography/mass spectrometry analysis of exhaled leukotrienes in asthmatic patients. *Thorax*, Vol. 59, No. 6, (June 2004), pp. 465-470, ISSN 1468-3296

Daussant, J. & Desvaux, F. X. (2007). *Introduction to Immunochemical Techniques for Medical Diagnosis, Food Quality Control and Environmental Testing*, J. Daussant (Ed.), ICT Prague, ISBN 978-80-7080-641-8, Prague, Czech Republic

Debley, J.S.; Hallstrand, T.S.; Monge, T.; Ohanian, A.; Redding, G.J. & Zimmerman, J. (2007). Methods to improve measurement of cysteinyl leukotrienes in exhaled breath condensate from subjects with asthma and healthy controls. *Journal of Allergy and Clinical Immunology*, Vol. 120, No. 5, (November 2007), pp. 1216-1217, ISSN 0091-6749

Dekhuijzen, P.N.; Aben, K.K.; Dekker, I.; Aarts, L.P.; Wielders, P.L.; van Herwaardne, C.A. & Bass, A. (1996). *American Journal of Respiratory and Critiacal Care Medicine*, Vol. 154, No. 3, (September 1996), pp. 813, ISSN 0002-9378

Dworski, R.; Stoke Peebles, R. & Sheller, J.R. (2004). *New perspectives in monitoring lung inflamation. Analysis of exhaled breath condensate*, P. Montuschi, (Ed.), 149-165, CRC press, ISBN 0-415-32465-3, Boca Raton, Florida

Effros, R.M.; Biller, J.; Dunning, M. & Shaker, R. (2004). *New perspectives in monitoring lung inflamation. Analysis of exhaled breath condensate*, P. Montuschi, (Ed.), 31-52, CRC press, ISBN 0-415-32465-3, Boca Raton, Florida

Emylyanov, A.; Fedoseev, G.; Abulimity, A.; Rudinski, K.; Fedoulov, A.; Karabanov, A. & Barnes, P.J. (2001). Elevated concentrations of exhaled hydrogen peroxide in asthmatic patients. *Chest*, Vol. 120, No. 4, (October 2001), pp. 1136-1139, ISSN 1931-3543

Fauler, J.; Tsikas, D.; Holch, M.; Seekamp, A.; Nerlich, M.L.; Sturm, J. & Frolich, J.C. (1991). Enhanced urinary excretion of leukotriene E4 by patients with multiple trauma with or without adult respiratory distress syndrome. *Clinical Science*, Vol. 80, No. 5, (May 1991), pp. 497-504, ISSN 1470-8736.

Ferretti, A.; Flanagan, V.P. & Maida, E.J. (1992). GC/MS/MS quantification of 11-dehydrothromboxane B2 in human urine. *Prostaglandins, Leukotrienes & Essential Fatty Acids*, Vol. 46, No. 4, (August 1992), pp. 271-275, ISSN 0952-3278

Gaber, F.; Acevedo, F.; Delin, I.; Sundblad, B-M.; Palmberg, L.; Larsson, K.; Kumlin M. & Dahle´n, S-E. (2006). Saliva is one likely source of leukotriene B4, in exhaled breath condensate. *European Respiratory Journal*, Vol. 28, No. 6, (December 2006), pp. 1229–1235, ISSN 1399-3003

Gerritsen, W.B.; Zanen, P.; Bauwens, A.A.; van den Bosch, J.M. & Hass, F.J. (2005). Validation of a new method to measure hydrogen peroxide in exhaled breath condensate. *Respiratory Medecine*, Vol. 99, No. 9, (September 2005), pp. 1132-1137, ISSN 0945-6111

Gessner, Ch.; Hammerschmidt, S.; Kuhn, H.; Seyfarth, H.J.; Sack, U.; Engelmann, L.; Schauer, J. & Wirtz, H. (2003). Exhaled breath condensate acidification in acute lung injury. *Respiratory Medecine*, Vol. 97, No. 11, (November 2003), pp. 1188-1194, ISSN 0945-6111

GINA (2010) Global Initiative for Asthma Prevention and Management, December 2010. Available from <http://www.ginasthma.org>

Goldbart, A.D.; Krishna, J.; Li, R.C.; Serpero, L.D. & Gozal, D. (2006). Inflammatory Mediators in Exhaled Breath Condensate of Children With Obstructive Sleep Apnea Syndrome. *Chest*, Vol. 130, No. 1, (July 2006), pp. 143-148, ISSN 1931-3543

Green, R.H.; Brightling, Ch.E.; Mc Kenna, S.; Hargadon, B.; Parker, D.; Bradding, P.; Wardlaw, A.J. & Pavord, I.D. (2002). Asthma exacerbations and sputum eosinophil counts: a randomised controlled trial. *The Lancet*, Vol. 360, No. 9347, (November 2002), pp. 1715-1721, ISSN 0140-6736

Hatipoglu, U. & Rubinstein, I. (2004). *New perspectives in monitoring lung inflamation. Analysis of exhaled breath condensate*, P. Montuschi, (Ed.), 123-138, CRC press, ISBN 0-415-32465-3, Boca Raton, Florida

Henden, T.; Strand, H.; Borde, E.; Semb, A.G. & Larsen, T.S. (1993). Measurements of leukotrienes in human plasma by solid phase extraction and high performance liquid chromatography. *Prostaglandins, Leukotrienes and Essential Fatty Acids*, Vol. 49, No. 5, (November 1993), pp. 851-854, ISSN 0952-3278

Higashi, N.; Taniguchi, M.; Mita, H.; Kawagishi, Y.; Ishii, T.; Higashi, A.; Osame, M. & Akiyama, K. (2004). Clinical features of asthmatic patients with increased urinary leukotriene E4 excretion (hyperleukotrienuria) Involvement of chronic hyperplastic rhinosinusitis with nasal polyposis. *Journal of Allergy and Clinical Immunology*, Vol. 113, No. 2, (August 2004), pp. 277-283, ISSN 0091-6749

Hoffmeyer,F.; Raulf-Heimsoth, M.; Harth, V.; Bünger, J. & Brüning, T. (2009). Comparative analysis of selected exhaled breath biomarkers obtained with two different temperature-controlled device. *BMC Pulmonary Medicine*, Vol. 9, (November 2009), pp. 48, ISSN 1471-2466

Hofmann, U.; Holzer, S. & Meese, C.O. (1990). Pentafluorophenyldiazoalkanes as novel derivatization reagents for the determination of sensitive carboxylic acids by gas chromatography-negative-ion mass spectrometry. *Journal of Chromatography*, Vol. 508, No. 2, (1990), pp. 349-356, ISSN 0021-9673

Holz, O.; Kips, J. & Magnussen, H. (2000). Update on sputum methodology. *European Respiratory Journal*, Vol. 16, No. 2, (August 2000), pp. 355–359, ISSN 1399-3003

Horváth, I.; Donnelly, L.E.; Kiss, A.; Kharitonov, S.A; LIM, S.; Fan Chung & Barnes, P.J. (1998). Combined use of exhaled hydrogen peroxide and nitric oxide in monitoring asthma. *American Journal of Respiratory and Critiacal Care Medicine,* Vol. 158, No. 4, (July 1998), pp. 1042-1046, ISSN 0002-9378

Horváth, I.; Hunt, J. & Barnes, P.J. (2005). Exhaled breath condensate: methodological recommendations and unresolved questions. *European Respiratory Journal*, Vol. 26, No. 3, (September 2005), pp. 523-548, ISSN 1399-3003

Howarth. P.H. (2000). Leukotrienes in rhinitis. *American Journal of Respiratory and Critiacal Care Medicine*, Vol. 161, No. 2, (Febuary 2000), pp. s133–s136, ISSN 1535-4970

Hunt, J.F.; Fang, K.; Malik, R.; Snyder, A.; Malhotra, N.; Platts- Mills, T.A. & Gaston, B. (2000). Endogenous Airway Acidification. Implications for Asthma Pathophysiology. *American Journal of Respiratory and Critiacal Care Medicine*, Vol. 161, No. 3, (March 2000), pp. 694-699, ISSN 0002-9378

Huwyler, J. & Gut, J. (1990). Single-step organic extraction of leukotrienes and related compounds and their simultaneous analysis by high-performance liquid chromatography. *Analytical Biochemistry: Methods in the Biological Sciences*, Vol. 188, No. 2, (August 1990), pp. 374-382, ISSN 0003-2697

Hyslop, P.A. & Sklar, L.A. (1984). A quantitative fluorimetric assay for the determination of oxidant production by polymorphonuclear leukocytes: Its use in the simultaneous fluorimetric assay of cellular activation processes. *Analytical biochemistry: Methods in the Biological Sciences*, Vol. 141, No. 1, (August 1984), pp. 280-286, ISSN 0003-2697

Izumi, T.; Yokomizo,T.; Obinata, H.; Ogasawara, H. & Shimizu, T. (2002). Leukotriene Receptors: Classification, Gene Expression, and Signal Transduction. *The journal of Biochemistry*, Vol. 132, No. 1, (July 2002), pp. 1-6, ISSN 1756-2651

Jarjour, N.N.; Peters, S.P.; Djukanovic, R. & Calhoun, W.J. (1998). Investigative Use of Bronchoscopy in Asthma. *American Journal of Respiratory and Critiacal Care Medicine*, Vol. 157, No. 3, (March 1998), pp. 692–697, ISSN 1535-4970

Jeffery, P.K.; Laitinen, A. & Venge, P. (2000). Biopsy markers of airway inflammation and remodelling. *Respiratory Medicine*, Vol. 94, No. Supplement 6, (July 2000), pp. S9–S15, ISSN 0954-6111

Kazani, S. & Israel, E. (2010). Exhaled breath condensates in asthma: Diagnostic and therapeutic implications. *Journal of Breath Research*, Vol. 4, No. 4, (December 2010), pp. 0407001, ISSN 1752-7163

Kharitonov, S.A. & Barnes, P.J. (2001). Exhaled markers of pulmonary disease. *American Journal of Respiratory and Critiacal Care Medicine*, Vol. 163, No. 7, (June 2001), pp. 1693-1722, ISSN 0002-9378

Klusáčková, P.; Lebedová, J.; Kačer, P.; Kuzma, M.; Brabec, M.; Pelclová, D.; Fenclová, Z. & Navrátil, T. (2008). Leukotrienes and 8-isoprostane in exhaled breath condensate in bronchoprovocation tests with occupational allergens. *Prostaglandins, Leukotrienes and Essential Fatty Acids*, Vol. 78, No. 4-5, (April-May 2008), pp. 281–292, ISSN 0952-3278

Kostikas. K.; Gaga, P.; Papatheodorou. G.; Karamanis, T.; Orphanidou, D. & Loukides, S. (2005). Leukotriene B4 in Exhaled Breath Condensate and Sputum Supernatant in Patients With COPD and Asthma. *Chest*, Vol. 127, No. 5, (May 2005), pp. 1553-1559, ISSN 1931-3543.

Kricka, L. J.; Master, S. R.; Joos, T. O. & Fortina, P. (2002). Current perspectives in protein array technology. *Annals of Clinical Biochemistry*, Vol. 43, No. 6, (2006), pp. 457-67, ISSN 0004-5632

Kullmann, T.; Barta, I.; Lázár,Z.; Szili, B.; Barát, E.; Valyon, M.; Kollai, M. & Horváth, I. (2007). Exhaled breath condensate pH standardised CO_2 partial pressure. *European Respiratory Journal*, Vol. 29, No. 3, (March 2007), pp. 496-501, ISSN 1399-3003

Lammers, J.W. (2001). Leukotrienes and cystic fibrosis. *Clinical and Experimental Allergy Reviews*, Vol. 1, No. 2, (July 2001), pp. 175-177, ISSN 1472-9733

Lee, K.-B.; Park, So-J.; Mirkin, Ch. A.; Smith, J. C. & Mrksich, M. (2002). Protein Nanoarrays Generated By Dip-Pen Nanolithography. *Science*, Vol. 295, No. 8, (March 2002), pp. 1702-1705, ISSN 1095-9203

Lemiere, C. (2007). Induced sputum and exhaled nitric oxide as noninvasive markers of airway inflammation from work exposures. *Current Opinion in Allergy and Clinical Immunology*, Vol. 7, No. 2, (April 2007), pp. 133–137, ISSN 1528-4050

Leung, T. F.; Li, Ch. Y.; Yung, E.; Liu, E.K.H.; Lam, Ch.W.K. & Wong, G.W.K. (2006). Clinical and Technical Factors Affecting pH and Other Biomarkers in Exhaled Breath Condensate. *Pediatric Pulmonology*, Vol. 41, No. 1, (January 2006), pp. 87–94, ISSN 1099-0496

Lindgren, J.A.; Hammerstrom, S. & Goetzl E. J. (1983). A sensitive and specific radioimmunoassay for leukotriene C4. *FEBS Lett*, Vol. 152, No. 1, (Febuary 1983), pp. 83-88, ISSN 0014-5793

Marzinzig, M.; Nussler, A.K.; Stadler, J.; Marzinzig, E.; Barthlen, W.; Nussler, N.C.; Beger, H.G.; Morris, S.M.Jr. & Brückner, U.B. (1997). Improved Methods to Measure End Products of Nitric Oxide in Biological Fluids: Nitrite, Nitrate, and S-Nitrosothiols. *Nitric Oxide: Biology and Chemistry*, Vol. 1, No. 2, (April 1997), pp. 177-189, ISSN: 1089-8603

McKinney, E.T.; Shouri, R.; Sean Hunt, R.; Ahokas, R.A. & Sibai, B.M.M (2000). Plasma, urinary, and salivary 8-epi-prostaglandin F2α levels in normotensive and preeclamptic pregnancies. *American Journal of Obstetrics and Gynecology*, Vol. 183, No. 4, (October 2000), pp. 874–877, ISSN 0002-9378

Misso, N. L. A.; Aggarwal, S.; Phelps, S.; Beard, R. & Thompson, P. J. (2004). Urinary leukotriene E_4 and 9α, 11β-prostaglandin F_2 concentrations in mild, moderate and severe asthma, and in healthy subjects. *Clinical & Experimental Allergy*, Vol. 34, No. 4, (April 2004), pp. 624-631, ISSN 1365-2222.

Mizugaki, M.; Hishinuma, T. & Suzuki, N. (1999). Determination of leukotriene E4 in human urine using liquid chromatography-tandem mass spectrometry. *Journal of Chromatography B*, Vol. 729, No. 1-2, (1999), pp. 279-285, ISSN 1570-0232

Montuschi P. (2004). *New perspectives in monitoring lung inflamation. Analysis of exhaled breath condensate*, P. Montuschi, (Ed.), 11-30, CRC press, ISBN 0-415-32465-3, Boca Raton, Florida

Montuschi P. (2009). LC/MS/MS analysisi of leukotriene B4 and other eicosaniods in exhaled breath condensate for assessing lung inflammation. *Journal of Chromatography B*, Vol. 877, No. 13, (May 2009), pp. 1272-1280, ISSN 1570-0232

Montuschi, P. & Barnes, P.J. (2002a). Analysis of exhaled breath condensate for monitoring airway inflammation. *Trends in Pharmacological Sciences*, Vol. 23, No. 5, (May 2002), pp. 232-237, ISSN 0165-6147

Montuschi, P. & Barnes P.J. (2002b). Exhaled leukotrienes and prostaglandins in asthma. *The Journal of Allergy and Clinical Immunology*, Vol. 109, No. 4, (April 2002), pp. 615-620, ISSN 0091-6749

Montuschi, P.; Kharitonov, S.; Ciabattoni, G.; Corradi, M.; van Rensen, L.; Geddes, D.; Hodson, M. & Barnes, P.J. (2000). Exhaled 8-isoprostane as a new non-invasive biomarker of oxidative stress in cystic fibrosis. *Thorax*, Vol. 55, No. 3, (March 2000), pp. 205–209, ISSN 1468-3296

Murugan, A.; Prys-Picard, C. & Calhoun, W.J. (2009). Biomerkes in athma. *Current opinions in pulmonary in medicine*, Vol. 15, No. 1, (January 2009), pp. 12-8, ISSN 1531-6971

Nguyen, T.A.; Woo-Park, J.; Hess, M.; Goins, M.; Urban, P.; Vaughan, J.; Smith, A. & Hund, J. (2005). Assaying all of the nitrogen oxides in breath modifies the interpretation of exhaled nitric oxide. *Vascular Pharmacology*, Vol. 43, No. 6, (December 2005), pp. 379-384, ISSN 1537-1891

Niimi, A.; Nguyen, L.T.; Usmani, O.; Mann, B. & Chung, K.F. (2004). Reduced pH and chloride levels in exhaled breath condensate of patients with chronic cough. *Thorax*, Vol. 59, No. 7, (July 2004), pp. 608-612, ISSN 1468-3296

Nowak, D.; Kasielski, M.; Antczak, A.; Pietras, T. & Bialasiewicz, P. (1999). Increased content of thiobarbituric acid-reactive substances and hydrogen peroxide in the expired breath condensate of patients with stable chronic obstructive pulmonary disease: no significant effect of cigarette smoking. *Respiratory Medecine*, Vol. 93, No. 6, (June 1999), pp. 389-396, ISSN 0945-6111

Nowak, D.; Kalucka, S.; Bialasiewicz, P. & Król, M. (2001). Exhalation of H_2O_2 and thiobarbituric acid reactive substances (TBARs) by healthy subjects. *Free Radical Biology & Medicine*, Vol. 30, No. 2, (January 2001), pp. 178, ISSN 0891-5849

Ohanian, A.S.; Zimmerman, J. & Debley, J.S. (2010). Effects of sample processing, time and storage condition on cysteinyl leukotrienes in exhaled breath condensate. *Journal of Breath Research*, Vol. 4, No. 4, (December 2010), pp. 046002, ISSN 1752-7163

Ojoo, J.C.; Mulrennan, S.A.; Kastelik, J.A.; Morice, A.H. & Redington, A.E. (2005). Exhaled breath condensate pH and exhaled nitric oxide in allergic asthma and in cystic fibrosis. *Thorax*, Vol. 60, No. 1, (January 2005), pp. 22-26, ISSN 1468-3296

Paget-Brown, A.O.; Ngamtrakulpanit, L.; Smith, A.; Bunyan, D.; Hom, S.; Nquyen, A. & Hunt, J.F. (2006). Normative data for pH of exhaled breath condensate. *Chest*, Vol. 129, No. 2, (Febuary 2006), pp. 426-430, ISSN 1931-3543

Peters-Golden, M. & Brock, T.G. (2003). 5-Lipoxygenase and FLAP. *Prostaglandins, Leukotrienes and Essential Fatty Acids*, Vol. 69, No. 2-3,(August -September 2003), pp. 99–109, ISSN 0952-3278

Piotrowski, W. J.; Antczak, A.; Marczak, J.; Nawrocka, A.; Kurmanowska, Z. & Górski, P. (2007). Eicosanoids in Exhaled Breath Condens and BAL Fluid of Patients With Sarcoidosis. *Chest*, Vol. 132, No. 2, (August 2007), pp.589-596, ISSN 1931-3543

Reynolds H.Y. (2000). Use of Bronchoalveolar Lavage in Humans-Past Necessity and Future Imperative. *Lung*, Vol. 178, No. 5, (September 2000), pp. 271–293, ISSN 1432-1750

Ricciardolo, F.L.; Di Stefano, A.; Sabatini, F. & Folkerts, G. (2006). Reactive nitrogen species in the respiratory tract. *European Journal of Pharmacology*, Vol. 533, No. 1-3, (March 2006), pp. 240-252, ISSN 0014-2999

Rosa, L.G. & Liang J. (2009). Atomic force microscope nanolithography: dip-pen, nanoshaving, nanografting, tapping mode, electrochemical and thermal nanolithography. *Journal of Physics Condensed Matter*, Vol. 21, No. 48, (December 2009), pp. 483001, ISSN 1361-648X

Rozy, A.; Czerniawska, J.; Stepniewska, A.; Wozbinska, B.; Goljan, A.; Puscinska, E.; Gorecka, D. & Chorostowska-Wynimko, J. (2006). Inflammatory markers in the exhaled breath condensate of patients with pulmonary sacroidosis. *Journal of Physiology and Pharmacology*, Vol. 57, No. Suppl 4, (September 2006), pp. 335, ISSN 0867-5910

Ruch, W.; Cooper, P.H. & Baggiolini, M. (1983). Assay of H_2O_2 production by macrophages and neutrophils with homovanillic acid and horse-radish peroxidise. *Journal of Immunological Methods*, Vol. 63, No. 3, (1983), pp. 347-357, ISSN 0022-1759.

Salari, H. & Steffenrud, S. (1986). Comparative study of solid phase extraction techniques for isolation of leukotrienes from plasma. *Journal of Chromatography B*, Vol. 378, (1986), Pages 35-44, ISSN 1570-0232

Samitas, K.; Chorianopoulos, D.; Vittorakis, S.; Zervas, E.; Economidou, E.; Papatheodorou, G.; Loukides, S. & Gaga, G. (2009). Exhaled cysteinyl-leukotrienes and 8-isoprostane in patients with asthma and their relation to clinical severity. *Respiratory Medicine*, Vol. 103, No. 5, (May 2009), pp. 750-756, ISSN 0954-6111

Sanak, M.; Gielicz, A.; Nagraba, K.; Kaszuba, M.; Kumik, J. & Szczeklik, A. (2010). Targeted eicosanoids lipidomics of exhaled breath condensate in healthy subjects. *Journal of Chromatography B*, Vol. 878, No. 21, (July 2010), pp. 1796-1800, ISSN 1570-0232

Shindo, K.; Hirai, Y.; Fukumura, M. & Koide, K. (1997). Plasma levels of leukotriene E_4 during clinical course of chronic obstructive pulmonary disease. *Prostaglandins, Leukotrienes and Essential Fatty Acids*, Vol. 56, No. 3, (March 1997), pp. 213-217, ISSN 0952-3278

Soyer, O. U.; Dizdar, E. A.; Keskin, O.; Lilly, C. & Kalayci, O. (2006). Comparison of two methods for exhaled breath condensate collection. *Allergy*, Vol. 61, No.8, (August 2006), pp. 1016–1018, ISSN 1398-9995

Svensson, S.; Olin, A.C.; Larstad, M.; Ljungkvist, G. & Torén, K. (2004). Determination of hydrogen peroxide in exhaled breath condensate by flow injection analysis with fluorescence detection. *Journal of Chromatography B*, Vol. 809, No. 2, (October 2004), pp. 199-203, ISSN 1570-0232

Syslová, K.; Kačer, P.; Kuzma, M.; Pankrácová , A.; Fenclová, Z. ; Vlčková, Š.; Lebedová, J. & Pelclová, D. (2010). LC-ESI-MS/MS method for oxidative stress multimarker screening in the exhaled breath condensate of asbestosis/silicosis patients. *Journal of Breath Research*, Vol. 4, No. 1, (March 2010), pp. 017104, ISSN 1752-7163

Syslová, K.; Kačer, P.; Vilhanová, B.; Kuzma, M.; Lipovová, P.; Fenclová, Z.; Lebedová, J. & Pelclová, D. (2011). Determination of cysteinyl leukotrienes in exhaled breath condensate: Method combining immunoseparation with LC–ESI-MS/MS. *Journal of Chromatography B*, Vol. 879, No. 23, (August 2011), pp. 2220-2228, ISSN 1570-0232

Tate. S.; MacGregor, G.; Davis, M.; Innes, J.A. & Greening, A.P. (2002). Airways in cystic fibrosis are acidified: detection by exhaled breath condensate. *Thorax*, Vol. 52, No. 11, (November 2002), pp. 926-929, ISSN 1468-3296

Thanachasai, S.; Rokutanzono, S.; Yoshida, S. & Watanabe, T. (2002). Novel Hydrogen Peroxide Sensors Based on Peroxidase-Carrying Poly{pyrrole-co-[4-(3-pyrrolyl)-butanesulfonate]} Copolymer Films. *Analytical Sciences*, Vol. 18, No. 7, (July 2002), pp. 773, ISSN 1348-2246

Tufvesson, E.; van Weele, L.J.; Ekedahl, H. & Bjermer, L. (2010). Levels of cysteinyl-leukotrienes in exhaled breath condensate are not due to saliva contamination. *Clinical Respiratory Journal*, Vol. 4, No. 2, (July 2010), pp. 83-88, ISSN 1752699X

Usery J.B.; Self, T.H.; Muthiah, M.P. & Finch, Ch. K. (2008). Potential Role of Leukotrienes Modifiers in the Treatment of Chronic Obstructive Pulmonary Disease. *Pharmacotherapy*, Vol. 28, No. 9, (September 2008), pp. 1183-1187, ISSN 1472-9733

Wan, Ch.; Kim-Chun, L.; Ning, L.; Ricky, N.S.W.; Huwei, L. & Zongwei, C. (2008). Liquid chromatography/mass spectrometry for metabonomics investigation of the biochemical effects induced by aristolochic acid in rats: the use of information-dependent acquisition for biomarker identification. *Rapid Communications in Mass Spectrometry*, Vol. 22, No. 6, (March 2008), pp. 873–880, ISSN 0951-4198

WHO, (30.11.2010). Health topics Asthma, In: World Health Organization, 1.7.2011, Available from: <http://www.who.int/topics/asthma/en/>

Yang, J.; Schmelzer, K.; Georgi, K. & Hammock, B.D. (2009). Quantitative Profiling Method for Oxylipin Metabolome by Liquid Chromatography Electrospray Ionization Tandem Mass Spectrometry. *Analytical Chemistry*, Vol. 81, No. 19, (October 2009), pp. 8085-8093, ISSN 0003-2700

Zakrzewski, J.T.; Barnes, N.C.; Costello, J.F. & Piper, P.J. (1987). Lipid mediators in cystic fibrosis and chronic obstructive pulmonary disease. *American Review of Respiratory Diseases*, Vol. 136, No. 3, (September 1987), pp. 779–782, ISSN 0003-0805

Zappacosta, B.; Persichilli, S.; Mormile, F.; Minucci, A.; Russo, A.; Giardina, B. & De Sole, P. (2001). A fast chemiluminescent method for H_2O_2 measurement in exhaled breath condensate. *Clinica Chimica Acta*, Vol. 310, No. 2, (August 2001), pp. 187-191, ISSN 0009-8981.

Zhao, J.J.; Shimizu, Y.; Dobashi, K.; Kawata, T.; Ono, A.; Yanagitani, N.Y.; Kaira, K.; Utsugi, M.; Hisada, T.; Ishizuka, T. & Mori, M. (2008).The relationship between oxidative stress and acid stress in adult patients with mild asthma. *Journal of Investigational Allergology and Clinical Immunology*, Vol. 18, No. 1, (January 2008), pp. 41-45, ISSN 1018-9068

Part 2

Immunological Mechanisms in the Development and Progression of Asthma

4

Immune Mechanisms of Childhood Asthma

T. Negoro et al.*
Department of Pharmacogenomics, Showa University School of Pharmacy, Japan

1. Introduction

Asthma is the syndrome defined with chronic airway inflammation and hypersensitivity. Asthma is classified into two phenotypes, atopic with IgE antibodies for specific allergens and nonatopic without IgE antibodies. Unlike adults, 90-95% of pediatric asthma patients exhibit an atopic phenotype (Japanese Society of Pediatric Allergy and Clinical Immunology [JSPACI], 2008). In addition, there are several significant differences between adult and childhood asthma such as duration of disease, extent of lung and immunological development, and duration of inhaled corticosteroid (ICS) use.

The phenotype of airway inflammation is caused by a complex network of various immunocytes; such as T helper 2 (Th2) cells, T helper 17 (Th17) cells, eosinophils, basophils etc (Broide et al., 2011). Typically, it is known that Th2 cells can promote eosinophil activation and IgE production by B cells, while recently Th17 cells have been thought to play a part in exacerbation of asthma, due to their ability to recruit neutrophils following neutrophil activation at an inflammatory site (Molet et al., 2001; Barczyk et al., 2003; Zhao et al., 2008).

Regulatory $CD4^+CD25^+$ T (Treg) cells, which are characterized by their anergy and immune-regulatory functions, can control allergic responses such as airway eosinophilia and airway hypersensitivity. To date, several reports have indicated that reduced numbers of Treg cells or functionally impaired Treg cells are implicated in asthma, rheumatoid arthritis and Kawasaki disease, among others (de Kleer et at., 2004; Furuno et al., 2004; Karlsson et al., 2004; Haddeland et al., 2005., Orihara et al., 2007; Schaub et al., 2008; Ly et al., 2009). Consistent with these reports, our own data suggested that Treg cells from childhood asthma patients were impaired in their suppressive functions (Yamamoto et al., 2011).

* Y. Yamamoto[2, 3], S. Shimizu[4], A. H. Banham[5], G. Roncador[6], H. Wakabayashi[1], T. Osabe[1], T. Yanai[1], H. Akiyama[1], K. Itabashi[3] and Y. Nakano[1]
1 Department of Pharmacogenomics, Showa University School of Pharmacy, Japan,
2 Department of Pediatrics,
Tokyo Metropolitan Health and Medical Treatment Corporation Ebara Hospital, Japan,
3 Department of Pediatrics, Showa Universtiry School of Medicine, Japan,
4 Department of Pathophysiology, Showa University School of Pharmacy, Japan,
5 Nuffield Department of Clinical Laboratory Sciences, University of Oxford, UK,
6 Monoclonal Antibodies Unit, Biotechnology Program,
Centro Nacional de Investigaciones Oncologicas (CNIO), Spain.

Coincident with the reduced regulatory functions of Treg cells, the ratio of Th17 cells also increased in childhood asthma patient (Yamamoto et al., 2010). Furthermore, single nucleotide polymorphisms of *FOXP3* have been associated with childhood allergy (Bottema et al., 2009).

Treg cells are anergic in both the resting state and after activation by TCR stimulation. Murine Tregs showed a low Ca^{2+} level accompanying their anergic state (Gavin et al., 2002) and our recent human Treg data imply that it the same low Ca^{2+} level accompanies their anergy (Yamamoto et al., 2011). The Ca^{2+} channel on the cell surface of T cells that responds to TCR stimulation is called the calcium release-activated Ca^{2+} (CRAC) channel. We have hypothesized that, in contrast to naïve T cells, the CRAC channel in resting Treg cells may not open easily in response to TCR stimulation and thus the regulation of the CRAC channel may be impaired in Treg cells from asthma patients. This impaired Ca^{2+} regulation in Treg cells may then partly contribute to reduce their regulatory functions.

2. Immune and inflammatory pathology in childhood asthma

Airway inflammation plays a critical role in the pathogenesis of asthma in both adults and during childhood (Warner et al., 1998; Wenzel, 2006; Broide et al., 2011). The immune mechanisms underlying adult asthma derive from the infiltration and activation of immune cells such as eosinophils, mast cells, T cells, basophils and neutrophils, and the activation of parenchymal cells like epithelial cells. It is also generally known that there are different inflammatory phenotypes in adult asthma such as those with a neutrophilic or an eosinophilic predominance (Wenzel, 2006). The airway inflammatory pattern of eosinophilic asthma is characterized by mast cell activation and increasing numbers of activated eosinopils and T cells. Neutrophilic asthma, which is dominanted by neutrophil infiltration and activation in the airways, is related to the severity of adult asthma and steroid-resistant disease (Wenzel et al., 1997). Almost all pediatric asthma has a similar basis to chronic asthma in adults. However, broncho-alveolar lavage cell profiles and induced sputum in childhood asthma revealed increasing numbers of eosinophils and neutrophils compared with controls (Warner et al., 1998). The number of neutrophils in childhood asthma was correlated with the frequency of symptoms and with positive bacterial cultures from the alveolar lavage. In the case of childhood asthma, the increasing neutrophil infiltration appears not to be an exacerbating factor related to disease severity, in contrast to such findings in adult asthma.

Human lung development can be broken down into four prenatal phases including *the embryonic phase* (up to the sixth week of gestation), *pseudoglandular phase* (from the seventh to the sixteenth week of gestation), *canalicular phase* (from the 16th to the 26th week of gestation), and *saccular phase* (from the 24th to the 26th week of gestation) (DiFiore & Wilson, 1994; Jeffery et al., 1998; Bolt et al., 2001). The development persists postnatally as *the alveolar phase,* during the formation of alveoli by 2yrs of age and the further development until adulthood, i.e., suggesting that the respiratory system in children is immature (Schittny et al., 1998; Bolt et al., 2001).

Likewise, development of the immune system is very important in early childhood and a significant body of evidence suggests that antigen reactivity could be initiated by the fetal immune system after approximately 22 weeks of gestation (Jones et al., 1996; Szépfalusi et al., 2000). Immunotoxin exposure during pregnancy through causes such as maternal smoking, folate intake, heavy metals, antibiotics and environmental estrogens etc is a particular concern at a period from mid-gestation until 2 years after birth (Dietert & Zelikoff, 2008). Furthermore, maternal exposure to allergens can induce the fetus to respond specifically to the allergens at birth (Prescott et al., 1998, 1999); implying that allergen sensitization could be determined prenatally. Both innate and acquired immune responses are still immature in infancy, for instances poor T cell responses due to defective functions of antigen presenting cells (APC) (Delespesse et al., 1998; Levy et al., 2004; Maródi, 2006; Lappalainen et al., 2009). Interestingly, the germ-free status of intrauterine environment favors Th2 responses, and a Th2-skewed response at birth in the human has been demonstrated (Prescott et al., 1998).

Asthma is an inflammatory disease that features a Th2 type immune response caused by inhaled allergens. The immune response is characterized by Th2 type cytokines such as IL-4, IL-13 and allergen-specific IgE. IL-4 and IL-13 play a role in class switching of B cell to produce allergen-specific IgE antibodies that bind to specific receptors on mast cells and basophils. IL-4 also promotes differentiation of naïve T cells into Th2 cells (Robinson et al., 1992; Constant et al., 2000).

Recently, Th17 cells, which are considered to be developmentally distinct from Th1 and Th2 cells, were found to be a subset of Th cells closely connected with the increased prevalence of allergies and asthma (Molet et al., 2001; Laan et al., 2002; Barczyk et al., 2003; Oboki et al., 2008). IL-17 gives rise to production of IL-6, IL-8 and CXCL1 from bronchial fibroblasts or epithelial cells, consequently inducing a positive neutrophil chemotaxis followed by chronic airway inflammation (Kawaguchi et al., 2001; Molet et al., 2001). In some cases, Th17 cells were able to secrete both Th2 and Th17 type cytokines and the cells increased in the peripheral blood from asthma patients (Cosmi et al., 2010). In addition, human eosinophils constantly expressed IL-17- and IL-23-receptors and IL-23 stimulated eosinophils to produce both chemokines (CXCL1, CXCL8, and CCL4) and cytokines (IL-1β, IL-6 and IL17/IL-23) (Cheung et al., 2008).

Our preliminary data have suggested that pediatric asthma patients exhibited a higher frequency of Th17 cells within the peripheral $CD4^+$ T cell population (Yamamoto et al., 2010). Th17 cells appeared during an early stage at the onset of child asthma and the increased frequency of Th17 cells in the peripheral blood could reflect the presence of their symptoms of asthma, but it could not be connected with the severity of asthma. The data implies that early neutrophil infiltration in the airways of children with asthma may be attributed to the high frequency of Th17 cells. In line with our results, polymorphisms of the *IL-17A* gene were also associated with the incidence of pediatric asthma (Wang et al., 2009). In contrast, the presence of elevated numbers of Th17 cells in adult airways was related to the severe type of asthma and the neutrophilic inflammation, such as an occur in steroid-resistant asthma (Zhao et al., 2010). The role of Th17 cells may thus be similar between childhood and adult asthma. Furthermore, a negative correlation between the frequency of Th17 cells and Treg cells was shown in a moderate type of child asthma and in autoimmunity (Bettelli et al., 2006; Yamamoto et al., 2010). Neutrophilic inflammation therefore seems to be ascribed to the increased activation of Th17 cells and the decline in the number and activity of Treg cells.

3. The role of Treg cells in childhood asthma

Allergy is a hyper-immunoresponse to specific antigens that also emerges as a consequence of perturbed immune tolerance. Since immune functions are initiated very early in life, the onset of allergic reactivity also appears before birth. Reflecting such a situation, the cytokine profiles such as the ratio of T helper 1 (Th1)/Th2 and elevated IgE levels in cord blood may predict those individuals who are at risk of developing allergic diseases later in life (Hinz et al., 2010). The germ-free status of the intrauterine environment favors Th2 responses, and a Th2-skewed response at birth in humans has been demonstrated (Prescott et al., 1998). A stronger maternal Th2 immune response has also been connected with childhood wheezing and atopy (Kim et al., 2008). Furthermore, reduced production of the Th2 antagonist IFN-γ during pregnancy has been associated with increasing IL-13 production in the child (Kopp et al., 2001). Maternal cells could cross the placenta and affect the regulation of immune responses after birth (Mold et al., 2008). Taken together, these results suggested that the perturbation of immune tolerance is initiated *in utero* and as a result specific responses to allergens emerge in early in life.

There are several reports implicating reductions in the numbers and functionality of $CD4^+CD25^+$ Treg cells in both human and mouse allergies; although the regulatory ability of Treg cells is still controversial in a mouse model of ovalbumin sensitized airway hypersensitivity (Suto et al., 2001; Hadeiba & Locksley, 2003; Jaffar et al., 2004). As previously noted, many studies have shown that the reduced number and the dysfunction of Treg cells were related with asthma. In adult humans, the regulatory function of Treg cells was reduced in symptomatic hay fever subjects during the pollen season but not in asymptomatic status from the same population outside of the pollen season (Ling et al., 2004). Ca^{2+} signaling is very important for lymphocyte functions and our own data have indicated that impaired Ca^{2+} regulation within $CD4^+CD25^+CD45RO^+$ Treg cells correlated with child asthma symptoms (Yamamoto et al., 2011). We showed that anergy, one of the defining human Treg cell features, is dependent on intra-cellular calcium. Importantly, intra-cellular Ca^{2+} influx in Treg cells identifies those populations that lack anergic status and may have a role in impairing their regulatory functions. Moreover, pulmonary $CD4^+CD25^{high}$ Treg cells were also functionally impaired in childhood asthma (Hartl et al., 2007). A diminished number of Treg cells were also observed in the peripheral blood of children subjects with symptomatic food allergy and atopic dermatitis implicating these cells in yet further allergic reactions (Bellinghausen et al., 2003; Karlsson et al., 2004). It has been proposed that reduced numbers of maternal Treg cells and increased production of Th2 cytokines during pregnancy might play a significant role in enhancing the allergy risk in children (Hinz et al., 2010).

Forkhead box P3 (FOXP3) is a forkhead transcription factor that has been shown to be a master regulator of Treg cell development and functions, and thereby is considered as the one of the most specific markers of Treg populations (despite its transient induction in activated human effector $CD4^+$ T cells). Human naïve and memory T cells can be distinguished by the reciprocal expression of CD45 isoforms (RA^+: naïve, RO^+: memory) (Michie et al., 1992). Human $FOXP3^+CD4^+$ Treg cells in adult peripheral blood are classified into three distinct subpopulations, namely $CD45RA^+FOXP3^{low}$, $CD45RA^-FOXP3^{high}$ and $CD45RA^-FOXP3^{low}$ T cells (Miyara et al., 2009). $CD45RA^+FOXP3^{low}$ and $CD45RA^-FOXP3^{high}$ Treg cells are resting and activated cells respectively, and both cell populations have functional suppressor activity *in vitro*. The $CD45RA^-FOXP3^{low}$ Treg cells are cytokine secreting non-suppressive cells. $CD45RA^+$ (naïve) subset in $FOXP3^+$ Treg cells from umblical blood is far greater than $CD45RO^+$ (memory) subset, because the fetus receives little stimulation from environmental factors such as bacteria, viruses and allergens (Thornton et al., 2004). We identified two subsets of $CD4^+CD25^+$ Treg cells, $CD45RO^-FOXP3^{low}$ (nearly equal in numbers to the $CD45RA^+$ population) and $CD45RO^+FOXP3^{high}$ (nearly equal in numbers to the $CD45RA^-$ population) T cells in peripheral blood from children (Yamamoto et al., 2011). However, our data indicated that $CD45RO^+$ Treg population did not have the distinctly different FOXP3 expression levels seen in the adult subsets and Ca^{2+} unresponsiveness in the cells seemed to be similar at different FOXP3 expression levels in children. This population seems to be anergic but the suppressive function may vary with FOXP3 expression levels, like the adult Treg cells subsets, since Treg cells with low level FOXP3 remained anergic but their suppressive activities was greatly impaired (Wan & Flavell, 2007). Furthermore, intra-cellular Ca^{2+} concentration in response to TCR activation also seemed to be different between $CD45RO^-FOXP3^{low}$ and $CD45RO^+FOXP3^{high}$ Treg cells from children, suggesting that the two populations were not equally functional. Furthermore, $CD45RA^+$ Treg cells from newborns were reported to lack Treg capability (Ly et al., 2009). That is, it may be different in the functions of $CD45RO^-$ Treg cells in children unlike the adult Treg cells subsets.

What kind of factors impair the functions of Treg populations? Tumor necrosis factor-α (TNF-α) has been reported to contribute to dysfunction of Treg cells and consequent breakdown of immunological self-torelance in Rheumatoid Arthritis (RA) (Nadkarni et al., 2007). TNF-α is one of main causative factors in RA, and anti-TNF treatment (infliximab etc) led to the elevated number of Treg cells and restored the partly impaired suppressive functions. TNF-α was able to inhibit the suppressive activity of $CD45RA^-$ Treg cells, via TNF-α receptor 2 (TNFR2) on their surface, in human RA subjects (Nagar et al., 2010). In childhood asthma, escalation of TNF-α level in allergen stimulated-peripheral blood mononuclear cells (PBMC) and in asthmatic airway has also seemed to be related to the functional insufficiency of Treg cells (Lin et al., 2008). Furthermore, the frequency of $FOXP3^+$ cells in $CD4^+CD25^{high}$ Treg cells in the subjects was significantly reduced and TNF-α treatment *in vitro* compromised the function of Treg cells, which was also associated with increased TNFR2 expression. $CD45RA^+$ Treg cells can promote human Th17 differentiation, which is impaired by TNF-α (Baba et al., 2010), but $CD45RO^+CD25^{high}$ Treg cells inhibit the function of murine Th17 (Bettelli et al., 2006). In childhood asthma, $CD45RO^-FOXP3^{low}$ (nearly equal in numbers to the $CD45RA^+$ population) Treg cells may accelerate Th17 development in addition to impairing the functions of $CD45RO^+FOXP3^{high}$ (equally $CD45RO^+CD25^{high}$) Treg cells.

4. Different mechanisms of determining anergic status in Treg cells

In response to TCR activation, under some conditions, T cells can be led to an unresponsive status termed anergy. Anergic cells do not transcribe the *IL-2* gene or proliferate in response to TCR activation, even in the presence of costimulation (Fathman & Lineberry, 2007; Zheng et al., 2008; Wells, 2009). Generally, when T cells are activated via TCR and CD28 costimulation molecule, phospholipase Cγ (PLCγ), protein kinase Cθ (PKCθ) and Ras can be activated very quickly. Subsequently, the activation of the major signal transduction pathways such as MAPK, JNK, RSK and IκB kinase (IKK) and intra-cellular Ca^{2+} influx are provoked. Finally, transcription factors (NFAT, AP1 and NFκB etc), which are essential for the transcription of *IL-2*, are activated (Kane et al., 2002; Wells, 2009).

The induction of anergy is observed both *in vitro* and *in vivo*. There are several methods for the induction of *in vitro* anergy; including antigen presentation by chemically fixed antigen presenting cells (APC), ionomycin stimulation, anti-CD3 stimulation without co-stimulation, etc (Lamb et al., 1983; Jenkins & Schwartz, 1987). Likewise there are several models of *in vivo* anergy induction, systemic delivery of superantigens, administration of soluble peptide antigen into TCR transgenic mice, etc (Rammensee et al., 1992; Rellahan et al., 1990; Kawabe & Ochi, 1990). Under these conditions, the *in vitro* induced clonal anergic cells produce less IL-2, proliferate poorly, and can be long-lived and stable for weeks if they escape from apoptosis. However, Ca^{2+} influx in these T cells is normal and subsequently induces the activation of nuclear factor of activated T cells (NFAT) when the cells are re-stimulated (Fathman & Lineberry, 2007). Cyclosporin A, an inhibitor of the immediate upstream activator of NFAT, can inhibit the induction of T cell anergy (Jenkins et al., 1990). Since NFAT (the Ca^{2+}-calcineurin signal) promotes *IL-2* transcription and cooperates with Fos/Jun dimers (AP-1) (the CD28-MAPK signal). Mutation of NFAT, which prevents its binding to AP-1, also induces an anergic phenotype (Macián et al., 2002). Excessive calcium-calcineurin-NFAT signaling without AP-1 induces the negative regulatory factors for TCR/CD28 dependent signaling such as the transcription factors, early growth response (Egr) 2, Egr3 and the lipid kinase, diacylglycerol kinase-α (DGK-α) etc (Safford et al., 2005; Zheng et al., 2008). In contrast, *in vivo* adaptive tolerance models showed a defect in TCR-induced calcium influx (Chiodetti et al., 2006). *In vitro* induced anergic cells also showed the same results but a short rest period of 1-2 days after anergy induction resulted in recovery of a normal calcium flux (Gajewski et al., 1994, 1995). As mentioned above, the *in vitro* clonal anergy model showed that Ca^{2+}-calcineurin-NFAT signal functions were normal but the MAPK-AP1 signal was impaired, whereas the *in vivo* adaptive tolerance model showed Ca^{2+}-calcineurin-NFAT signal was significantly impaired. These systems thus operate at quite different mechanisms at the molecular level.

In contrast to effector T cells, $CD4^+CD25^+$ Treg cells produce less IL-2, proliferate poorly, and exhibit a low level of Ca^{2+} influx in response to TCR stimulation (Gavin et al., 2002; Yamamoto et al., 2011). The decline of *IL-2* transcription in Treg cells is mainly attributed to the master regulator FOXP3, which is able to inhibit the function of NFAT by competing with its binding to AP-1 (Wu et al., 2006). Although anergy is one of the key Treg features, the molecular mechanisms by which this phenotype are achieved are quite different from those mentioned above in the *in vitro* clonal anergy and *in vivo* adaptive tolerance models. FOXP3 acts as both a transcriptional repressor and activator, regulating the transcription of a diverse array of target genes (Marson et al., 2007; Zheng et al., 2007). Low level of Ca^{2+} influx in response to TCR activation may be either directly or indirectly regulated by FOXP3. One possible explanation for the low level of Ca^{2+} influx in Tregs is that several molecules involved in the regulation of intra-cellular Ca^{2+} concentration may be controlled by FOXP3. Intra-cellular Ca^{2+} influx, in response to TCR activation, in T cells depends on the CRAC channel, comprising the subunits ORAI1 and STIM1 etc (Zhang et al., 2005; Prakriya et al., 2006). Intra-cellular Ca^{2+} signaling events in T cells are as follows: Engagement of the TCR brings about ZAP70 phosphorylation and is followed by PLCγ1 activation. Activated PLCγ1 cleaves membrane phospholipids into two different second messengers, inositol triphosphate (IP_3) and diacylglycerol (DAG). IP_3 interacts with IP_3Rs (Ca^{2+} channel) on endoplasmic reticulum (ER) and triggers this to release Ca^{2+} from the ER via IP_3Rs. Increasing intra-cellular Ca^{2+} concentration induces Ca^{2+} influx through a pore-forming unit of CRAC channels involving ORAI1 on plasma membrane (Zweifach & Lewis, 1993). Down regulation of any component of this signaling cascade offers the possibility to reduce the Ca^{2+} influx in Treg cells. Notably, ZAP70 is one of target genes reported to be repressed by FOXP3 (Marson et al., 2007). However, the exact molecular mechanisms of low level of Ca^{2+} influx in response to TCR activation remain obscure in Treg cells.

5. Conclusion

Immunopathology of childhood asthma seems to have little difference in terms of neutrophilic inflammation when compared to the adult disease. Impaired Ca^{2+} regulation in Treg cells from asthma patients appears to compromise their regulatory functions, consequently increasing the number of Th17 cells and neutrophils. Consistent with these data, Ca^{2+} elevation in immunocytes induced by several stimuli also seems to have a key role for aggravation of airway inflammation in asthma. The intra-cellular Ca^{2+} elevation may then result in production of IL-2 via NFAT activation in asthma Treg cells. These data imply that dysregulation of Ca^{2+} unresponsiveness was concurrent with the impaired regulatory functions in Treg cells from asthma patients (Fig.1). Moreover, our Ca^{2+} analysis is a useful tool for the evaluation of Treg functions that proves particularly valuable when only small blood samples are available for study.

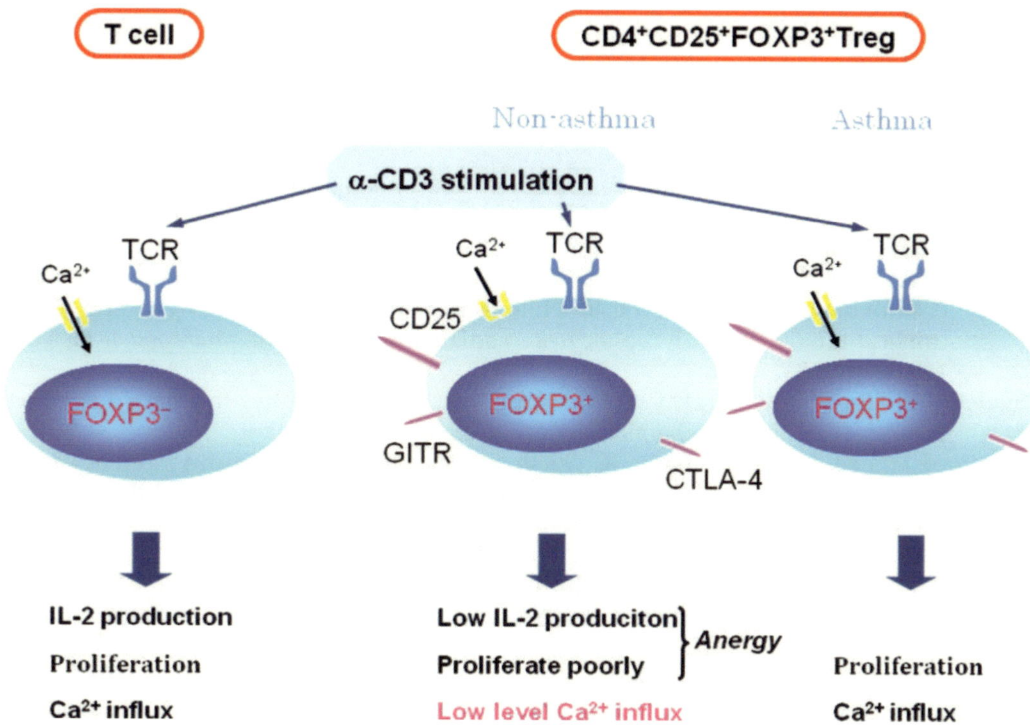

Fig. 1. Characteristics of CD4+CD25+FOXP3+ Treg cells.

In response to TCR activation, FOXP3⁻ T cell (effector T cell, left), FOXP3+ Treg cells from non-asthma (middle) and from asthma (right) are compared in terms of anergy status (low IL-2 production and proliferation poorly) and Ca^{2+} response.

6. Acknowledgment

This work was supported in part by a Grant-in-Aid from the Ministry of Education, Culture, Sports, Science, and Technology (MEXT) of Japan (#21591288), "High-Tech Research Center" Project for Private Universities: matching fund subsidy from MEXT of Japan, 2005-2009, and 2010-2012.

7. References

Baba, N., Rubio, M. & Sarfati, M. (2010). Interplay between CD45RA^{+} regulatory T cells and TNF-α in the regulation of human Th17 differentiation, *Int Immunol* 22(4): 237-44.

Barczyk, A., Pierzchala, W. & Sozańska, E. (2003). Interleukin-17 in sputum correlates with airway hyperresponsiveness to methacholine, *Respir Med* 97(6): 726-33.

Bellinghause, I., Klostermann, B., Knop, J. & Saloga, J. (2003). Human CD4+CD25+ T cells derived from the majority of atopic donors are able to suppress TH1 and TH2 cytokine production, *J Allergy Clin Immunol* 111(4): 862-8.

Bettelli, E., Carrier, Y., Gao, W., Kom, T., Strom, T.B., Oukka, M., Weiner, H.L. & Kuchroo, V.K. (2006). Reciprocal developmental pathways for the generation of pathogenic effector TH17 and regulatory T cells, *Nature* 441(7090): 235-8.

Bolt, R.J., van Weissenbruch, M.M., Lafeber, H.N. & Delemarre-van de Waal, H.A. (2001). Glucocorticoids and lung development in the fetus and preterm infant, *Pediatr Pulmonol* 32(1): 76-91.

Bottema, R.W., Kerkhof, M., Reijmerink, N.E., Koppelman, G.H., Thijs, C., Stelma, F.F., Smit, H.A., Brunekreef, B., van Schayck, C.P. & Postma, D.S. (2009). X-chromosome Forkhead Box P3 polymorphisms associate with atopy in girls in three Dutch birth cohorts, *Allergy* 65(7): 865-74.

Broide, D.H., Finkelman, F., Bochner, B.S. & Rothenberg, M.E. (2011). Advances in mechanisms of asthma, allergy, and immunology in 2010, *J Allergy Clin Immunol* 127(3): 689-95.

Cheung, P.F., Wong, C.K. & Lam, C.W. (2008). Molecular mechanisms of cytokine and chemokine release from eosinophils activated by IL-17A, IL-17F, and IL-23: implication for Th17 lymphocytes mediated allergic inflammation, *J Immunol* 180(8): 5625-35.

Chiodettli, L., Choi, S., Barber, D.L. & Schwartz, R.H. (2006). Adaptive tolerance and clonal anergy are distinct biochemical states, *J Immunol* 176(4): 2279-91.

Constant, S.L., Lee, K.S. & Bottomly, K. (2000). Site of antigen delivery can influence T cell priming: pulmonary environment promotes preferential Th2-type differentiation, *Eur J Immunol* 30(3): 840-7.

Cosmi, L., Maggi, L., Santarlasci, V., Capone, M., Cardilicchia, E., Frosali, F., Querci, V., Angeli, R., Matucci, A., Fambrini, M., Liotta, F., Parronchi, P., Maggi, E., Romagnani, S. & Annunziato, F. (2010). Identification of a novel subset of human circulating memory CD4(+) T cells that produce both IL-17A and IL-4, *J Allergy Clin Immunol* 125(1): 222-30.

De Kleer, I.M., Wedderburn, L.R., Taams, L.S., Patel, A., Varsani, H., Klein, M., de Jager, W., Pugayung, G., Giannoni, F., Rijkers, G., Albani, S., Kuis, W. & Prakken, B. (2004). CD4+CD25bright regulatory T cells actively regulate inflammation in the joints of patients with the remitting form of juvenile idiopathic arthritis, *J Immunol* 172(19): 6435-43.

Delespesse, G., Yang, L.P., Ohshima, Y., Demeure, C., Shu, U., Byun, D.G. & Sarfati, M. (1998). Maturation of human neonatal CD4+ and CD8+ T lymphocytes into Th1/Th2 effectors, *Vaccine* 16(14-15): 1415-9.

Dietert, R.R. & Zelikoff, J.T. (2008). Early-life environment, developmental immunotoxicology, and the risk of pediatric allergic disease including asthma, *Birth Defects Research (Part B)* 83(6): 547-560.

DiFiore, J.W. & Wilson, J.M. (1994). Lung development, *Semin Pediatr Surg* 3(4): 221-32.

Fathman, C.G. & Lineberry, N.B. (2007). Molecular mechanisms of $CD4^{+}$ T-cell anergy, *Nat Rev Immunol* 7(8): 599-609.

Furuno, K., Yuge, T., Kusuhara, K., Takada, H., Nishio, H., Khajoee, V., Ohno, T. & Hara, T. (2004). CD25+CD4+ regulatory T cells in patients with Kawasaki disease, *J Pediatr* 145(3): 385-90.

Gajewski, T.F., Qian, D., Fields, P. & Fitch, F.W. (1994). Anergic T-lymphocyte clones have altered inositol phosphate, calcium, and tyrosine kinase signaling pathways, *Proc Natl Acad Sci* USA 91(1): 38-42.

Gajewski, T.F., Fields, P. & Fitch, F.W. (1995). Induction of the increased Fyn kinase activity in anergic T heler type 1 clones requires calcium and protein synthesis and is sensitive to cyclosporine A, *Eur J Immunol* 25(7): 1836-42.

Gavin, M.A., Clarke, S.R., Negrou, E., Gallegos, A. & Rudensky, A. (2002). Homeostasis and anergy of CD4(+)CD25(+) suppressor T cells in vivo, *Nat Immunol* 3(1): 33-41.

Haddeland, U., Karstensen, A.B., Farkas, L., Bø, K.O., Pirhonen, J., Karlsson, M., Kvåvik, W., Brandtzaeq, P. & Nakstad, B. (2005). Putative regulatory T cells are impaired in cord blood from neonates with hereditary allergy risk, *Pediatr Allergy Immunol* 16(2): 104-12.

Hadeiba, H. & Lockslev, R.M. (2003). Lung CD25CD4 regulatory T cells suppress type 2 immune responses but not bronchial hyperreactivity, *J Immunol* 170(11): 5502-10.

Hartl, D., Koller, B., Mehlhorn, A.T., Reinhardt, D., Nicolai, T., Schendel, D.J., Griese, M. & Krauss-Etschmann, S. (2007). Quantitative and functional impairment of pulmonary CD4+CD25hi retulatory T cells in pediatric asthma, *J Allergy Clin Immunol* 119(5): 1258-66.

Hinz, D., Simon, J.C., Maier-Simon, C., Milkova, L., Roder, S., Sack, U., Borte, M., Lehmann, I. & Herberth, G. (2010). Reduced maternal regulatory T cell numbers and increased T helper type 2 cytokine production are associated with elevated levels of immunoglobulin E in cord blood, *Clin Exp Allergy* 40(3): 419-26.

Jaffar, Z., Sivakuru, T. & Roberts, K. (2004). CD4+CD25+ T cells regulate airway eosinophilic inflammation by modulating the Th2 cell phenotype, *J Immunol* 172 (6): 3842-9.

Jeffrey, P.K. (1998). The development of large and small airway, *Am J Respir Crit Care Med* 157(5 Pt 2): S174-80.

Jenkins, M.K. & Schwartz, R.H. (1987). Antigen presentation by chemically modified splenocytes induces antigen-specific T cell unresponsiveness in vitro and in vivo, *J Exp Med* 165(2): 302-19.

Jenkins, M.K., Chen, C.A., Jung, G., Mueller, D.L. & Schwartz, R.H. (1990). Inhibition of antigen-specific proliferation of type 1 murine T cell clones after stimulation with immobilized anti-CD3 monoclonal antibody, *J Immunol* 144(1): 16-22.

Jones, A.C., Miles, E.A., Warner, J.O., Colwell, B.M., Bryant, T.N. & Warner, J.A. (1996). Fetal peripheral blood mononuclear cell proliferative responses to mitogenic and allergenic stimuli during gestation, *Pediatr Allergy Immunol* 7(3): 109-16.

Kane, L.P., Lin, J. & Weiss, A. (2002). It's all Rel-ative: NF-κB and CD28 costimulation of T-cell activation, *Trends Immunol* 23(8): 413-20.

Karlsson, M.R., Rugtvit, J. & Brandtzaeg, P. (2004). Allergen-responsive CD4+CD25+ regulatory T cells in children who have outgrown cow's milk allergy, *J Exp Med* 199(12): 1679-88.

Kawabe, Y. & Ochi, A. (1990). Selective anergy of $V\beta8^+$, $CD4^+$ T cells in Staphycoccus enterotoxin B-primed mice, *J Exp Med* 172(4): 1065-70.

Kawaguchi, M., Kokubu, F., Kuga, H., Matsukura, S., Hoshino, H., Leki, K., Imai, T., Adachi, M. & Huang, S.K. (2001). Modulation of bronchial epithelial cells by IL-17, *J Allergy Clin Immunol* 108(5): 804-9.

Kim J.H., Kim, K.H., Woo, H.Y. & Shim, J.Y. (2008). Maternal cytokine production during pregnancy and the development of childhood wheezing and allergic disease in offspring three years of age, *J Asthma* 45(10): 948-52.

Kopp, M.V., Zehle, C., Pichler, J., Szépfalusi, Z., Moseler, M., Deichmann, K., Forster, J. & Kuehr, J. (2001). Allergen-specific T cell reactivity in cord blood: the influence of maternal cytokine production, *Clin Exp Allergy* 31(10): 1536-43.

Lamb, J.R., Skidmore, B.J., Green, N., Chiller, J.M. & Feldmann, M. (1983). Induction of tolerance in influenza virus-immune T lymphocyte clones with synthetic peptides of influenza hemagglutinin, *J Exp Med*, 157(5): 1434-47.

Lappalainen, M., Roponen, M., Pekkanen, J., Huttunen, K. & Hirvonen, M-R. (2009). Maturation of cytokine-producing capacity from birth to 1 yr of age, *Pediatr Allergy Immunol* 20(8): 714-25.

Levy, O., Zarember, K.A., Roy, R.M., Cywes, C., Godowski, P.J. & Wessels, M.R. (2004). Selective impairment of TLR-mediated innate immunity in human newborns: neonatal blood plasma reduces monocyte TNF-alpha induction by bacterial lipopeptides, lipopolysaccharide, and imiquimod, but preserves the response to R-848, *J Immunol* 173(7): 4627-34.

Ling, E.M., Smith, T., Nguyen, X.D., Pridgeon, C., Dallman, M., Arbery, J., Carr, V.A. & Robinson, D.S. (2004). Relation of CD4+CD25+ regulatory T-cell suppression of allergen-driven T-cell activation to atopic status and expression of allergic disease, *Lancet* 363(9409): 608-15.

Lin Y.-L., Shieh, C.C. & Wang, J.Y. (2008). The functional insufficiency of human $CD4^+CD25^{high}$ T-regulatory cells in allergic asthma is subjected to TNF-α modulation, *Allergy* 63(1): 67-74.

Ly, N.P., Ruiz-Perez,B., McLoughlin, R.M., Visness, C.M., Wallace, P.K., Cruikshank, W.W., Tzianabos, A.O., O'Connor, G.T., Gold, D.R & Gern, J.E. (2009). Characterization of regulatory T cells in urban newborns, *Clin Mol Allergy* 8(7): 8.

Macián, F., García-Cózar, F., Im, S.H., Horton, H.F., Byrne, M.C. & Rao, A. (2002). Transcriptional mechanisms underlying lymphocyte tolerance, *Cell* 109(6): 719-31.

Maródi, L. (2006). Innate cellular immune responses in newborns, *Clin Immunol* 118(2-3): 137-44.

Marson, A., Kretschmer, K., Frampton, G.M., Jacobsen, E.S., Polansky, J.K., Maclsaac, K.D., Levine, S.S., Fraenkel, E., von Boehmer, H. & Young, R.A. (2007). Foxp3 occupancy and regulation of key target genes during T-cell stimulation, *Nature* 445(7130): 931-5.

Michie, C.A., McLean, A., Alcock, C. & Beverley, P.C. (1992). Lifespan of human lymphocyte subsets defined by CD45 isoforms, *Nature* 360(6401): 264-5.

Miyara, M., Yoshioka, Y., Kitoh, A., Shima, T., Wing, K., Niwa, A., Parizot, C., Taflin, C., Heike, T., Valeyre, D., Mathian, A., Nakahata, T., Yamaguchi, T., Nomura, T., Ono, M., Amoura, Z., Gorochov, G. & Sakaguchi, S. (2009). Functional delineation and differentiation dynamics of human CD4+ T cells expressing the FoxP3 transcription factor, *Immunity* 30(6): 899-911.

Mold, J.E., Michaëlsson, J., Burt, T.D., Muench, M.O., Beckeman, K.P., Busch, M.P., Lee, T.H., Nixon, D.F. & McCune, J.M. (2008). Maternal alloantigens promote the development of tolerogenic fetal regulatory T cells in utero, *Science* 322(5907): 1562-5.

Molet, S., Hamid, Q., Davoine F., Nutku, E., Taha, R., Pagé, N., Olivenstein, R., Elias, J. & Chakir, J. (2001). IL-17 is increased in asthmatic airways and induces human bronchial fibroblasts to produce cytokines, *J Allergy Clin Immunol* 108(3): 430-38.

Nadkarni, S., Mauri, C. & Ehrenstein, M.R. (2007). Anti-TNF-alpha therapy induces a distinct regulatory T cell population in patients with rheumatoid arthritis via TGF-beta, *J Exp Med* 204(1): 33-9.

Nagar, M., Jacob-Hirsch, J., Vernitsky, H., Berkun, Y., Ben-Horin, S., Amariglio, N., Bank, I., Kloog, Y., Rechavi, G. & Goldstien, I. (2010). TNF activites a NF-κB-regulated cellular program in human CD45RA^{-} regulatory T cells that modulates their suppressive function, *J Immunol* 184(7): 3570-81.

Nishimuta, T., Nishima, S. & Morikawa, A. (Ed(s).)(2008). *Japanese Pediatric Guideline for the Treatment and Management of Asthma 2008*, Kyowa Kikaku, ISBN978-4877941154, Tokyo, Japan.

Orihara, K., Narita, M., Tobe, T., Akasawa, A., Ohya, Y., Matsumoto, K. & Saito, H. (2007). Circulating Foxp3+CD4+ cell numbers in atopic patients and healthy control subjects, *J Allergy Clin Immunol* 120(4): 960-2.

Prakriya, M., Feske, S., Gwack, Y., Srikanth, S., Rao, A. & Hogan, P.G. (2006). Orai1 is an essential pore subunit of the CRAC channel, *Nature* 443(7108): 230-3.

Prescott, S.L., Macaubas, C., Holt, B.J., Smallacombe, T.B., Loh, R., Sly, P.D. & Holt, P.G. (1998). Transplacental priming of the human immune system to environmental allergens: Universal skewing of initial T cell responses toward the Th2 cytokine profile, *J Immunol* 160(10): 4730-7.

Prescott, S.L., Macaubas, C., Smallacombe, T., Holt, B.J., Sly P.D. & Holt, P.G. (1999). Development of allergen-specific T-cell memory in atopic and normal children, *Lancet* 353(9148): 196-200.

Rammensee H.G., Kroschewski, R. & Frangoulis, B. (1989). Clonal anergy induced in mature Vβ6^{+} T lymphocytes on immunizing Mls-1^{b} mice with Mls-1^{a} expressing cells, *Natue* 339(6225): 541-4.

Rellahan, B.L., Jones, L.A., Kruisbeek, A.M., Fry, A.M. & Matis, L.A. (1990). In vivo induction of anergy in peripheral Vβ8^{+}T cells in staphylococcal enterotoxin B, *J Exp Med* 172(4): 1091-100.

Robinson, D.S., Hamid, Q., Ying, S., Tsicopoulos, A., Barkans, J., Bentley, A.M., Corrigan, C., Durham, S.R. & Kay, A.B. (1992). Predominant TH2-like bronchoalveolar T-lymphocyte population in atopic asthma, *N Engl J Med* 326(5): 298-304.

Safford, M., Collins, S., Lutz, M.A., Allen, A., Huang, C.T., Kowalski, J., Blackford, A., Horton, M.R., Drake, C., Schwartz, R.H. & Powell, J.D. (2005). Egr-2 and Egr-3 are negative regulators of T cell activation, *Nat Immunol* 6(5): 472-80.

Schaub, B., Liu, J., Hoppler, S., Haug, S., Sattler, C., Lluis, A., Illi, S. & Mutius, E. (2008). Impairment of T-regulatory cells in cord blood of atopic mothers, *J Allergy Clin Immunol* 121(6): 1492-9.

Schittny, J.C., Djonov, V., Fine, A. & Burri, P.H. (1998). Programmed cell death contributes to postnatal lung development, *Am J Respir Cell Mol Biol* 18(6): 786-93.

Suto, A., Nakajima, H., Kagami, S.I., Suzuki, K., Saito, Y. & Iwamoto, I. (2001). Role of CD4(+)CD25(+) regulatory T cells in T helper 2 cell-mediated allergic inflammation in the airways, *Am J Respir Crit Care Med* 164(4): 680-7.

Szépfalusi, Z., Pichler, J., Elsässer, S., van Duren, K., Ebner, C., Bernaschek, G. & Urbanek, R. (2000). Transplacental priming of the human immune system with environmental allergens can occur early in gestation, *J Allergy Clin Immunol* 106(3): 530-6.

Thornton, C.A., Upham, J.W., Wikström, M.E., Holt, B.J., White, G.P., Sharp, M.J., Sly, P.D. & Holt, P.G. (2004). Functional maturation of CD4+CD25+CTLA4+CD45RA+ T regulatory cells in human neonatal T cell responses to environmental antigens/allergens, *J Immunol* 173(5): 3084-92.

Yamamoto, Y., Negoro, T., Wakagi, A., Hoshi, A., Banham, A.H., Roncador, G., Akiyama, H., Tobe, T., Susumu, S., Nakano, Y. & Itabashi, K. (2010). Participation of Th17 and Treg cells in pediatric bronchial asthma, *J Health Sci* 56(5): 589-97.

Yamamoto, Y., Negoro, T., Hoshi, A., Wakagi, A., Shimizu, S., Banham, A.H., Ishii, M., Akiyama, H., Kiuchi, Y., Sunaga, S., Tobe, T., Roncador, G., Itabashi, K. & Nakano, Y. (2011). Impaired Ca^{2+} regulation of $CD4^{+}CD25^{+}$ regulatory T cells from pediatric asthma, *Int Arch Allergy Immunol* 156(2):148-58.

Wan, Y.Y. & Flavell, R.A. (2007). Regulatory T-cell functions are subverted and converted owing to attenuated Foxp3 expression, *Nature* 445(7129): 766-70.

Wang, J.Y., Shyur, S.D., Wang, W.H., Liou, Y.H., Lin, C.G.J., Wu, Y.J. & Wu, L.S.H. (2009). The polymorphisms of interleukin 17A (IL17A) gene and its association with pediatric asthma in Taiwanese population, *Allergy* 64(7): 1056-60.

Warner, J.O., Marguet, C., Rao,R., Roche, W.R. & Pohunek, P. (1998). Inflammatory mechanisms in childhood asthma, *Clin Exp Allergy* 28(5): 71-5.

Wells, A.D. (2009). New insights into the molecular basis of T cell anergy: Anergy factores, avoidance sensors, and epigenetic imprinting, *J Immunol* 182(12): 7331-41.

Wenzel, S.E., Szefler, S.J., Leung, D.Y.M., Sloan, S.I., Rex, M.D. & Martin, R.J. (1997). Bronchoscopic evaluation of severe asthma: persistent inflammation despite high dose glucocorticoids, *Am J Resp Crit Care Med* 156(3 Pt 1): 737-43.

Wenzel, S.E. (2006). Asthma: Defining of the persistent adult phenotypes, *Lancet* 368(9537):804-13.

Wu, Y., Borde, M., Heissmeyer, V., Feuerer, M., Lapan, A.D., Stroud, J.C., Bates, D.L., Guo, L., Han, A., Ziegler, S.F., Mathis, D., Benoist, C., Chen, L. & Rao, A. (2006). FOXP3 controls regulatory T cell function through cooperation with NFAT, *Cell* 126(2): 375-87.

Zhang, S.L., Yu, Y., Roos, J., Kozak, J.A., Deerinck, T.J., Ellisman, M.H., Stauderman, K.A. & Cahalan, M.D. (2005). STIM1 is a Ca^{2+} sensor that activates CRAC channels and migrates from the Ca^{2+} store to the plasma membrane, *Nature* 437(7060): 902-5.

Zhao, Y., Yang, J., Gao, Y-D. & Guo, W. (2010). Th17 immunity in patients with allergic asthma, *Int Arch Allergy Immunol* 151(4): 297-307.

Zheng, Y., Josefowicz, S.Z., Kas, A., Chu, T.T., Gavin, M.A. & Rudensky, A.Y. (2007). Genome-wide analysis of Foxp3 target genes in developing and mature regulatory T cells, *Nature* 445(7130): 936-40.

Zheng, Y., Zha, Y. & Gajewski, T.F. (2008). Molecular regulation of T-cell anergy, *EMBO Rep* 9(1): 50-5.

Zweifach, A. & Lewis, R.S. (1993). Mitogen-regulated Ca^{2+} current of T lymphocytes is activated by depletion of intracellular Ca^{2+} stores, *Proc Natl Acad Sci USA* 90(13): 6295-9.

5

Allergic Asthma and Aging

Gabriele Di Lorenzo[1], Danilo Di Bona[2,3],
Simona La Piana[2], Vito Ditta[4] and Maria Stefania Leto-Barone[1]
[1]*Dipartimento di Medicina Interna e Specialistica (DIMIS), Università degli Studi di Palermo*
[2]*Dipartimento di Dipartimento di Biopatologia e Biotecnologie Mediche e Forensi, Università degli Studi di Palermo*
[3]*Unità Operativa di Immunoematologia e Medicina Trasfusionale, Azienda Ospedaliera, Universitaria Policlinico di Palermo*
[4]*Centro Trasfusionale ASP- Palermo. P.O. San Raffaele G. Giglio Cefalù, Palermo*
Italia

1. Introduction

Chronic obstructive pulmonary disease (COPD) and asthma are the result of particular inflammatory processes that occur over time. Both of these diseases can lead to chronic obstructive airway abnormalities and contribute to a significant social and economic burden on the patient, family, and healthcare system. Distinguishing between COPD and asthma is important because the therapy and expected progression and outcomes of the two conditions are different. Respiratory disease misdiagnosis is common: up to 25% of patients over 40 years of age who are labeled as having asthma actually have COPD. Conversely, many patients in primary care are labeled as having COPD when they in fact have asthma.

Asthma in the elderly is an increasingly serious health issue. Due to the worldwide population trend to enhanced longevity, the number of elderly with asthma will rise in the coming years.

The definition of atopic conditions like asthma, is based on the ability to mount an IgE response to common allergens. Traditionally, the atopy has been associated with atopic asthma and other diseases of childhood and adolescence, which seemed less important at older ages. The allergic asthmatics, who lived through the atopic epidemic between 1970 and 1980, today are older, and now many of them are age ≥ 64 years. Entering the third millennium, physicians must embrace the new demographic challenge. Therefore the atopic diseases, as asthma, in the elderly will be an increasingly serious health issue. Physicians who treat patients with asthma are well aware that there is considerable variability in the course of the disease. Some asthmatics seem to recover completely. Others have long remissions with occasional mild relapses. Most seem to continue unchanged for many years. Asthma may persist from childhood or have its onset in adult life. The presence of atopy increases the incidence of asthma in children and young adults. This observation had promoted the concept that atopy decreases with age and hence asthma also decreases.

Elderly asthmatic patients mainly include those who have acquired the disease during childhood or adolescence and whose disease has progressed over time or is recurrent after periods of remission (elderly asthmatics, long life), but the first manifestations of asthma can occur even in late adulthood or after 65 years of age (the elderly, asthmatics, late-onset). These considerations, taken in isolation, have resulted in asthma being under-diagnosed and under-treated in elderly patients, which may be due to diagnostic misclassification. Underestimation of the prevalence of asthma may be due to confusion with COPD.

In this chapter, after describing the basics of atopy and immune alteration of the immune system in the elderly, we will examine the flow characteristics of the pathophysiology of asthma and COPD, establish the basis for correct diagnosis of asthma, highlighting the confounding factors of diagnosis, and the importance of monitoring the clinical course, identifying areas for improvement.

2. Definition of asthma

Scientific knowledge has changed the definition of bronchial asthma and is now defined as reported by the National Institutes of Health (NIH) [1]. Asthma is defined as an inflammatory disorder of the airway associated with airflow obstruction and bronchial hyper-responsiveness, This definition replaces the previous definition of asthma in which only the airflow obstruction and the bronchial hyper-responsiveness was emphasized [2].

2.1 Epidemiology

The overall prevalence of asthma in children and adults varies in European countries, with estimates of 15%–18% in the United Kingdom, 7% in France and Germany, 4.4 Italy and of 1.9 in Albania [3].

Long considered a disease of childhood or young adulthood, its prevalence is now known to be similar in older people [4].

The incidence of newly diagnosed asthma in patients ≥ 65 years is 0.1%/years in a population based study done on Rochester residents [5].

Asthma may persist from childhood or have its onset in adult life. The primary variable for persistence and severity of asthma identified in longitudinal studies is the severity in childhood. However, common sense and everyday experience tell us that continued exposure to relevant indoor allergens is also important [6,7].

The studies also suggest that sensitization and exposure to outdoor allergens, result in more persistent and severe asthma [8]. The presence of atopy increases the incidence of asthma in children and may also increase the incidence in young adults.

A cohort of college students evaluated for hay fever or asthma were followed up 23 years later. At the age of 40 years, about half of subjects who had asthma as freshmen continued to have asthma. Of these subjects, half (a quarter of the entire group) reported that they continued to have about the same frequency and severity of symptoms; very few were worse. During these 23 years, 5.2% of subjects who did not have asthma as freshmen developed asthma subsequently; the yearly incidence rate was 0.23%. The presence of positive skin test results or hay fever as freshmen did not affect the incidence of new cases of asthma as these subjects grew older. Unfortunately, skin tests were not performed at the 23-year follow-up of middle-aged adults, so it is not known whether these new case of asthma were allergic [9].

The incidence of asthma is the same in patients age 65 to 84 years as it is in younger adults [10]. However the disease may be more likely to persist and progress in severity. A cross-sectional study of 242 patients with asthma age 65 and older found that 80% had irreversible obstruction; 20% of them were unable to achieve an FEV1 greater than 50% predicted. The authors concluded that only a part of this irreversibility is the result of airway remodeling from asthmatic inflammation [10].

The diagnosis of asthma may be more difficult in the elderly because of the high prevalence of other disorders that can have similar symptoms, and because airflow obstruction is often caused by chronic obstructive pulmonary disease [11].

2.2 The problems of asthma

Under-diagnosis of asthma may occur in older people because they attribute breathlessness to normal aging and because common symptoms are often dismissed by doctors as being 'normal'. Physicians commonly underestimate the severity of breathlessness and even when breathlessness is seen as a 'problem' the possibility of asthma is often not considered [12]. The differential diagnosis of breathlessness includes not only asthma but also other conditions common in older people including chronic obstructive pulmonary disease (COPD), heart failure and obesity. Identifying the asthmatic patients from the one-third of the older population with significant breathlessness is quite a challenge [13]. A Dutch investigation has estimated that the identification of new cases of asthma or chronic obstructive pulmonary disease in an adult population subjected to a screening program cost $500–1000 per case [14].

Wheeze and sensation of bronchospasm are the symptoms which suggest the diagnosis of asthma, but they may be absent in older asthmatic patients. Furthermore, the perception of bronchoconstriction in asthmatic patients falls throughout adulthood [15]. In elderly patients there is a close relationship between the severity of wheezing complaints and impairment of the forced expiratory volume in 1 second (FEV1). Elderly patients with long-standing asthma have more severe airway obstruction than patients with recently acquired disease but patients with newly diagnosed asthma experienced a more rapid rate of decline FEV1 than patients with chronic asthma [16,17].

The asthmatic symptoms such as wheeze and sensation of bronchospasm, can have more than one cause in one elderly individual. In addition, in older patients co-morbidities may be present, such as senile dementia, which may alter the clinical presentation of asthma [18]. Several recent reviews have recommended the need for a global multidimensional assessment of obstructive airway diseases, i.e. asthma and COPD, in older people. [19,20]

3. Differential diagnosis of asthma in older patients

The differential diagnosis of asthma from other obstructive airway diseases, should include cardiac disease, tumors (laryngeal, tracheal, lung), bronchiectasis, foreign body, interstitial lung disease, pulmonary emboli, aspiration, vocal cord dysfunction, hyperventilation, anaphylactic reactions, (uncommon in the elderly unless atopic), obesity and some medications.

3.1 Obstructive airway diseases

Emphysema and chronic bronchitis are encompassed within the term COPD. COPD should be considered in any patient >35 years of age with risk factors, usually smoking, who presents with dyspnoea on exertion, chronic cough, frequent winter 'bronchitis' or wheeze. [21]. None of these symptoms are specific to COPD, and several other disorders may present with similar symptoms, signs and spirometry results, such as asthma, bronchiectasis, congestive cardiac failure and carcinoma of the bronchus. COPD is defined by the presence of airflow limitation that is "not fully reversible and does not change markedly over several months" [21]. Traditionally measurement of the degree of reversibility using bronchodilators or corticosteroids has been used to confirm the diagnosis and in particular to try to separate patients with asthma from those with COPD [22]. However, the same study in patients with fixed airflow obstruction diagnosed as having COPD, on the basis of the clinical history has shown that the clinical diagnosis was correct as assessed by the basis of the pattern of inflammation seen on the differential cell counts in induced sputum findings. Reversibility testing was unable to differentiate patients with COPD from patients with asthma [22].

3.2 Left ventricular failure

Left ventricular failure (LVF) can sometimes be very difficult to differentiate from asthma as signs can be unreliable in older people. The following characteristics are present both in LVF and in asthma: airways obstruction, bronchial hyper-reactivity and episodic nocturnal dyspnoea. A history of ischemic heart disease is suggestive of heart failure, but not necessarily so, as diseases can co-exist [23].

Levels of B-type natriuretic peptide (BNP), a neurohormone secreted by the left ventricle in response to volume-elevated left ventricular pressure, are higher in acute and chronic heart failure. Measurement of plasma BNP proved to be a useful diagnostic test in differentiating HF from other causes in patients who presented with dyspnea [24].

3.3 Gastro-esophageal reflux disease (GERD)

The incidence of gastro-esophageal reflux disease (GERD) increases with age and leads to broncho-constriction via microaspiration and vagal stimulation. Methylxanthines used to treat asthma can reduce lower esophageal pressure and cause aspiration. GERD should be considered in elderly patients with heartburn or nocturnal symptoms occurring early at night [25].

3.4 Aspiration

Conditions resulting in reduced conscious level, such as dementia, Parkinson's disease and stroke as well as use of medications such as sedatives, alcohol and antipsychotics, and immobility increase the risk of aspiration [26].

3.5 Tumors (laryngeal, tracheal, lung)

Tumors that affect the central airways, i.e. cancers of tracheal or of the proximal bronchus, and the bronchogenic carcinoma, or mediastinal lymphadenopathy may present with cough, wheeze and dyspnoea, all symptoms of asthma. Also the gastric and breast cancer spread via lymphatics and can produce wheeze [27,28].

3.6 Pulmonary embolism (PE)

In PE breathless and tachipnoeic (> 20 breaths/min) are the most prominent signs, while bronchoconstriction is less often present. Differentiating asthma from PE, in the absence of pleuritic chest pain, is very difficult. However, computed tomographic pulmonary angiography is usually recommended for the diagnosis of PE [29]. A blood D-dimer test can be useful [30].

3.7 Drugs

Polypharmacy is common in outpatients and has been identified as a major risk factor for drug-drug interactions (DDIs), which are an important cause of adverse drug reactions [31]. Therefore a detailed drug history is essential. β-adrenoceptor antagonist drugs [32], aspirin and NSAIDs, may worsen asthma control by inducing bronchospasm[33]. ACE inhibitors can cause cough [34]. Methylxanthines can reduce lower esophageal sphincter tone, increase GERD and cause 'uncontrolled' asthma [35].

4. Definition of Chronic obstructive pulmonary disease

Chronic obstructive pulmonary disease (COPD) is a lung disease characterized by chronic obstruction of lung airflow that interferes with normal breathing and is not fully reversible. The more familiar terms 'chronic bronchitis' and 'emphysema' are no longer used, but are now included within the COPD diagnosis [36].

While asthma features obstruction to the flow of air out of the lungs, usually, the obstruction is reversible. Between "attacks" of asthma the flow of air through the airways typically is normal. These patients do not have COPD. However, if asthma is left untreated, the chronic inflammation associated with this disease can cause the airway obstruction to become fixed. That is, between attacks, the asthmatic patient may then have abnormal air flow. This process is referred to as lung remodeling. These asthma patients with a fixed component of airway obstruction are also considered as having COPD [22].

Often patients with COPD are labeled by the symptoms they are having at the time as an exacerbation of their disease. For instance, if they present with mostly shortness of breath, they may be referred to as emphysema patients. While if they have mostly cough and mucus production, they are referred to as having chronic bronchitis. In reality, it is better to refer to these patients as having COPD since they can present with a variety of lung symptoms. There is frequent overlap among COPD patients. Thus, patients with emphysema may have some of the characteristics of chronic bronchitis and vice a versa [37].

4.1 Causes of COPD

4.1.1 Smoking

Smoking is responsible for 90% of COPD [36]. Although not all cigarette smokers will develop COPD, it is estimated that 15% will. Smokers with COPD have higher death rates than nonsmokers with COPD [38]. They also have more frequent respiratory symptoms (coughing, shortness of breath, etc.) and more rapid deterioration in lung function than non-smokers [36]. It is important to note that when COPD patients stop smoking, their decline in lung function slows to the same rate as nonsmokers [36,39]. Therefore, it is never "too late" to quit.

Effects of passive smoking or "second-hand smoke" on the lungs are not well understood; however, evidence suggests that respiratory infections, asthma, and symptoms are more common in children who live in households where adults smoke [2]. Cigarette smoking damages the lungs in many ways. For example, the irritating effect of cigarette smoke attracts cells to the lungs that promote inflammation. Cigarette smoke also stimulates these inflammatory cells, predominantly neutrophils, to release elastase, an enzyme that breaks down all components of the extracellular matrix including the elastic fibers in lung tissue [40].

4.1.2 Air pollution

Air pollution can cause problems for persons with lung disease, but it is unclear whether outdoor air pollution contributes to the development of COPD. However, in the non-industrialized world, the most common cause of COPD is indoor air pollution. This is usually due to indoor stoves used for cooking [41,42].

4.1.3 Occupational pollutants

Some occupational pollutants such as silica and cadmium do increase the risk of COPD. Persons at risk for this type of occupational pollution include coal miners, construction workers, metal workers, cotton workers, etc. Most of this risk is associated with cigarette smoking and these occupations, an issue not well controlled for. These occupations are more often associated with the pneumoconioses than are the interstitial lung diseases. Nevertheless, the adverse effects of smoking cigarettes on lung function are far greater than occupational exposure [43].

4.1.4 Alpha-1 antitrypsin

Another well-established cause of COPD is a deficiency of alpha-1 antitrypsin (AAT). AAT deficiency is a rare genetic (inherited) disorder that accounts for less than 1% of the COPD in the United States.

Normal function of the lung is dependent on elastic fibers surrounding the airways and in the alveolar walls. Elastic fibers are composed of a protein called elastin. An enzyme called neutrophil elastase that is found even in normal lungs (and is higher in cigarette smokers) can break down the elastin and damage the airways and alveoli. Another protein called alpha-1 antitrypsin (AAT) (produced by the liver and released into the blood) is present in normal lungs and can block the damaging effects of elastase on elastin. It does this on a one molecular basis, so that one molecule of ATT inhibits one molecule of neutrophil elastase, preventing elastase related destruction of surrounding tissue (proteolysis).

The manufacture of AAT by the liver is controlled by genes which are contained in DNA-containing chromosomes that are inherited. Each person has two AAT genes, one inherited from each parent. There are multiple inherited single nucleotide polymorphisms which alter the tertiary structure of the AAT protein, and can alter its release from liver cells (causing liver damage in some case, and can alter the levels of AAT in blood. Individuals who inherit two copies of the most defective AAT polymorphism (PiZ) (one from each parent) have both low amounts of AAT in the blood and AAT that does not function properly as it forms strings of joined proteins (polymers) which cannot inibit elastase and are pro-inflammatory in their own right. The reduced action of AAT in these individuals allows the destruction of tissue in the lungs by elastase to continue unopposed. This causes emphysema by age 30 or 40. Cigarette smoking accelerates the destruction and results in an even earlier onset of COPD.

Individuals with one normal and one defective AAT gene have AAT levels that are lower than normal but higher than individuals with two defective genes. These individuals may have an increased risk of developing COPD if they do not smoke cigarettes; however, their risk of COPD probably is higher than normal if they smoke. Though their Alpha-1 antitrypsin blood levels may be in the normal range, the function of this enzyme is impaired relative to normal patients. Some may even develop bronchiectasis instead of emphysema [44,45].

5. Symptoms of COPD

Typically, after smoking 20 or more cigarettes a day for more than twenty years, patients with COPD develop a chronic cough, shortness of breath (dyspnea), and frequent respiratory infections [36]. In patients affected predominantly by emphysema, shortness of breath may be the major symptom. Dyspnea usually is most noticeable during increased physical activity, but as emphysema progresses, dyspnea occurs at rest. In patients with chronic bronchitis as well as bronchiectasie, chronic cough and sputum production are the major symptoms [46]. The sputum is usually clear and thick. Periodic chest infections can cause fever dyspnea, coughing, production of purulent (cloudy and discolored) sputum and wheezing. (Wheezing is a high pitched noise produced in the lungs during exhalation when mucous, bronchospasm, or loss of lung elasticity obstructs airways.) Infections occur more frequently as bronchitis and bronchiectasis progress.

In advanced COPD, patients may develop cyanosis (bluish discoloration of the lips and nail beds) due to a lack of oxygen in blood. They also may develop morning headaches due to an inability to remove carbon dioxide from the blood. Weight loss occurs in some patients, due to combination of reduced intake of food, the additional energy that is required to breathe and the cachectic consequences of inflammation, in particular excessive Tumor Necrosis Factor alfa (TNFα) acting via leptin. In advanced COPD, small blood vessels in the lungs are destroyed, and this blocks the flow of blood through the lungs. As a result, the heart must pump with increased force and pressure to get blood to flow through the lungs. The elevated pressure in the blood vessels of the lungs develops pulmonary hypertension. If the heart cannot manage the additional work, right heart failure also known as Cor pulmonale results and leads to swelling of the feet and ankles.

Patients with COPD may cough up blood (hemoptysis). Usually hemoptysis is due to damage to the inner lining of the airways and the airways' blood vessels; however, occasionally, hemoptysis may signal the development of lung cancer [47,48].

6. Diagnosis of COPD

COPD is usually diagnosed on the basis of a medical history, the symptoms of COPD and the physical examination which reveals signs of COPD [22, 49]. The tests to diagnose COPD include tests of lung function (spirometry), the measurement of carbon dioxide, oxygen levels in the blood, chest X-ray and computerized tomography (CT) scan of the chest. The medical history of patients with COPD is often suspected in chronic smokers who develop shortness of breath with or without exertion [22, 36]. These patients have chronic persistent cough with sputum production, and frequent infections of the lungs. Sometimes COPD is first diagnosed after a patient develops a respiratory illness necessitating hospitalization. Some physical findings of COPD include enlarged chest cavity and wheezing. Faint and distant breath sounds are heard when listening to the chest with a stethoscope. Air is trapped in the lungs from the patient's inability to empty their lungs with exhalation. This extra air dampens the sounds heard and results in the overinflated chest cavity. In patients affected predominantly with emphysema, the chest X-ray may show an enlarged chest cavity and decreased lung markings reflecting destruction of lung tissue and enlargement of air-spaces. In patients with predominantly chronic bronchitis, the chest X-ray may show increased lung markings which represent the thickened, inflamed and scarred airways. CT scans of the chest show the abnormal lung tissue and airways in COPD. Chest X-rays and CT scans of the chest are also useful in excluding lung infections (pneumonia) and cancers. CT of the chest usually is not necessary for the routine diagnosis and management of COPD, but can be helpful in evaluating the extent of emphysematous change as well as detecting early lung cancers [36].

Spirometry is a test which quantitates the amount of airway obstruction and its reversibility after bronchodilator. Oxygen and carbon dioxide levels are measured in samples of arterial blood. A noninvasive method to measure oxygen levels in the blood is the pulse oximetry. Another very effective and simple test used to monitor COPD is called the six minute walking test (6MWT) [50]. The patient is asked to walk on a level surface at their own pace for six minutes. There is a very detailed script that is utilized when performing this test. The patient is informed about the time left to complete the test, but no encouragement is offered. The patient may stop and rest at any time during the study. The distance traveled is measured and is a very accurate index of the state of health and effectiveness of therapy.

7. Differences between asthma and COPD

Asthma and COPD are very different in terms of cellular mechanisms, inflammatory mediators, inflammatory effects, and response to therapy. Both diseases are characterized by airflow obstruction and a chronic persistent inflammatory process, but the nature of the inflammation differs markedly between these diseases [51, 52].

7.1 Inflammatory cells

Airway inflammation in asthma is characterized by an eosinophilic inflammation, with an increase in activated and degranulating eosinophils in bronchial biopsies, BAL, and in induced sputum [22, 53]. There is also an increase in CD4 T lymphocytes (T-helper type 2 cells) that appear to orchestrate the eosinophilic inflammation and degranulated mast cells that underlie the rapid and episodic bronchoconstrictor responses that are so characteristic of asthma. Airway inflammation in asthma is characterized by an eosinophilic inflammation, with an increase in activated and degranulating eosinophils in bronchial biopsies, BAL, and in induced sputum [54]. Epithelial shedding is a common feature of biopsies from asthmatic airways and may be a consequence of eosinophilic inflammation. Inflammation affects all of the airways in asthma and does not involve the lung parenchyma. Fibrosis is remarkable by its absence, and although much has been made of the subepithelial fibrosis, this is trivial in amount and is seen even in patients with very mild asthma of short duration. Airway hyper-responsiveness is the characteristic physiological abnormality in asthma, and although its mechanism is uncertain, it is linked to eosinophilic inflammation [54].

The pathology of COPD differs clearly from that of asthma [55]. In larger airways, there is evidence of neutrophil rather than an eosinophilic inflammation, as judged by increased numbers of neutrophils in BAL [54,55]. Induced sputum shows a characteristic increase in the proportion of neutrophils that is much greater in patients with COPD than in smokers without obstruction. Granulocyte markers of neutrophil inflammation, namely myeloperoxidase and human neutrophil lectin, are actively degranulating [56]. The eosinophils can be present in the induced sputum of patients with COPD. However, the eosinophils aren't activated [22]. The neutrophils transit rapidly from the circulation into the airway lumen, as demonstrated by the bronchial biopsies that have demonstrated an infiltration with mononuclear cells, CD8+ T lymphocytes, rather than neutrophils. A similar inflammatory aspect has been shown in bronchial biopsies of ex-smokers, confirming that inflammation may persist in the airway once established [57].

In the lung parenchyma a predominance of macrophages and CD8+ T cells have been found at sites of parenchymal destruction [53, 55, 57]. Finally in COPD, a squamous metaplasia can be present. In contrast to asthma, most of the pathologic changes are found in peripheral airways, where there is also fibrosis, resulting in an obliterative bronchiolitis [53].

In patients with COPD the airway hyper-responsiveness is not a common feature. Furthermore, in COPD, unlike asthma, patients do not constrict with indirect bronchial challenges, such as exercise [55].

Cigarette smoking and/or other inhaled irritants may initiate an inflammatory response in the peripheral airways and lung parenchyma. It is likely that neutrophil chemotactic factors are released from activated macrophages and also from epithelial cells and CD8+ T lymphocytes [53, 57].

Although both COPD and asthma involve chronic inflammation of the respiratory tract, the pattern of inflammation is markedly different between these two diseases (Table 1). Mild asthma is characterized by eosinophilic inflammation driven by TH2 cells and DCs, and is associated with mast-cell sensitization by IgE, and by the release of multiple bronchoconstrictors. By contrast, COPD is characterized by neutrophilic inflammation that can be driven by a marked increase in the number of lung-resident macrophages, which also attract CD4+ and CD8+ T cells to the lungs. This lymphocytic infiltration can also be driven by chronic stimulation by viral and bacterial antigens or by autoantigens released following lung injury. Mast cells and DCs, which have such a key role in asthma, have little or no known involvement in COPD. However, these distinctions between asthma and COPD may not be as clear as previously believed, as in patients with severe asthma and in asthmatic individuals who smoke there is a neutrophilic pattern of inflammation, and acute exacerbations of asthma and of COPD have similar inflammatory features [54]

	Asthma			COPD		
	Mild	Severe	Exacerbation	Mild	Severe	Exacerbat
Steroid response	++++	++	+	0	0	0
Neutrophils	0	++(?)	++++*	++	++++	++++
Eosinophils	+	+++	+++	0	0	0
T cells	Th_2 cells ++	Th_1 cells + Th_2 cells +	?	Th_1 cells +	Th_1 cells +++	?
B-cells	IgE producing	IgE producing	?	+	+++	?
Mast cells	++	+++	?	0	0	0
Macrophages	+	+	?	+++	++++	++++
Dendritic cells	+	?	?	?	?	?
Cytokines	IL4 +++, IL5 +++, IL13 ++	TNF ++	?	TNF +	TNF ++	TNF ++
Chemokines	CCL11+	CXCL8+	CXCL8++	CXCL8+	CXCL8++	CXCL8+-
Lipid mediators	PD_2 +, LTC_4,D_4,E_4 ++	PD_2 +, LTB_4 ++	?	LTB_4 +	LTB_4 ++	LTB_4 ++
Eosinophil proteins	0	ECP +++ MBP ++	ECP +++	0	0	0
Oxidative stress	0	+	+++	++	+++	++++

0 = no response; + to ++++, magnitude response; ? = uncertain

Table 1. The pattern of inflammation and the response to steroid in asthma and COPD

7.2 Inflammatory mediators

More than 50 inflammatory mediators have been found in asthma [58]. In table 1 we reported the cells and mediators that characterized asthma and COPD. Histamine, prostaglandin and kinins derive from mast cells and basophils. Cysteinyl-leukotrienes derive from mast cells and eosinophils. These inflammatory mediators, particularly kinins, could activate the cholinergic reflex. In contrast, there are likely to be few bronchoconstrictor mediators released in COPD airways, and cholinergic tone is likely to be the only reversible component. This explains why anticholinergic drugs are relatively more effective in COPD and may be even more effective than β2-agonists [58].

In induced sputum of patients with COPD elevated levels of Leukotriene-B4 (LTB4) have been found, which it is a potent neutrophil chemoattractant [59]. The cytokines of asthma: interleukin (IL)-4 and IL-13, are likely to be important, as they are necessary for IgE formation, whereas IL-5 is critical for eosinophilic inflammation [60].

Eosinophil chemotactic cytokines (CC chemokines), such as eotaxin and RANTES, are also important in asthmatic inflammation and selectively recruit primed eosinophils from the circulation into the airways [58].

IL-8 is a selective attractant of neutrophils and its levels in induced sputum are correlated with the extent of neutrophilic inflammation and with disease severity (% predicted FEV1) of COPD [56, 59] Other CXC chemokines, such as GRO-a, may also be involved in neutrophil recruitment in COPD. Also, Tumor necrosis factor-α is present in high concentration in the sputum of COPD patients, and may activate the transcription of nuclear factor-kB which switches on the transcription of the IL-8 gene [61].

Markers of oxidative stress are higher in COPD. This is likely to be because of the large increase in activated macrophages and neutrophils in COPD, and the effects of cigarettes, which provide high oxidative stress [62].

7.3 Enzymes

The predominant inflammatory enzyme involved in asthma is the typtase that is produced by the mast cell. Tryptase plays an important role in AHR and in some aspects of airway remodeling in asthma [63].

COPD proteinase/antiproteinase imbalance

Excessive activity of proteases, and an imbalance between proteases and endogenous antiproteases is the characteristic of COPD.

The destruction of lung parenchymal is due to several proteases. Neutrophil elastase, a neutral serine protease, is the major constituent of lung elastolytic activity and also potently stimulates mucus secretion [64]. In the patient's α1-antitrypsin deficiency this enzyme activity is likely to be the major mechanism mediating elastolysis, and may not be the major elastolytic enzyme in smoking-related COPD [65]. It is important to consider other enzymes as targets for inhibition, including cathepsins, collagenase (MMP-1), gelatinase B (MMP-9) and matrix metalloproteinases (MMPs). MMPs are produced by several inflammatory cells, including macrophages and neutrophils [65]. Some metalloproteinases, MMP-2 and MMP-9, have been found in the parenchyma of patients with emphysema. The levels of MMPs are lower in patients with asthma and may be derived predominantly from eosinophils; this is not surprising since parenchymal destruction is not a feature of asthma [66]. CD8+ (cytotoxic or Tc cells) may also contribute to parenchymal destruction through the release of proteolytic perforins and granzymes.

COPD oxidant/antioxidant imbalance

The lung is susceptible to oxidative injury by virtue of myriads of reactive forms of oxygen species and free radicals. Reactive oxygen species and reactive nitrogen species are highly unstable due to unpaired electrons that are capable of initiating oxidation. As a part of their normal physiology and external challenges posed by various microorganisms and chemicals, biological systems continuously generate reactive oxygen/nitrogen species to ward off these agents and in turn are exposed to the deleterious effects of these reactive species. Free radical species may be endogenously produced by metabolic reactions (e.g. from mitochondrial electron transport during respiration or during activation of phagocytes) or exogenously, such as air pollutants or cigarette smoke [67]. Antioxidants are major *in vivo* and *in situ* defence mechanisms of the cells against oxidative stress. Two classes of antioxidants are recognized: (a) non-enzymatic antioxidants such as Vitamins E, Vitamin C, β-carotene, GSH and (b) enzymatic antioxidants such as GSH redox system comprising of glutamate cysteine ligase, glutathione reductase, glutathione peroxidase, glucose-6-phosphate dehydrogenase, and in addition superoxide dismutases, catalase, heme oxygenase-1, peroxiredoxins, thioredoxins and glutaredoxins. The two classes of antioxidants often work in tandem with each other and are involved in redox recycling process. The human lungs and different inflammatory cells exhibit diverse antioxidant profiles. Depending on the status of the antioxidants in a particular region and the specific burden, a specific disease process may be initiated. All the major varieties of inflammatory lung diseases, asthma, chronic obstructive pulmonary disease, idiopathic pulmonary fibrosis, acute respiratory distress syndrome, interstitial lung diseases and bronchopulmonary dysplasia share a common feature of impaired oxidant/antioxidant ratio. The localization of specific antioxidant enzymes in various sub-compartments of lung tissue, particularly during lung diseases remains largely unclear. It may be possible that various antioxidant enzymes are expressed in a cell-specific manner depending upon the milieu of deleterious reactive oxygen species generated. Emerging data indicate that various antioxidant enzymes are upregulated at the level of mRNA expression but actually have low enzyme activity or low levels of proteins [68].

8. Immune-senescence and asthma

The last clinical manifestation of asthma is generally considered the arrival of atopic march. The atopic march is generally characterized by the progression of atopic dermatitis to asthma and allergic rhinitis during the first years of life. The putative mechanism is the skin, which acts as the site of primary sensitization through possible defects in the epidermal barrier with later sensitization in the airways [69].

The typical inflammation of allergic asthma and other allergic diseases, as allergic rhinitis, consists of predominantly Th2 lymphocytes and cytokines, e.g. IL-4, IL-5, and IL-13 [54]. Studies of induced sputum, bronchoalveolar fluid, and bronchial biopsies have shown an inflammation that consists of T-cells and eosinophils. [70,71]. In addition to these cells, the expression of a number of inflammatory mediators including cytokines, chemokines, and lipids (prostaglandins and leukotrienes) are significantly higher in the airway, see paragraph *6.0 Differences beteween asthma and COPD* [58]. The IL-13 and leukotriene LTC4, can directly induce the pathophysiological hallmarks of asthma, including airway hyper-responsiveness, goblet cell hyperplasia, mucus secretion, and smooth muscle cell hypertrophy [72,73]. It is recognized as a more severe asthma phenotype with a greater degree of airflow obstruction, more frequent exacerbations, and a greater rate of lung function decline. In a study comparing patients with asthma of long duration and patients with asthma of short duration, it was found that the duration of asthma is associated with the degree of airflow limitation [4].

An important "trigger" of asthma exacerbations is upper respiratory tract viral infection. Estimates suggest that up to 80% of asthma exacerbations in adults are caused by viral upper respiratory infections [74]. Because immune function is important for the resolution of respiratory infections, question arise regarding the impact of immune-senescence on the clinical features of asthma in the elderly [75].

Numerous studies suggest that immune function declines with aging, a phenomenon frequently referred to as "immunosenescence" [76]. This is thought to contribute to more frequent infections [77], an increased incidence of autoimmune disease [78], and increased incidence of malignancy due to impaired immune surveillance [79]. Immunosenescence has been described for both adaptive and innate components of the immune response.

The most extensively studied component of the immune system with regard to immunosenescence is the T-cell population. The involution of the thymus gland begins shortly after birth and undergoes replacement by fatty tissue that is nearly complete by 60 years of age. Consequently, a decline in the numbers of circulating naïve T-cells gradually occurs, and memory T-cells (CD45RO+) eventually predominate [80]. Additionally, the T-cell receptor repertoire diversity appears to diminish, and T helper cell activity declines [81]. Other observations of the T-cell population with aging include reduced proliferative responses [82], a shift of Th1 to Th2 cytokine profiles upon stimulation with PHA (phytohaemoagglutinin) [83,84] and a decline in Fas-mediated T-cell apoptosis [85]. Whether any of these age-related changes is more or less pronounced in specific inflammatory disorders, such as allergic diseases or asthma, is not known.

Also a decreased production of B-cells with aging has been observed. More specifically, there is a transition from the presence of naïve B-cells to "antigen-experienced" B-cells [86]. In addition, the quality of antibody produced is altered with lower affinity and avidity for antigen [87, 88]. The ability of neutrophils to kill phagocytosed organisms is diminished in the elderly compared to younger individuals [89]. We studied the superoxide production, chemotaxis and the expression of the apoptosis-related molecule APO1/Fas (CD95) on neutrophils (PMN) from young and old subjects. We have also measured the basal natural killer (NK) activity of young and elderly subjects comparing the number of CD16+ cells as well. We observed a significant age-related decrease both of formation of O_2^- and chemotaxis, whereas no significant correlation between age and the expression of CD95 on granulocyte membrane was demonstrated, suggesting that an age-related increase of CD95-linked apoptosis of PMN should not be an important determinant in the decreased PMN function. We also observed a significant correlation between age and NK activity. The decreased NK cell function was not due to a decreased number of NK cells in effector cell preparations since the number of CD16+ cells was significantly higher in old subjects [89].

In a study examining age-related changes in eosinophil function, it was found that peripheral blood eosinophils from older asthma subjects exhibited decreased degranulation in response to cytokine stimulation and displayed a trend for decreased superoxide production [90]. However, eosinophils may have an altered or diminished role in the airway inflammation of older asthma patients and the production of IL-5 is not defective in old subjects [22, 90]. These observations strengthen the suggestions of the existence of Th-2 shift in elderly [91-93].

9. Treatment of asthma in older patients

We performed computer-assisted searches of the medical literature to identify information on the treatment of asthma in individuals over 65 years old. We reviewed the articles identified as matches for our search criteria and tabulated the data from them. We searched the PubMed/MEDLINE databases, and included citations from 1966 to 2010. Our search strategy combined medical subject headings or the text words for *asthma, humans, English, aged (65+ years)* and treatment.

As regards the treatment in older asthmatics using all databases, we found 2 controlled studies that focused exclusively on asthma in patients aged over 65 years: 1 on a β2-agonist and the other on a leukotriene receptor antagonist [94,95]. In the other published randomized, controlled treatment trials of asthma, the numbers of individuals aged over 65 years were small. Finally the diagnosis of asthma was approximate, many patients included were patients with both asthma and COPD. Thus, the information to follow was, for the most part, derived from less rigorous data, in part to the systematic exclusion of the elderly from clinical trials of asthma therapy [96]. However, only in 2007 in the Expert Panel Report a section, "Special Issues for Older Adults," specifically addressed asthma in seniors [2]. Because of the high prevalence of chronic bronchitis and emphysema among the elderly, a 2- to 3-week trial of systemic corticosteroids was suggested to detect "significant reversibility of airway disease" in patients thought to have asthma who fail to demonstrate reversibility on pulmonary function testing [22]. Because seniors have decreased awareness of bronchoconstriction, decreased physiologic responses to hypoxemia and hypercapnia, and more advanced airway obstruction than younger asthmatic patients, pulmonary function testing could be more appropriate to use than symptoms as the primary guide for treatment [4, 22]. The lack of an evidence-based approach to asthma in the elderly was attributed in part to the systematic exclusion of the elderly from clinical trials of asthma therapy [97]. Therefore the therapeutic approach to asthma in older patients does not differ from what is recommended for young patients. Treatment protocols use step-care pharmacologic therapy based on the asthma symptoms and the clinical response to these interventions. As symptoms and lung function worsen, step-up or add-on therapy is given. As symptoms improve, therapy can be ''stepped down.'' Several factors must be taken into consideration when considering appropriate pharmacological therapy in older patients who have asthma and special attention should also be given to the potential adverse effects of commonly used medications [98].

9.1 Anti-inflammatory

9.1.1 Corticosteroids

Because asthma is an inflammatory disease any patients with persistent asthma should receive daily anti-inflammatory therapy to control and suppress the airway inflammation [2]. The anti-inflammatory therapy of asthma is the corticosteroids [2, 99]. They have been used by Boardley et al. at Johns Hopkins University, in 1949 in patients with asthma, demonstrating good results. Subsequently, oral cortisone, widely used at that time to treat several inflammatory diseases, was shown to be an effective replacement for the injections, in patients with difficult-to-control asthma. In 1956, the first multicenter trial of cortisone placebo-controlled trial in asthma patients was done. The results of this trial were disappointing compared to Boardley's data. However, the reasons can be traced to the low dose of cortisone used, the lack of objective measurements of lung function and the inclusion of many patients who had COPD [100,101]. However, despite this poor result, oral steroids were used in patients with severe asthma, but it was clear that side effects, stunting of growth in children, osteoporosis and metabolic disturbances, were a major problem of this treatment. A way of reducing systemic side effects was to give corticosteroids by inhalation. The first two molecules of inhalator corticosteroids used were cortisone and dexamethasone. Beclomethasone dipropionate (BDP) was used successfully.

Inhaled BDP was very effective in reducing the need for oral corticosteroids and in many patients achieved better control. The authors observed that the patients who did best had high numbers of eosinophils in their sputum [102]. This observation has been confirmed in other subsequent studies and the use of inhaled corticosteroids in asthma has been the major reason why asthma morbidity and mortality have fallen [103].

There is now a search for inhaled corticosteroids with improved therapeutic ratios and less systemic side effects.

The newer inhaled corticosteroids i.e. budesonide, fluticasone propionate and mometasone fuorato, have improved therapeutic ratios and less systemic side effects, because oral bioavailability has been reduced [104-106]. The last inhaled corticosteroid is the cliclosonide, which is a prodrug, activated by esterases in the lower airways [107].

There has recently been a much better understanding of the molecular mechanisms involved in the anti-inflammatory effects of corticosteroids in asthma, with particular emphasis on the effects of corticosteroids on chromatin remodeling through increased recruitment of histone deacetylase-2 to activated inflammatory genes [108, 109].

Does the prescribing of ICS to older patients increase the risk of bone fractures? A study of patients aged 56-91 years demonstrated that women who took ICS had a modest decrease in BMD compared to women who did not take corticostcroids [110]. A retrospective evaluation of 800,000 women aged >66 years found that systemic, but not inhaled, corticosteroids were associated with an increased risk of hip fractures [111]. Finally it has been demonstrated that long-term use of inhaled and nasal corticosteroids at the usual recommended doses is not associated with a risk of fracture in older patients with respiratory disease [112]. Budesonide, fluticasone propionate and mometasone have <1% oral bioavailability, whereas the oral bioavailability of beclometasone. triamcinolone and flunisolide is >10% [113]. The role of bisphosphonates in preventing fractures in patients taking ICS is controversial and studies have reported mixed results [114-115]. Observational studies in the elderly have suggested that use of ICS is associated with a small but significant risk of subcapsular and nuclear cataracts [116, 117] and development of glaucoma [118, 119]. However no randomized controlled trials have been performed to establish these aspects.

9.1.2 Chromones

Chromones are extracted from the medicinal plant Amni visnaga. The researchers of Fisons Pharmaceuticals identified the most active compounds, leading eventually to the synthesis of a bischromone, disodium cromoglycate (DSCG). DSCG was orally inactive and had to be given by a dry powder inhaler device. This drug inhibited not only antigen challenge but also challenges due to exercise and irritant gases. However, DSCG had a short duration of action, prompting the search for compounds of longer duration or that were orally active. Nedocromil sodium was introduced as a slightly longer-acting inhaled chromone but had little advantage over DSCG. Chromones have now largely been replaced by inhaled corticosteroids [120, 121].

9.2 Bronchodilating medications

9.2.1 Muscarinic receptor antagonist

Jimson weed or thorn apple, which were smoked in India for several centuries as a treatment for respiratory disorders (including asthma), contain a muscarinic receptor antagonist, atropine. The Egyptians also inhaled the vapour of heated henbane alkaloid, scopolamine, for the treatment of asthma-like conditions. These therapies were available until well into the last century. An important advance in the use of muscarinic receptor antagonists for asthma was the development of quaternary ammonium derivatives, which did not pass the blood–brain barrier and thus were devoid of the central side effects, such as hallucinations, of naturally occurring atropine-like compounds. They are effective when inhaled and ipratropium bromide, a synthetic quaternary antimuscarinic compound, is still used as a bronchodilator in patients with severe asthma.

The antimuscarinic agents have turned out to be the bronchodilators of choice in the treatment of COPD, where the only reversible component appears to be cholinergic tone in the airways. The recognition of distinct muscarinic receptor subtypes, which have different functions and distribution, has been a turning point. The recognition is that M3 receptors mediate the bronchoconstrictor effect of cholinergic tone, whereas M2 receptors function as feedback inhibitory receptors (autoreceptors) in human airways [122]. The clinical consequence is that the nonselective muscarinic antagonists, such as atropine and ipratropium, will also increase acetylcholine production from cholinergic nerves by blocking the M2 autoreceptors and may thus overcome the blockade of the M3 receptors on airway smooth muscle cells. This led to the idea that M3-selective antagonists may be more effective as bronchodilators. Indeed, tiotropium has a kinetic selectivity for M3 receptors as it dissociates much more slowly from M3 receptors than from M2 receptors. New developments include more long-acting muscarinic antagonists which will be used alone and in combination with long-acting β2-agonists, mainly for COPD patients [123]. Glycopyrrolate, used for many years by anesthetists to dry upper airway secretions, has recently been found to have pharmacological properties similar to tiotropium, with kinetic selectivity for M3 receptors and a long duration of action when given by inhalation [124]. One report has suggested that the use of ipratropium bromide in elderly asthmatics was associated with a slight increase in mortality, a finding that the investigators concluded was secondary to these patients having more severe asthma compared to those patients not receiving ipratropium bromide [125]. However. anticholinergics, because of their atropine-like effects may produce adverse effects in the elderly, including dry mouth, urinary hesitancy, constipation and exacerbation of glaucoma [126].

9.2.2 β2-agonist

Chinese medicine used a derivative of the Ephedra plant, ephedrine. In 1969 ephedrine was tested in humans [127]. Isoetharine, like isoprenaline was short-lived in its effects, due to rapid metabolism of the catechol ring [127]. In 1968, the first β2-selective agonist with a longer duration of action than isoprenaline was discovered: salbutamol [128]. Since then, salbutamol has been a reference molecule in the treatment of asthma [129]. The next step was to extend the duration of action of salbutamol by substitution in the side chain and the result was salmeterol, the first long-acting β2-agonist with a bronchodilator action of over 12h [130]. Inhaled salmeterol was introduced into clinical practice in 1990. Another long-acting β2-agonist, formoterol, was initially used in tablet form in Japan. Later formoterol was given by inhalation to asthmatic patients and shown to have a similar duration of action to salmeterol [131]. Both salmeterol and formoterol have found an important place in the management of asthma in combination with a corticosteroid. The combination inhalers, salbutamol/fluticasone propionate and formoterol/budesonide, and recently form formoterol/beclometasone dipropionate are the most effective asthma therapies currently available, as the long-acting β2-agonist and corticosteroids exert complementary actions and, in some situations, can show synergism [132].

The most recent development being the synthesis of even longer acting β2-agonists, such as indacaterol, which has a duration of over 24h making it suitable for once-daily dosing [133].

9.2.3 Theophylline

A methyl xanthine, theophylline, was isolated from tea at the end of the 19th century. It had bronchodilator effect as reported by Hirsch [134]. Aminophylline is a soluble ethylene diamine salt of theophylline, which can be administered for intravenous and was shown to be very effective in acute severe asthma, particularly in patients who had not responded well to adrenaline [134].

Intravenous aminophylline remained a standard treatment for acute exacerbations of asthma until displaced by nebulised β2-agonists over the last 20 years. It is still used in occasional patients who fail to respond to adrenergic bronchodilators [35]. The main limitations of theophylline are its side effects, such as nausea, headache and diuresis, which occurred within the therapeutic range and occasionally the very serious adverse effects of cardiac arrhythmias and seizures.

This led to several studies relating the efficacy and side effects of theophylline to plasma concentrations. It has been demonstrated that the bronchodilator effect of theophylline was related to plasma concentration between 5 and 20 μgl/mL, but above 20 μgl/mL, and side effects were very common. This led to recommendations for a therapeutic range of 10-20 μgl/mL. Plasma monitoring became routine, particularly in view of the variable pharmacokinetics of theophylline and the multiplicity of factors that affected plasma concentrations. Oral theophylline was a very popular treatment which was inexpensive, but presented the limitation of a short duration of action. This limitation led to the formulation of slow-release theophylline and aminophylline preparations that could be given once or twice daily, which were successful due to their convenience and greater tolerability. Side effects limited the use of theophylline as a bronchodilator, and inhaled β2-agonists were introduced as bronchodilators that are more effective and better tolerated. The bronchodilator effect of theophylline appears to be due to inhibition of phosphodiesterases (principally PDE3 and PDE4) in airway smooth muscle and this may also account for the nausea, headaches and some of the cardiovascular side effects, explaining why these side effects are commonly seen at bronchodilator doses Theophylline acts as a functional antagonist in airway smooth muscle and has greater efficacy than β2-agonists when airway smooth muscle is strongly contracted [135]. Theophylline is also an adenosine receptor antagonist at relatively high concentrations and this may account for serious side effects such as cardiac arrhythmias and seizures. However, there is increasing evidence that at lower plasma concentrations (5-10 μg/mL) theophylline has nonbronchodilator effects that include anti-inflammatory actions and immunomodulatory effects. These effects seem to correlate to activate the nuclear enzyme histone deacetylase [136].

9.2.4 Antagonists of inflammatory mediators

There are many mediators implicated in asthma, making it unlikely that blocking a single mediator would have a major clinical effect. Histamine is the first mediator implicated in the pathophysiology of asthma. However, it has been demonstrated that intravenous and inhaled histamine caused bronchoconstriction only in patients with asthma but not in normal subjects. In the same study the airway hyperresponsiveness in patients with asthma was demonstrated, which is the defining physiological abnormality of this disease and remains an important target of asthma therapy [137]. The use of antihistamines for asthma is theoretical, since these drugs tested in asthma have demonstrated disappointing results. Even with the development of much more potent nonsedating H1-receptor antagonists, there is no clinical benefit in patients with asthma. However, in patients with allergic rhinitis and concomitant asthma it has been reported that unlike many other second-generation histamine H1-receptor antagonists, desloratadine provides the added benefit of efficacy against nasal obstruction in SAR [138].

On human isolated bronchus preparations, the cysteinyl leukotrienes [i.e. leukotriene C4 (LTC4) and leukotriene D4 (LTD4) and leukotriene E4 (LTE4)] are at least 1000 times more potent than histamine in causing smooth muscle contraction, with a long duration of action [139]. However, the concentration required to achieve a given bronchoconstrictor response varies considerably between individuals [140]. Although the airways of asthmatic patients *in vivo* are more responsive to LTC4, LTD4 and LTE4 than those of non-asthmatics [141]. Leukotrienes are produced by neutrophils, macrophages, basinophils, eosinophils and monocytes. Two sub-groups of CysLT receptors have been recognized. Those blocked by known antagonists are termed CysLT1 receptors, and those that are resistant to blockade are known as CysLT2 receptors. In human airway smooth muscle, LTC4, LTD4 and LTE4 all activate CysLT1 receptors [142].

However, no correlation is found between clinical asthma severity, as measured by the degree of airflow obstruction or bronchial hyper-responsiveness, and the level of LTE, in the urine of stable asthmatic subjects [143]. The current leukotriene antagonists act at CysLT1 receptors, i.e. montelukast, no specific blockers of CysLT2 receptors have yet been identified [144].

Elderly patients with mild bronchial asthma classified as steps 1 and 2, treated with pranlukast monotherapy, a leukotriene receptor antagonist sold in Japan, presented a superior compliance to inhaled bronchial steroid therapy and it would produce an equivalent level of clinical efficacy to the monotherapy with inhaled bronchial steroid therapy [95].

9.2.5 Allergen specific Immunotherapy

In younger patients that have persistent symptoms despite medical treatment, allergen specific immunotherapy (ASI') may be considered [145]. Allergen immunotherapy involves the subcutaneous and more recently, sublingual, administration of antigens to which the patient is sensitized. Most studies of immunotherapy for treatment of respiratory allergic disease have excluded older patients because of safety concerns, e.g. risks of developing anaphylaxis, particularly in patients taking a β-adrenoceptor antagonist who may not respond to rescue adrenaline. However, according to the latest update of the American Academy of Allergy, Asthma & Immunology (AAAAI), of the American College of Allergy, Asthma & Immunology (ACAAI); and of the Joint Council of Allergy, Asthma & Immunology, there is no absolute upper age limit for initiation of immunotherapy.

Using the following terms: elderly, immunotherapy, allergic rhinitis, asthma, we found one article in PubMed [146], and one abstract in Google [147]. ASI can be considered an effective therapeutic option in otherwise healthy elderly patients with a short disease duration whose symptoms cannot be adequately controlled by drug therapies alone [146].

10. Conclusions

Although allergic diseases, as asthma, are commonly thought of as pediatric diseases. Asthma is common in older patients but is frequently under diagnosed or diagnosed as chronic obstructive pulmonary disease. The first step in the treatment of asthma in older patients is to consider differential diagnosis. Although diagnostic techniques are generally the same in younger and older patients, in the latter age groups several other diseases must be considered in the differential diagnosis. Treatment of asthma in older patients is complicated by the presence potential for other co-morbid conditions and for the possible drug interactions. Furthermore, research on pathogenesis and guidelines for therapy of allergic diseases in older patients are limited, making treatment more difficult. These disorders can interfere with the patient's quality of life and in the case of asthma can cause significant morbidity and mortality. Therefore as the study of population ages it is critical to understand how to diagnose and treat asthma in older patients.

11. Financial and competing interests dislousure

This chapter was supported by grants from MIUR (Italian University and Research Ministry) (former 60% funds) to Gabriele Di Lorenzo. Maria Stefania Leo-Barone is a PhD student of Pathobiology PhD Course (directed by Calogero Caruso, full Professor at Palermo University, and this work is submitted in partial fulfillment of the requirement for the PhD degree.

No support was received from the pharmaceutical and diagnostic industry. The authors no other relevant affiliations or financial involvement with any organization or entity with a financial interest in or financial conflict with the subject or material discussed in the manuscript a part those disclosed. No writing was utilized in the production of the chapter.

12. References

[1] Fletcher CM, Pride NB. Definitions of emphysema, chronic bronchitis, asthma, and airflow obstruction: 25 years on from the Ciba symposium. Thorax. 1984; 39: 81-5.

[2] NIH. NIH Expert Panel Report 2. Clinical practice guidelines: guidelines for the diagnosis and management of asthma. NIH Publication 1997: 97-4051 [online]. Available from URL: http://www.nhlbi.nih.gov/guidelines/asthma/asthgdln.pdf [Accessed 2005 Oct 18.

[3] Masoli M, Fabian D, Holt S, Beasley R; Global Initiative for Asthma (GINA) Program. The global burden of asthma: executive summary of the GINA Dissemination Committee report. Allergy. 2004;59:469-78.

[4] Cassino C, Berger KI, Goldring RM, Norman RG, Kammerman S, Ciotoli C, Reibman J. Duration of asthma and physiologic outcomes in elderly nonsmokers. Am J Respir Crit Care Med. 2000; 162: 1423-8.

[5] Bauer BA, Reed CE, Yunginger JW, Wollan PC, Silverstein MD. Incidence and outcomes of asthma in the elderly. A population-based study in Rochester, Minnesota. Chest. 1997; 111: 303-10.

[6] Phelan PD, Robertson CF, Olinsky A. The Melbourne Asthma Study: 1964-1999. J Allergy Clin Immunol 2002;109:189-94.

[7] Townley RG, Ryo UY, Kolotkin BM, Kang B. Bronchial sensitivity to methacholine in current and former asthmatic and allergic rhinitis patients and control subjects. J Allergy Clin Immunol. 1975 Dec;56(6):429-42.

[8] Di Lorenzo G, Mansueto P, Melluso M, et al. Non-specific air way hyperresponsiveness in mono-sensitive Sicilian patients with allergic rhinitis. Its relationship to total serum IgE levels and blood eosinophils during and out of the pollen season. Clin Exp Allergy. 1997; 27: 1052-9.

[9] Settipane GA, Greisner WA III, Settipane RJ. Natural history of asthma: a 23-year followup of college students. Ann Allergy Asthma Immunol 2000;84:499-503.

[10] Reed CE. The natural history of asthma in adults: the problem of irreversibility. J Allergy Clin Immunol 1999;103:539-47.

[11] Dow L, Fowler L, Phelps L, Waters K, Coggon D, Kinmonth AL, Holgate ST. Prevalence of untreated asthma in a population sample of 6000 older adults in Bristol, UK. Thorax. 2001; 56: 472-6.

[12] Ho SF, O'Mahony MS, Steward JA, et al. Dyspnoea and quality of life in older people at home. Age Ageing 2001; 30: 155-9

[13] Wolfenden LL, Diette GB, Krishnan JA, et al. Lower physician estimate of underlying asthma severity leads to undertreatment. Arch Intem Med 2003; 163: 231-6

[14] Van den Boom, van Schayck CP, Rutten-van Molken PMH, et al. Active detection of chronic obstructive pulmonary disease and asthma in the general population. Am J Respir Crit Care Med 1998;158:1730–8.

[15] Connolly MJ, Crowley JJ, Charan NB, Nielson CP, Vestal RE. Reduced subjective awareness of bronchoconstriction provoked by methacholine in elderly asthmatic and normal subjects as measured on a simple awareness scale. Thorax. 1992; 47: 410-3.

[16] Weiner P, Magadle R, Waizman J, Weiner M, Rabner M, Zamir D. Characteristics of asthma in the elderly. Eur Respir J. 1998; 12: 564-8.

[17] Ulrik CS, Lange P. Decline of lung function in adults with bronchial asthma. Am J Respir Crit Care Med. 1994 Sep;150(3):629-34.

[18] Lieberman J, Schleissner L, Tachiki KH, Kling AS. Serum alpha 1-antichymotrypsin level as a marker for Alzheimer-type dementia. Neurobiol Aging. 1995; 16: 747-53.

[19] Marks GB, Poulos LM, Jenkins CR, Gibson PG. Asthma in older adults: a holistic, person-centred and problem-oriented approach. Med J Aust. 2009; 191: 197-9.

[20] Fabbri LM, Luppi F, Beghé B, Rabe KF. Complex chronic comorbidities of COPD. Eur Respir J. 2008; 31: 204-12.

[21] National Institute for Clinical Excellence (NICE). Management of chronic obstructive pulmonary disease in adults in primary and secondary care (clinical guideline 12). London: NICE; 2004 [online]. Available from URL: http://guidance.nice.org.uk/CG101/Guidance/pdf/English [Accessed 2010 June 23]

[22] Di Lorenzo G, Mansueto P, Ditta V, Esposito-Pellitteri M, Lo Bianco C, Leto-Barone MS, D'Alcamo A, Farina C, Di Fede G, Gervasi F, Caruso C, Rini G. Similarity and differences in elderly patients with fixed airflow obstruction by asthma and by chronic obstructive pulmonary disease. Respir Med. 2008; 102: 232-8.

[23] Ormiston TM, Salpeter SR. Beta-blocker use in patients with congestive heart failure and concomitant obstructive airway disease: moving from myth to evidence-based practice. Heart Fail Monit. 2003; 4: 45-54.

[24] Sirithunyanont C, Leowattana W, Sukumalchantra Y, Chaisupamonkollarp S, Watanawaroon S, Chivatanaporn B, Bhuripanyo K, Mahanonda N. Role of the plasma brain natriuretic peptide in differentiating patients with congestive heart failure from other diseases. J Med Assoc Thai. 2003; 86 (Suppl 1): S87-95.

[25] Pasina L, Nobili A, Tettamanti M, Salerno F, Corrao S, Marengoni A, Iorio A, Marcucci M, Mannucci PM; on behalf of REPOSI Investigators. Prevalence and appropriateness of drug prescriptions for peptic ulcer and gastro-esophageal reflux disease in a cohort of hospitalized elderly. Eur J Intern Med. 2011; 22: 205-210.

[26] Marik PE. Pulmonary aspiration syndromes. Curr Opin Pulm Med. 2011 Feb 9. [Epub ahead of print].

[27] Korycki J, Dobrowolski J. Primary tracheal cancer treated by restoring the patency. Wiad Lek. 1968; 21: 1239-42.

[28] Harada K, Noguchi T, Fujiwara S, Moriyama H, Kitano S, Kawahara K. Complete response in an elderly patient with advanced gastric cancer treated with TS-1. Gan To Kagaku Ryoho. 2007; 34: 427-30.

[29] Mamlouk MD, vanSonnenberg E, Gosalia R, Drachman D, Gridley D, Zamora JG, Casola G, Ornstein S. Pulmonary embolism at CT angiography: implications for appropriateness, cost, and radiation exposure in 2003 patients. Radiology. 2010; 256: 625-32.

[30] Lucassen WA, Douma RA, Toll DB, Büller HR, van Weert HC. Excluding pulmonary embolism in primary care using the Wells-rule in combination with a point-of care D-dimer test: a scenario analysis. BMC Fam Pract. 2010;11: 64.

[31] Lin CF, Wang CY, Bai CH. Polypharmacy, aging and potential drug-drug interactions in outpatients in Taiwan: a retrospective computerized screening study. Drugs Aging. 2011; 28: 219-25.

[32] Erdmann E. Safety and tolerability of beta-blockers: prejudices & reality. Indian Heart J. 2010; 62: 132-5.

[33] Lee RU, Stevenson DD. Aspirin-exacerbated respiratory disease: evaluation and management. Allergy Asthma Immunol Res. 2011; 3: 3-10.

[34] Irwin RS. Unexplained cough in the adult. Otolaryngol Clin North Am. 2010b; 43: 167-80.

[35] Di Lorenzo G, Morici G, Drago A, Pellitteri ME, Mansueto P, Melluso M, Norrito F, Squassante L, Fasolo A. Efficacy, tolerability, and effects on quality of life of inhaled salmeterol and oral theophylline in patients with mild-to-moderate chronic obstructive pulmonary disease. SLMT02 Italian Study Group. Clin Ther. 1998; 20: 1130-48.

[36] Global Initiative for Chronic Obstructive Lung Disease. Global strategy for the diagnosis, management, and prevention of chronic obstructive pulmonary disease. Updated 2009. Available from: www.goldcopd.com. Accessed 2010 May 12.

[37] von Scheele I, Larsson K, Dahlén B, Billing B, Skedinger M, Lantz AS, Palmberg L. Toll-like receptor expression in smokers with and without COPD. Respir Med. 2011; 105:1222-30.

[38] Bafadhel M, Umar I, Gupta S, Raj JV, Vara DD, Entwisle JJ, Pavord ID, Brightling CE, Siddiqui S. The role of computed tomography in multi-dimensional phenotyping of chronic obstructive pulmonary disease. Chest. 2011 Mar 31.

[39] Papadopoulos G, Vardavas CI, Limperi M, Linardis A, Georgoudis G, Behrakis P. Smoking cessation can improve quality of life among COPD patients: Validation of the clinical COPD questionnaire into Greek. BMC Pulm Med. 2011; 11: 13.

[40] Deslee G, Woods JC, Moore CM, Liu L, Conradi SH, Milne M, Gierada DS, Pierce J, Patterson A, Lewit RA, Battaile JT, Holtzman MJ, Hogg JC, Pierce RA. Elastin expression in very severe human COPD. Eur Respir J. 2009; 34: 324-31.

[41] Peacock JL, Anderson HR, Bremner SA, Marston L, Seemungal TA, Strachan DP, Wedzicha JA. Outdoor air pollution and respiratory health in patients with COPD. Thorax. 2011; 66: 591-6.

[42] Perez-Padilla R, Schilmann A, Riojas-Rodriguez H. Respiratory health effects of indoor air pollution. Int J Tuberc Lung Dis. 2010 Sep;14(9):1079-86.

[43] Roche N, Gaillat J, Garre M, Meunier JP, Lemaire N, Bendjenana H. Acute respiratory illness as a trigger for detecting chronic bronchitis in adults at risk of COPD: a primary care survey. Prim Care Respir J. 2010; 19 :371-7.

[44] Sifers RN. Intracellular processing of alpha1-antitrypsin. Proc Am Thorac Soc. 2010; 7: 376-80.

[45] Bals R. Alpha-1-antitrypsin deficiency. Best Pract Res Clin Gastroenterol. 2010; 24: 629-33.

[46] Sona A, Maggiani G, Astengo M, Comba M, Chiusano V, Isaia G, Merlo C, Pricop L, Quagliotti E, Moiraghi C, Fonte G, Bo M. Determinants of recourse to hospital treatment in the elderly. Eur J Public Health. 2011 Mar 31.

[47] Delage A, Tillie-Leblond I, Cavestri B, Wallaert B, Marquette CH. Cryptogenic hemoptysis in chronic obstructive pulmonary disease: characteristics and outcome. Respiration. 2010; 80: 387-92.

[48] Barker AF. Bronchiectasis. N Engl J Med. 2002; 346: 1383-93.

[49] Hancock DB, London SJ; CHARGE Pulmonary Function Working Group. Determinants of lung function, COPD, and asthma. N Engl J Med. 2011; 364: 86-7.

[50] Wong R, Sibley KM, Hudani M, Roeland S, Visconti M, Balsano J, Hill K, Brooks D. Characteristics of people with chronic lung disease who rest during the six-minute walk test. Arch Phys Med Rehabil. 2010; 91: 1765-9.

[51] Baldacci S, Omenaas E, Oryszczyn MP. Allergy markers in respiratory epidemiology. Eur Respir J. 2001; 17: 773-90.

[52] Terho EO, Koskenvuo M, Kaprio J. Atopy: a predisposing factor for chronic bronchitis in Finland. J Epidemiol Community Health. 1995; 49: 296-8.

[53] Fabbri LM, Romagnoli M, Corbetta L, Casoni G, Busljetic K, Turato G, et al. Differences in airway inflammation in patients with fixed airflow obstruction due to asthma or chronic obstructive pulmonary disease. Am J Respir Crit Care Med 2003; 167:418–24.

[54] Barnes PJ. Pathophysiology of asthma. Br J Clin Pharmacol 1996; 42:3–10.

[55] Jeffery PK. Structural and inflammatory changes in COPD: a comparison with asthma. Thorax 1998; 53:129–136.

[56] Keatings VM, Barnes PJ. Granulocyte activation markers in induced sputum: comparison between chronic obstructive pulmonary disease, asthma and normal subjects. Am J Respir Crit Care Med 1997; 155:449–453

[57] Turato G, Di Stefano A, Maestrelli P, et al. Effect of smoking cessation on airway inflammation in chronic bronchitis. Am J Respir Crit Care Med 1995; 152:1262–1267.

[58] Barnes PJ. Immunology of asthma and chronic obstructive pulmonary disease. Nat Rev Immunol. 2008; 8: 183-92.

[59] Barnes PJ. The cytokine network in chronic obstructive pulmonary disease. Am J Respir Cell Mol Biol. 2009; 41: 631-8.

[60] Di Lorenzo G, Pacor ML, Esposito Pellitteri M, et al. A study of age-related IgE pathophysiological changes. Mech Ageing Dev. 2003; 124: 445-8.

[61] Barnes PJ, Karin M. Nuclear factor-kB: a pivotal transcription factor in chronic inflammatory diseases. N Engl J Med 1997; 336:1066–1071.

[62] Cantin AM. Cellular response to cigarette smoke and oxidants: adapting to survive. Proc Am Thorac Soc. 2010; 7: 368-75.

[63] Royce SG, Tang ML. The effects of current therapies on airway remodeling in asthma and new possibilities for treatment and prevention. Curr Mol Pharmacol. 2009; 2: 169-81.

[64] Demkow U, van Overveld FJ. Role of elastases in the pathogenesis of chronic obstructive pulmonary disease: implications for treatment. Eur J Med Res. 2010; 15 (Suppl 2): 27-35.

[65] Tuder RM, Janciauskiene SM, Petrache I. Lung disease associated with alpha1-antitrypsin deficiency. Proc Am Thorac Soc. 2010; 7: 381-6.

[66] Lagente V, Boichot E. Role of matrix metalloproteinases in the inflammatory process of respiratory diseases. J Mol Cell Cardiol. 2010; 48: 440-4.

[67] Folkerts, G., Kloek, J., Muijsers, R.B.R., Nijkamp, F.P. Reactive nitrogen and oxygen species in airway inflammation. Eur. J. Pharmacol.2001; 429: 251–262.

[68] Rahman, I., MacNee, W., 2000. Oxidative stress and regulation of glutathione synthesis in lung inflammation. Eur. Respir. J. 2000; 16: 534–554.

[69] Spergel JM. From atopic dermatitis to asthma: the atopic march. Ann Allergy Asthma Immunol. 2010; 105: 99-106.

[70] Bousquet J, Chanez P, Campbell AM, Vignola AM, Godard P. Cellular inflammation in asthma. Clin Exp Allergy. 1995; 25 (Suppl 2): 39-42.

[71] Spanevello A, Vignola AM, Bonanno A, Confalonieri M, Crimi E, Brusasco V. Effect of methacholine challenge on cellular composition of sputum induction. Thorax. 1999; 54: 37-9.

[72] Wills-Karp M. Interleukin-13 in asthma pathogenesis. Immunol Rev. 2004; 202: 175-90.

[73] Busse W, Kraft M. Cysteinyl leukotrienes in allergic inflammation: strategic target for therapy. Chest. 2005; 127: 1312-26.

[74] Lopez-Souza N, Favoreto S, Wong H, Ward T, Yagi S, Schnurr D, Finkbeiner WE, Dolganov GM, Widdicombe JH, Boushey HA, Avila PC. In vitro susceptibility to rhinovirus infection is greater for bronchial than for nasal airway epithelial cells in human subjects. J Allergy Clin Immunol. 2009; 123: 1384-90.e2.

[75] Trogdon JG, Nurmagambetov TA, Thompson HF. The economic implications of influenza vaccination for adults with asthma. Am J Prev Med. 2010; 39: 403-10.

[76] Solana R, Pawelec G. Molecular and cellular basis of immunosenescence. Mech Ageing Dev. 1998 May 15;102(2-3):115-29.

[77] Tillett HE, Smith JW, Clifford RE. Excess morbidity and mortality associated with influenza in England and Wales. Lancet. 1980; 1: 793-5.

[78] Candore G, Di Lorenzo G, Mansueto P, et al. Prevalence of organ-specific and non organ-specific autoantibodies in healthy centenarians. Mech Ageing Dev. 1997; 94: 183-90.

[79] Derhovanessian E, Solana R, Larbi A, Pawelec G. Immunity, ageing and cancer.Immun Ageing. 2008; 5:11.

[80] Colonna-Romano G, Akbar AN, Aquino A. et al. Impact of CMV and EBV seropositivity on CD8 T lymphocytes in an old population from West-Sicily. Exp Gerontol. 2007; 42: 995-1002.

[81] Lio D, Candore G, Cigna D, et al. . In vitro T cell activation in elderly individuals: failure in CD69 and CD71 expression. Mech Ageing Dev. 1996; 89: 51-8.

[82] Candore G, Di Lorenzo G, Caruso C, et al. The effect of age on mitogen responsive T cell precursors in human beings is completely restored by interleukin-2. MechAgeing Dev. 1992; 63: 297-307.

[83] Candore G, Di Lorenzo G, Melluso M, Cigna D, Colucci AT, Modica MA, Caruso C. gamma-Interferon, interleukin-4 and interleukin-6 in vitro production in old subjects. Autoimmunity. 1993; 16: 275-80.

[84] Lio D, D'Anna C, Scola L, Di Lorenzo G, Colombo A, Listì F, Balistreri CR, Candore G, Caruso C. Interleukin-5 production by mononuclear cells from aged individuals: implication for autoimmunity. Mech Ageing Dev. 1999; 106: 297-304.

[85] Potestio M, Caruso C, Gervasi F, et al. Apoptosis and ageing. Mech Ageing Dev. 102: 221-37.

[86] Colonna-Romano G, Aquino A, Bulati M, Di Lorenzo G, Listì F, Vitello S, Lio D, Candore G, Clesi G, Caruso C. Memory B cell subpopulations in the aged. Rejuvenation Res. 2006; 9:149-52.

[87] Doria G, Dagostaro G, Poretti A. Age-Dependent Variations of Antibody Avidity. Immunology. 1978; 35: 601–611.

[88] Intonazzo V, La Rosa G, Di Lorenzo G, Sferlazzo A, Perna AM, Crescimanno G, Ingrassia, A. Immune response to a subunit trivalent influenza vaccine. Igiene Moderna. 1996; 96: 800-810.

[89] Di Lorenzo G, Balistreri CR, Candore G, Cigna D, Colombo A, Romano GC, Colucci AT, Gervasi F, Listì F, Potestio M, Caruso C. Granulocyte and natural killer activity in the elderly. Mech Ageing Dev. 1999; 108: 25-38.

[90] Lio D, D'Anna C, Scola L, Di Lorenzo G, Colombo A, Listì F, Balistreri CR, Candore G, Caruso C. Interleukin-5 production by mononuclear cells from aged individuals: implication for autoimmunity. Mech Ageing Dev. 1999; 106: 297-304.

[91] Caruso C, Candore G, Cigna D, DiLorenzo G, Sireci G, Dieli F, Salerno A. Cytokine production pathway in the elderly. Immunol Res. 1996; 15: 84-90.

[92] Pawelec G, Rehbein A, Haehnel K, Merl A and Adibzadeh M. Human T-cell clones as a model for immunosenescence. Immunol Rev 1997; 160: 31–43.

[93] Pawelec G, Mariani E, Bradley B, Solana R. Longevity in vitro of human CD4+ T helper cell clones derived from young donors and elderly donors, or from progenitor cells: age-associated differences in cell surface molecule expression and cytokine secretion. Biogerontology. 2000; 1: 247-54.
[94] Sitar DS, Aoki FY, Warren CP, Knight A, Grossman RF, Alexander M, Soliman S. A placebo-controlled dose-finding study with bambuterol in elderly patients with asthma. Chest. 1993; 103: 771-6.
[95] Horiguchi T, Tachikawa S, Kondo R, Miyazaki J, Shiga M, Hirose M, Kobayashi K, Hayashi N, Ohira D, Nasu T, Otake Y, Hata H. Comparative evaluation of the leukotriene receptor antagonist pranlukast versus the steroid inhalant fluticasone in the therapy of aged patients with mild bronchial asthma. Arzneimittelforschung. 2007; 57: 87-91.
[96] Busse PJ, Kilaru K. Complexities of diagnosis and treatment of allergic respiratory disease in the elderly. Drugs Aging. 2009; 26: 1-22.
[97] Braman SS, Hanania NA. Asthma in older adults. Clin Chest Med. 2007; 28: 685-702.
[98] Braman SS. Drug treatment of asthma in the elderly. Drugs 1996;51:415–23.
[99] Djukanović R, Wilson JW, Britten KM, Wilson SJ, Walls AF, Roche WR, Howarth PH, Holgate ST. Effect of an inhaled corticosteroid on airway inflammation and symptoms in asthma. Am Rev Respir Dis. 1992; 145: 669-74.
[100] Boardley JE, Carey RA, Harvey AM Preliminary observations on the effect of adrenocorticotropic hormone in allergic diseases. Bull. Johns. Hopkins. Hosp. 1949: 85: 396–410.
[101] Medical Research Council. Controlled trial of effects of cortisone acetate in status asthmaticus; report to the Medical Research Council by the subcommittee on clinical trials in asthma. Lancet, 1956; 271: 803–806.
[102] Brown HM, Storey G, George WH. Beclomethasone dipropionate: a new steroid aerosol for the treatment of allergic asthma. Br Med J. 1972; 1: 585-90.
[103] CONTROLLED trial of effects of cortisone acetate in status asthmaticus; report to the Medical Research Council by the subcommittee on clinical trials in asthma. Lancet. 1956; 271: 803-6.
[104] Ryrfeldt A, Andersson P, Edsbacker S, Tonnesson M, Davies D, Pauwels R. Pharmacokinetics and metabolism of budesonide, a selective glucocorticoid. European Journal of Respiratory Diseases. Supplement. 1982 122 (suppl): 86–95.
[105] Adams NP, Bestall JC, Lasserson TJ, Jones P, Cates CJ. Fluticasone versus placebo for chronic asthma in adults and children. Cochrane Database Syst Rev. 2008; 8: CD003135.
[106] Cowie RL, Giembycz MA, Leigh R. Mometasone furoate: an inhaled glucocorticoid for the management of asthma in adults and children. Expert Opin Pharmacother. 2009; 10: 2009-14.
[107] Korenblat PE. Ciclesonide and the treatment of asthma. Expert Opin Pharmacother. 2010; 11: 463-79.
[108] Barnes PJ, Adcock IM. How do corticosteroids work in asthma? Ann Intern Med. 2003; 139: 359-70.
[109] Baptist AP, Reddy RC. Inhaled corticosteroids for asthma: are they all the same? J Clin Pharm Ther. 2009; 34: 1-12.

[110] Maryslone JF. Barrett-Connor El., Vlorton DJ Inhaled and oral corticosteroids: their effects on bone nnnerul density in oldcr adults. Am J Public Health 1995: 85: 1693-5.
[111] Lau E, Mamdani M, Tu K. Inhaled or systemic corticosteroids and the risk of hospitalization for hip fracture among elderly women. Am J Med. 2003; 114: 142-5.
[112] Suissa S, Baltzan M, Kremer R, Ernst P. Inhaled and nasal corticosteroid use and the risk of fracture. Am J Respir Crit Care Med. 2004 Jan 1;169(1):83-8.
[113] Bernstein DI, Allen DB. Evaluation of tests of hypothalamic-pituitary-adrenal axis function used to measure effects of inhaled corticosteroids. Ann Allergy Asthma Immunol. 2007; 98: 118-27.
[114] Campbell IA, Douglas JG, Francis RM, Prescott RJ, Reid DM; Research Committee of the British Thoracic Society. Five year study of etidronate and/or calcium as prevention and treatment for osteoporosis and fractures in patients with asthma receiving long term oral and/or inhaled glucocorticoids. Thorax. 2004; 59: 761-8.
[115] Kasayama S, Fujita M, Goya K, Yamamoto H, Fujita K, Morimoto Y, Kawase I, Miyatake A. Effects of alendronate on bone mineral density and bone metabolic markers in postmenopausal asthmatic women treated with inhaled corticosteroids. Metabolism. 2005; 54: 85-90.
[116] Cumming RG, Mitchell P, Leeder SR. Use of inhaled corticosteroids and the risk of cataracts. N Engl J Med. 1997; 337: 8-14.
[117] Ernst P, Baltzan M, Deschênes J, Suissa S. Low-dose inhaled and nasal corticosteroid use and the risk of cataracts. Eur Respir J. 2006; 27: 1168-74.
[118] Garbe E, LeLorier J, Boivin JF, Suissa S. Inhaled and nasal glucocorticoids and the risks of ocular hypertension or open-angle glaucoma. JAMA. 1997; 277: 722-7.
[119] Mitchell P, Cumming RG, Mackey DA. Inhaled corticosteroids, family history, and risk of glaucoma. Ophthalmology. 1999; 106: 2301-6.
[120] Minette PA, Barnes PJ. Prejunctional inhibitory muscarinic receptors on cholinergic nerves in human and guinea pig airways. J Appl Physiol. 1988; 64: 2532-7.
[121] Cox JS. Disodium cromoglycate (FPL 670) ('Intal'): a specific inhibitor of reaginic antibody-antigen mechanisms. Nature. 1967; 216: 1328-9.
[122] Rodrigo G. Asthma in adults (acute). Clin Evid (Online). 2011 Apr 4; 2011.
[123] Ogoda M, Niiya R, Koshika T, Yamada S. Comparative characterization of lung muscarinic receptor binding after intratracheal administration of tiotropium, ipratropium, and glycopyrrolate. J Pharmacol Sci. 2011; 115: 374-82.
[124] Sin DD, Tu JV. Lack of association between ipratropium bromide and mortality in elderly patients with chronic obstructive airway disease. Thorax. 2000;55: 194-7.
[125] Newnham DM. Asthma medications and their potential adverse effects in the elderly: recommendations for prescribing. Drug Saf. 2001; 24: 1065-80.
[126] Fernández-Barrientos Y, Jiménez-Santos M, Martínez-de-la-Casa JM, Méndez-Hernández C, García-Feijoó J. [Acute angle-closure glaucoma resulting from treatment with nebulised bronchodilators]. Arch Soc Esp Oftalmol. 2006; 81: 657-60.
[127] Collier JG, Dornhorst AC. Evidence for two different types of beta-receptors in man. Nature. 1969; 223: 1283-4.
[128] Cullum VA, Farmer JB, Jack D, Levy GP. Salbutamol: a new, selective beta-adrenoceptive receptor stimulant. Br J Pharmacol. 1969; 35: 141-51.

[129] Di Lorenzo G, Morici G, Norrito F, Mansueto P, Melluso M, Purello D'Ambrosio F, Barbagallo Sangiorgi G. Comparison of the effects of salmeterol and salbutamol on clinical activity and eosinophil cationic protein serum levels during the pollen season in atopic asthmatics. Clin Exp Allergy. 1995; 25: 951-6.
[130] Ball DI, Brittain RT, Coleman RA, Denyer LH, Jack D, Johnson M, Lunts LH, Nials AT, Sheldrick KE, Skidmore IF. Salmeterol, a novel, long-acting beta 2-adrenoceptor agonist: characterization of pharmacological activity in vitro and *in vivo*. Br J Pharmacol. 1991;104: 665-71.
[131] Anderson GP. Pharmacology of formoterol: an innovative bronchodilator. Agents Actions Suppl. 1991;34: 97-115.
[132] Barnes PJ. Scientific rationale for inhaled combination therapy with long-acting beta2-agonists and corticosteroids. Eur Respir J. 2002; 19: 182-91.
[133] Cazzola M, Matera MG. Novel long-acting bronchodilators for COPD and asthma. Br J Pharmacol. 2008; 155: 291-9.
[134] Persson CG. On the medical history of xanthines and other remedies for asthma: a tribute to HH Salter. Thorax. 1985; 40: 881-6.
[135] Jenne JW. What role for theophylline therapy? Thorax. 1994;49:97-100.
[136] Ito K, Lim S, Caramori G, Cosio B, Chung KF, Adcock IM, Barnes PJ. A molecular mechanism of action of theophylline: Induction of histone deacetylase activity to decrease inflammatory gene expression. Proc Natl Acad Sci U S A. 2002; 99: 8921-6.
[137] Curry JJ. The action of histamine on the respiratory tract in normal and asthmatic subjects. J Clin Invest. 1946; 25: 785-91.
[138] Van Cauwenberge P. Advances in allergy management. Allergy. 2002; 57 (Suppl 75):29-36.
[139] Dahlén SE, Hedqvist P, Hammarström S, Samuelsson B. Leukotrienes are potent constrictors of human bronchi. Nature. 1980; 288: 484-6.
[140] Adelroth E, Morris MM, Hargreave FE, O'Byrne PM. Airway responsiveness to leukotrienes C4 and D4 and to methacholine in patients with asthma and normal controls. N Engl J Med. 1986; 315: 480-4.
[141] Davidson AB, Lee TH, Scanlon PD, Solway J, McFadden ER Jr, Ingram RH Jr, Corey EJ, Austen KF, Drazen JM. Bronchoconstrictor effects of leukotriene E4 in normal and asthmatic subjects. Am Rev Respir Dis. 1987; 135: 333-7.
[142] Chung KF. Leukotriene receptor antagonists and biosynthesis inhibitors: potential breakthrough in asthma therapy. Eur Respir J. 1995; 8: 1203-13.
[143] Smith CM, Hawksworth RJ, Thien FC, Christie PE, Lee TH. Urinary leukotriene E4 in bronchial asthma. Eur Respir J. 1992; 5:693-9.
[144] D'Urzo AD, Chapman KR. Leukotriene-receptor antagonists. Role in asthma management. Can Fam Physician. 2000; 46: 872-9.
[145] Cox L, Nelson H, Lockey R, Calabria C, Chacko T, Finegold I, Nelson M, Weber R, Bernstein DI, Blessing-Moore J, Khan DA, Lang DM, Nicklas RA, Oppenheimer J, Portnoy JM, Randolph C, Schuller DE, Spector SL, Tilles S, Wallace D. Allergen immunotherapy: a practice parameter third update. J Allergy Clin Immunol. 2011; 127 (1 Suppl): S1-55.
[146] Asero R. Efficacy of injection immunotherapy with ragweed and birch pollen in elderly patients. Int Arch Allergy Immunol. 2004; 135: 332-5.

[147] Eidelman F, Darzentas N. Efficacy of Allergy Immunotherapy in the Elderly. J Allergy Clin Immunol 2000; 105 (suppl 1): s 313.

6

Airway Smooth Muscle: Is There a Phenotype Associated with Asthma?

Gautam Damera and Reynold A. Panettieri, Jr.
Pulmonary, Allergy and Critical Care Division, Airways Biology Initiative, University of Pennsylvania, Philadelphia, PA, USA

1. Introduction

Increases in airway smooth muscle (ASM) mass characterize the pathology of patients who died of asthma. Recent studies also show that bronchial biopsies from individuals diagnosed with mild-to-moderate asthma also have increased ASM mass. As a consequence of such increases and the role of ASM in regulating bronchomotor tone, ASM plays a pivotal role in asthma pathophysiology. In the following review, we summarize the clinical and basic science evidence that suggests that ASM is a phenotypically distinct tissue whose therapeutic manipulation is critical for overall asthma management.

1.1 ASM and airway mechanics

In developed lungs, ASM modulates ventilation and perfusion dynamics and expedite clearing of foreign particulates from distal airways. As with other myocytes, ASM shortening is largely dependent upon Ca^{2+} homeostasis. Unlike cardiac and vascular myocytes, however, where membrane depolarization induces Ca^{2+} influx via voltage-dependent Ca^{2+} channels, the pharmacological inability of Ca^{2+} channel blockers to affect bronchoconstriction implies a limited capacity of extracellular Ca^{2+} sources in regulating excitation-contraction coupling. This unique contractile property of ASM could be due to outward rectification that counteracts membrane depolarization. Such rectifying currents are mediated by the opening of large conductance Ca^{2+}-activated and delayed rectifier K^+ channels, responsible for repolarizing or hyperpolarizing ion fluxes imparting electrical stability to ASM (Parameswaran et al., 2002).

Also integral to ASM are functional receptors for acetylcholine, cysteinyl leukotrienes, prostaglandins, thromboxanes, neurokinins, bradykinin, endothelin, thrombin and serotonin, whose pharmacological manipulation regulates airway contractile mechanics. Extracellular engagement of these receptors elicits intracellular inositol trisphosphate (IP_3) and diacylglycerol (DAG)-mediated biphasic Ca^{2+} responses. Post-stimulus, the primary phase tension development is modulated by IP_3R agonism at the sarcolemma, stimulating peak release of sarcoplasmic Ca^{2+} stores (Amrani, 2006; Deshpande & Penn, 2006). The secondary phase of tension is characterized by prolonged Ca^{2+} levels albeit lower than peak thresholds, regulated by PLC-β1-mediated production of IP_3 and DAG. The IP_3-induced release of Ca^{2+} complexes with calmodulin (CaM) activates the enzymatic domain of myosin light chain kinase (MLCK), in turn phosphorylating the regulatory 20 kDa light chain

(MLC_{20}) subunit of myosin. Sympathomimetics via cAMP/PKA-dependent mechanisms in part mitigate IP_3R-mediated Ca^{2+} mobilization altering airway hyperresponsiveness (AHR). In addition, recent studies show that enhanced expression of MLCK in disease or upstream manipulation of its activity by therapeutic engagement of β-adrenoceptor could also alter mediator-induced ASM contractility. Contractile agents such as acetylcholine (ACh) induce regenerative and propagative Ca^{2+} oscillations and airway narrowing. Once initiated in ASM cells, Ca^{2+} oscillations remain resistant to IP_3R antagonists, as shown by the limited ability of heparin to suppress methacholine (MCh)-induced bronchoconstriction in individuals with asthma. Interestingly, agonist-induced Ca^{2+} oscillations can be inhibited by antagonists of the SR-resident ryanodine receptor (RyR), such as ryanodine and ruthenium red. These observations imply that Ca^{2+} release through RyR channels cooperates with IP_3-mediated Ca^{2+} mobilization to integrate the Ca^{2+} responses of ASM triggered by contractile agonists. Mechanistic studies show that RyR channel-dependent Ca^{2+} oscillations are regulated by CD38, a cyclic ADP ribose hydrolase that catalyzes the conversion of β-NAD to cADPR (Jude et al., 2008). Formation of cADPR and its interactions with several accessory proteins including tacrolimus (FK506)-binding protein modulate RyR-mediated Ca^{2+} kinetics. Similarly, cADPR could stimulate CaM-mediated mechanisms leading to Ca^{2+}-induced Ca^{2+} release, enhancing the overall propagation of Ca^{2+} oscillations throughout the cytosol. Several extracellular stimuli enhance CD38 expression and cADPR generation in human ASM; however, the precise mechanism by which extracellular cADPR is shunted to Ca^{2+} intracellular stores remains unknown (Bara et al., 2010).

1.2 ASM as a structural cell immunomodulator

Cytokine secretions of $CD4^+$ Th2 subtypes play a pivotal role in integrating inflammation and hypercontractile responses in airways of individuals with asthma. Studies in sensitized knock-out or transgenic murine models illustrate Th2 cytokine prominence in regulating abnormal airway physiology. As structural and spatially organized tissue throughout the airways, ASM cells serve as effector cells for most cytokines. After cytokine stimulation, ASM alters pro-inflammatory gene expression in an autocrine-paracrine manner promoting inflammatory processes within airways (Damera et al., 2009b). In isolated ASM tissue, IL-4 or IL-13 stimulates eotaxin that is inhibited by anti-IL-4Rα antibodies and antisense oligonucleotides to STAT-6 (Hirst et al., 2002; Peng et al., 2004). Based on the demonstrated ability of several disease-specific mediators including tumor necrosis factor alpha (TNFα), IL-1β, transforming growth factor beta (TGFβ), thymic stromal lymphopoietin (TSLP), IL-17A, endothelin-1 and sphingosine-1-phosphate (S-1-P) to induce IL-6 secretion in ASM, airway myocytes may directly contribute to IL-6 production in asthma (Ammit et al., 2001; Iwata et al., 2009; McKay & Sharma, 2002; Shan et al., 2010; Tliba & Panettieri, 2009). Pharmacological inhibition of cellular ligand for herpes virus entry mediator and lymphotoxin receptor (LIGHT), a leukocyte expressed member of TNF family, reduces allergen-induced lung fibrosis, smooth muscle hyperplasia, cytokine levels (IL-13) and AHR in murine models of chronic asthma, despite having little effect on airway eosinophilia (Doherty et al., 2011). In a more complex role, TNFα induces interferon beta (IFNβ) secretion from ASM which, by its autocrine actions, alters TNFα-mediated IL-6 and regulated upon activation, normal T cell expressed and secreted (RANTES) secretion (Tliba et al., 2003). ASM in spatial proximity to epithelium also selectively enhances basal or TNFα-induced IL-6 and IP-10 secretion, with little effect on fractalkine levels (Damera et al., 2009c). Despite the lack of a membrane-adherent IL-6R in ASM, IL-6 induces eotaxin secretion via a soluble IL-6R (sIL-6Rα) receptor (Ammit et al., 2007). Evolving evidence also shows that conditioned serum from ASM cells treated with a combination of TNFα, IL-1β and IFNγ advances an eosinophilopoietic potential on CD34+ bone marrow-derived cells, a phenomenon ablated by neutralizing antibodies to IL-5 and granulocyte-macrophage colony-stimulating factor (GM-CSF) (Fanat et al., 2009). Modulating eosinophil activation and survival, ASM cells secrete GM-CSF in response to TNFα/IL-1β alone or in combination with serum, or mast cell-derived tryptase. Endothelin (ET-1) and TNFα also elicit GM-CSF and ET-1 secretion via an intricate mechanism sensitive to bosentan and specific inhibition of ET-R (Knobloch et al., 2009). Another constituent member of the IL-6 superfamily, oncostatin M (OSM), enhances IL-1R1 abundance and augments IL-1β-mediated VEGF, monocyte chemotactic protein-1 (MCP-1) and IL-6 secretion, or synergizes with IL-13 to augment eotaxin-1 expression in airway myocytes (Faffe et al., 2005a; Faffe et al., 2005b) as summarized in Table 1.

Mediator in Asthma	***In Vitro***	**Biopsies**	**Function**
Cytokines			
IL-6	Yes	Yes	Inflammation
IL-33	Yes	Yes	Inflammation
CX3CL-1		Yes	Mast cell chemotaxis
CCL-11	Yes		Eosinophil chemoattractant
CXCL-8	Yes		Neutrophil chemotaxis
CXCL-10	Yes	Yes	Mast cell chemotaxis
Peptide growth factors			
TGF-β1, LAP		Yes	ASM hyperplasia
Adhesion molecules			
CD51, CD44	Yes		Cell-ECM interactions
CD40, OX40, CD54	Yes		Cell-cell interaction
Integrin alpha(5)	Yes		ECM deposition
CD106		Yes	Leukocyte ligand
ECM components			
Collagen type I α1	Yes		Airway remodeling
Perlecan	Yes		Airway remodeling
Collagen III	Yes	Yes	Airway remodeling
Fibronectin	Yes		Airway remodeling
Transcription factors			
mtTFA, NRF-1, PGC-1 α	Yes		Mitochondrial biogenesis
Receptors			
E-prostanoid receptor 2/ 3	Yes		ASM hyperplasia
Proteases			
ADAM-33		Yes	Cell-matrix interaction

Table 1. Mediators expressed by airway myocytes from asthmatics *in vitro* and in biopsies. References are included within the text.

In individuals with severe asthma, airway neutrophil abundance correlates with enhanced CXCL-8 levels. Enhanced CXCL-8 in supernatants from ASM cultures activates CXCR-1 receptors and promotes mast cell trafficking. An increase in CXCL-8 secretion can also increase binding of nuclear factor kappa-light-chain-enhancer of activated B cells (NF-κB), CCAAT/enhancer-binding protein beta (C/EBPβ), and RNA polymerase 2 (RNA Pol II) transcriptional elements to CXCL-8 promoter (John et al., 2009) in ASM cells. Human ASM cells secrete IL-8 when treated exogenously with IL-1β, TNFα, or TGFβ (Chung, 2000). Likewise, phenotypic changes in ASM have been suggested to augment IL-8-dependent AHR and to enhance IgE-mediated IL-4 and IL-6 levels from ASM cells (Govindaraju et al., 2006; Govindaraju et al., 2008). Evoking a COPD-relevant phenotype, pro-inflammatory stimuli, such as TNFα and cigarette smoke, also synergize to induce IL-8 secretion from ASM (Oltmanns et al., 2005). Despite minimal effect in directly mediating ASM-derived cytokine secretion, IL-9 augments TNFα-induced IL-8- or IL-13-induced eotaxin secretion in cultured ASM cells (Baraldo et al., 2003). Further, IL-9 selectively and directly enhances eotaxin-1/CCL11 secretion that can promote airway eosinophilia (Yamasaki et al., 2010).

Leukocyte migration and retention, primarily regulated by selectins on endothelial cells, are subsequently mediated by timely expression of cell adhesion molecules (CAMs) on "primed" airway structural cells as shown in Figure 1.

Studies *in vitro* and *in vivo* show that expression of CAMs mediates cell-cell interactions during inflammation and tissue remodeling (Kelly et al., 2007). Expectedly, disease-relevant components such as cytokines, bacterial endotoxins and viral proteins enhance ASM resident intercellular adhesion molecule-1 (ICAM-1) expression (Tliba et al., 2008a). Cytokines including TNFα and IL-1β induce ICAM-1 and vascular cell adhesion molecule-1 (VCAM-1) in ASM via diverse signaling pathways enhancing localized inflammation. Others show that using blocking antibodies against ICAM-1 and VCAM-1 on ASM cells or activated T cell resident lymphocyte function-associated antigen 1 (LFA-1) and very late antigen-4 (VLA-4) greatly attenuated T cell adherence to ASM as compared to either anti-ICAM or anti-VCAM alone (Duplaa et al., 1997). Further, anti-CD44 antibodies (Abs) in combination with monoclonal Abs (mAbs) against LFA-1 and VLA-4 synergistically reduce the binding of activated T cells to the level observed for resting T cells (Lazaar et al., 1994). CAM expression could mediate T cell adherence to airways and alter airway bronchoconstriction and bronchodilation responses (Hakonarson et al., 2001; Hughes et al., 2000). In cultured ASM cells, the engagement of adhesion and immune receptors such as CD40, CD44 and VCAM-1 leads to signaling events that may be involved in proliferative responses (Lazaar et al., 1998). After successive antigen challenges, adoptive transfer of CD4+ T cells from sensitized rats induces proliferation and attenuates apoptosis of ASM in naive recipients. Concomitantly, modified CD4+ T cells expressing enhanced green fluorescent protein (GFP) were localized in juxtaposition to ASM cells conferring that cell-cell interaction participates in airway remodeling. In children or adults with asthma, respiratory viruses frequently trigger exacerbations of asthma symptoms. Empirical studies now show that replication-independent rhinovirus-15 (RV-15) induces ASM-derived IL-5 and IL-1β secretion via ASM-resident ICAM-1 molecules (Grunstein et al., 2001; Oliver et al., 2006). Expanding the role of CAMs in T lymphocyte trafficking, anti-ICAM-1 or anti-VCAM-1 depletes eosinophil and neutrophil adherence to ASM. Besides immune cells, mast cell infiltration of ASM tissue occurs via expression of a heterophilic adhesion molecule, tumor suppressor in lung cancer-1 (TSLC-1) (Yang et al., 2006). In an expanding role for

CAMs in airway inflammation, studies also determined a critical role for a β-galactoside-binding lectin, Galectin-3 (Gal-3), in eosinophil trafficking and recruitment (Ramos-Barbon et al., 2005). As compared to allergen-induced responses in Gal-$3^{+/+}$ mice, Gal-$3^{-/-}$ mice have altered CAM expression, lower AHR and Th2 responses (Zuberi et al., 2004).

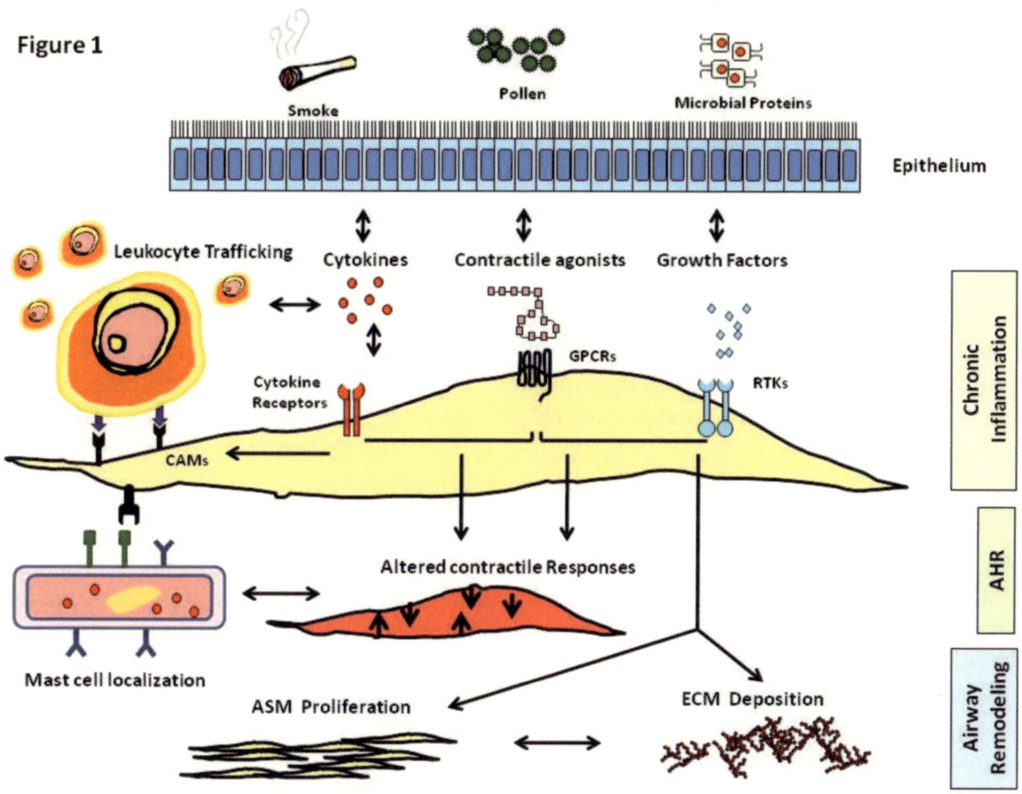

Fig. 1. Phenotypic modulation of airway smooth muscle (ASM) in asthma. Environmental stimuli induce chronic alterations in ASM characterized by hypertrophy and hyperplasia. Additionally, cytokines and growth factors modulate agonist-induced shortening of ASM that promotes airway hyperresponsiveness (AHR). Over time, ASM mass increases often in concert with extracellular matrix (ECM) deposition. The physiologic relevance of the increased ASM mass may relate to irreversible airflow obstruction. ASM also interacts directly with trafficking leukocytes and with mast cells and indirectly through the secretion of chemokines and cytokines. CAMs: cell adhesion molecules; GPCRs: G protein coupled receptors; RTKs: receptor tyrosine kinases

1.3 ASM phenotype switching

While increased ASM mass is a constitutive characteristic of remodeling in asthma, convincing studies by Ebina et al show that ASM mass increases are both physiologically discontinuous and subtype specific (Ebina et al., 1993). For instance, in some subjects with asthma, ASM mass was increased only in the central bronchi compared with others who manifested enhanced muscle thickness throughout the bronchi. In addition the number of smooth muscle nuclei in the central airways was increased, indicating the presence of ASM hyperplasia. In patients with increased mass throughout the bronchi, ASM cell volume was significantly increased, signifying ASM hypertrophy (Wenzel et al., 1999). Accordingly, examination of biopsies from patients with mild asthma shows significant increases in ASM numbers, with minimal alterations in cellular morphometry. Indeed, studies addressing the molecular mechanism inducing ASM mass in animals have convincingly shown that allergic sensitization enhances ASM mass. In murine models, ovalbumin (OVA)-induced sensitization and challenge promotes thickening of the peribronchial smooth muscle layer. Similarly, in guinea pigs, allergen challenge induces bromodeoxyuridine uptake into ASM layers, implying enhanced mitogenesis. Likewise, bronchoalveolar lavage (BAL) fluid derived from individuals with asthma enhances DNA synthesis and ASM cell numbers (Naureckas et al., 1999), implying that BAL soluble constituents likely promote ASM hyperplasia. Post-allergen challenge, quantitative increases in cytokines, enzymes including tryptases and matrix metalloproteinase (MMPs) and growth factors define airway pathology in animal studies; however, contradictory empirical outcomes limit the mitogenic potential of BAL cytokines. More prominent are the effects of airway-localized growth factors in stimulating ASM growth via the RTK-PI3K axis. Among asthma-relevant outcomes such as tissue maturation and epithelial mucin (MUC) gene expression, peptides that stimulate receptors for epidermal growth factor (EGF), insulin-like growth factors (IGFs), platelet-derived growth factor (PDGF), and fibroblast growth factor (FGF)-2 also induce ASM proliferation (Marwick et al., 2010).

Selected contractile agents such as histamine, ET-1, substance P, 5-HT, α-thrombin, thromboxane A_2 and LTD_4 also enhance ASM mitogenesis (Dekkers et al., 2009; Lazaar & Panettieri, 2005). Studies suggest that mediator-induced ASM proliferation is regulated by cell cycle proteins as surrogate markers of mitogenesis. While BAL fluid derived from subjects with asthma mediates ERK-mediated DNA synthesis in ASM, such responses are associated with increased cyclin D1 protein (Naureckas et al., 1999). Besides ERK, pharmacological inhibitors of PI3K also diminish cyclin D1 protein expression and DNA synthesis in ASM. Other studies identified two nuclear antigens, Ki67 and proliferating cell associated nuclear antigen (PCNA), as potential markers of proliferation. Investigators suggest that despite comparable mitogen-induced induction of PI3K-AKT axis, ASM proliferation results from diminished cell cycle inhibitory proteins such as C/EBPa elements. Others have shown that ASM proliferation is induced by overexpression of Src or PI3K alone, and inhibition of PI3K abrogated mitogen-induced ASM proliferation. Downstream PI3K stimulates S6K1-mediated translation of cell cycle proteins via rapamycin-sensitive events (Scott et al., 1996). Importantly, sustained activation of PI3K and S6K1 at 12h discriminated ASM mitogens from non-mitogenic agonists that otherwise equally potentiate ERK1/2 at 1h (Krymskaya et al., 2000). Similar upstream pathways also induce ASM hypertrophy via mammalian target of rapamycin (mTOR), 4E-binding protein (4E-BP), the transcription factor eIF4E and S6 kinase or the inhibition of glycogen synthase kinase (GSK)-3β (Bara et al., 2010; Berger et al., 2005)

Myofibroblasts are α-smooth actin-positive mesenchymal precursors that transiently undergo reversible phenotypic differentiation to/from a variety of resident structural populations including ASM cells (Begueret et al., 2007; Brewster et al., 1990; Gizycki et al., 1997). These cells may migrate and differentiate into resident populations within ASM bundles, thus mediating hyperplasia. In support of this phenomenon, studies show that bone marrow-derived, $CD34^{+}$-Collagen-1^{+}-α-SMA^{+} circulating fibrocytes migrate towards ASM bundles during inflammatory challenge. Post allergen challenge, increased presence of myofibroblasts in the submucosa has led some to postulate that ASM cells could migrate from airway bundles towards epithelium, explaining diminished space between smooth muscle and epithelium in asthmatic airways. Varied mediators including PDGF, TGF-β and chemokines such as CCL-11 and CXCL-8 induce chemotaxis of ASM cells *in vitro* (Govindaraju et al., 2006; Hirst et al., 2004; Ito et al., 2009; Joubert & Hamid, 2005; Mukhina et al., 2000). Similarly, migration of ASM *in vitro* could be enhanced by coating with collagens III and V and fibronectin as compared with collagen I, elastin and laminin (Bullimore et al., 2011), implying that disease-specific matrix alteration could also mitigate this process. In line with *in vitro* studies, Thomson and Schellenberg hypothesized that the presence of collagen deposition in and around ASM bundles may contribute to the overall increase in the ASM content (Thomson & Schellenberg, 1998).

The overall functional impact of enhanced ASM mass on asthma symptoms including AHR seems heterogeneous and remains unclear. During proliferation, ASM cells likely manifest a phenotypic switch characterized by compromised contractile characteristics as shown after mitogen treatment or cultured on diverse ECM (Dekkers et al., 2007; Halayko et al., 2008; Halayko et al., 2006). Predictably, such alterations correlate with quantitative increases in synthetic pathways for protein and lipids and mitochondrial function with a diminished abundance of contractile proteins. Compared to specific proteins that mark pro-contractile characteristics, such as smooth muscle myosin heavy chain, SM22, calponin and smooth muscle α-actin, proliferating ASM shows increased non-muscle myosin heavy chain (MHC), caldesmon, vimentin, α/β-protein kinase C (PKC) and CD44 homing cellular adhesion molecule (Halayko et al., 2008; Hirota et al., 2009). Others appreciate the expression and accumulation of dystrophin glycoprotein complex (DGC), a multimeric sarcolemma complex that regulates caveoli organization, with altered ASM contractility (Sharma et al., 2008).

2. Is ASM different in asthma?

2.1 ASM mass and airway remodeling

Using anatomically matched bronchial samples derived from inflated lungs, Hossain and Heard show that thickness of ASM is enhanced in patients with fatal asthma (Hossain & Heard, 1970). Pursuing alternate procedures to inflate lungs via pulmonary vasculature, Dunnill et al. show that increased ASM mass accounts for $11.4 \pm 3.4\%$ of wall thickness in asthmatic airways, as compared to $4.6 \pm 2.2\%$ in normal airways (Dunnill et al., 1969). Others explain that expression of α-smooth muscle actin and myosin light-chain kinase negatively correlates with prebronchodilator and postbronchodilator FEV_1 values in patients with severe asthma (Benayoun et al., 2003). Similarly, quantitative structural analysis of peripheral airways showed that, in addition to increased luminal occlusion and immune cell infiltrates, bronchioles of subjects with fatal asthma showed enhanced smooth muscle presence (Saetta et al., 1991). In addition to acknowledged effects in fatal asthma, discontinuous increases in ASM numbers distinguish airway physiology within asthma subtypes (Ebina et al., 1993). Owing to challenges in obtaining biopsies that encompass the full thickness of ASM, few studies could define growth of ASM in patients with non-fatal asthma. In studies by Carroll et al, analysis of similarly identified central airways samples from inflated lungs of all asthma severities showed that the area of smooth muscle in large bronchioles was greater in fatal and non-fatal cases than in control cases, but there were no differences between fatal and non-fatal cases of asthma (Carroll et al., 1993). Accordingly, comprehensive evaluation of endobronchial biopsies by quantitative morphometry, laser capture microdissection, and RT-PCR also shows a two-fold increase in ASM numbers in individuals with mild asthma. These studies concluded that ASM hyperplasia and not hypertrophy is a pathologic characteristic in airways of individuals with mild-to-moderate asthma, and that gene expression of contractile proteins considered markers of a hypercontractile phenotype are not increased across asthma populations (Woodruff et al., 2004). Studying ASM growth in steroid-resistant asthmatics, Pegorier et al report that epithelium resident endothelin (EDN1) and IL-8/CXCL8 levels negatively correlate with pre and postbronchodilator FEV_1 values, and positively relate to ASM area and thickness of subepithelial basement membrane (Pegorier et al., 2007).

2.2 ASM function and AHR

Since airway smooth muscle (ASM) is the pivotal effector tissue controlling bronchomotor tone, it is suggested that ASM dysfunction contributes directly towards AHR in asthma. Mutually distinct lines of evidence show that increases in the shortening velocity of ASM could mediate AHR (Antonissen et al., 1979; Mitchell et al., 1993; Seow et al., 1998; Solway & Fredberg, 1997). Following induced bronchoconstriction, deep inspiration causes airways of both normal and asthmatic individuals to dilate transiently; yet, the subsequent reconstriction is more prompt in asthmatics (Jackson et al., 2004; Jensen et al., 2001; Pellegrino et al., 1996). Empirical evidence *in vitro* shows that bronchial ASM cells from asthmatic patients have increased shortening velocity relative to controls (Ma et al., 2002). Likewise animal models of innate and allergic AHR manifest enhanced ASM shortening (Bullimore et al., 2011). Such increase in muscle-shortening velocity may be due to augmented MLCK activity in asthmatic ASM (Ammit et al., 2000). Concurrently, others propose that altered cytosolic calcium handling within ASM could induce AHR in ASM from subjects with asthma (Janssen, 1998). Indeed, ASM $[Ca^{2+}]_i$ levels are greater in hyperresponsive Fisher rats as compared to less responsive Lewis rats (Tao et al., 1999). Since diverse excitatory stimuli, such as leukotrienes, acetylcholine, ozone, acroleins and cytokines, provoke AHR by mobilizing cytoplasmic calcium concentration, it is conceivable that the calcium handling in the smooth muscle *per se* is altered (Parameswaran et al., 2002). ASM contractility is hormone-responsive, leading some to focus on gender disparities in asthma epidemiology. Preliminary studies now suggest that oxytocin levels are enhanced in BAL fluid from asthmatic individuals and that selected cytokines (IL-13) amplify oxytocin's effects by increasing the expression of functional oxytocin receptor within ASM (Amrani et al., 2010).

As with TNFα and IL-13, pro-inflammatory cytokines modulate intracellular Ca^{2+} responses and AHR via expression of CD38. Compared to $CD38^{-/-}$ mice, airway myocytes isolated from wild-type mice exhibit higher agonist-induced intracellular Ca^{2+} responses *in vitro* while $CD38^{+/+}$ mice develop a higher magnitude of AHR after allergen challenge (Gally et al., 2009; Guedes et al., 2008; Guedes et al., 2006). Later studies in human ASM imply that differential expression of CD38 by heightened induction of common signaling cascades likely mediates AHR in asthma (Jude et al., 2010). Clinical evidence shows that ASM derived from subjects who died of asthma has enhanced immunoreactivity to receptors for receptor tyrosine kinases (RTKs) and that such increases correlate with disease severity (Chanez et al., 1995; Perkett, 1995; Polosa et al., 2002; Puddicombe et al., 2000; Yamanaka et al., 2001). Increased expression of EGFR and PDGFR ligands can be triggered by factors that modulate asthma etiology including allergens, pro-inflammatory cytokines, environmental tobacco smoke, and virus infection (Ingram & Bonner, 2006; Le Cras et al., 2011). Expectedly, EGFR ligands are elevated in samples from asthmatic airways, and mechanistic studies show that EGFR activation elicits augmented mitogenic responses in asthmatic ASM (Amishima et al., 1998). Such proliferative responses are accompanied by inhibition of cyclic AMP (cAMP) effectors such as protein kinase A (PKA) and exchange protein directly activated by cAMP (Epac), entailing a phenotypic switch characterized by diminished expression of contractile proteins including smooth muscle actin, myosin and calponin (Roscioni et al., 2011). As seen in biopsies of severe asthmatics, empirical studies show that ASM mitogens enhanced expression of defined GTPase-accelerating proteins (GAPs) called RGS (Damera et al., 2010). Given the ability to interact with Gα subunits of GPCR and p85α-PI3K, expression of RGS molecules could induce a hypocontractile and hyperproliferative ASM phenotype reminiscent of severe asthma (Bansal et al., 2008; Liang et al., 2009).

2.3 ASM markers of chronic inflammation

As repeatedly illustrated by mechanistic studies *in vitro*, ASM-expressed cytokines, peptide growth factors, ECM proteins and adhesion molecules extensively regulate airway pathology (Damera et al., 2009b; Tliba & Panettieri, 2008). Predictably, bronchial biopsies from asthmatic individuals show a greater role of ASM in inflammation and remodeling; however, the ability of isolated ASM cells to retain this phenotype in culture has led some to propose a genetic etiology. Although functionally ambiguous, a disintegrin and metalloproteinase-33 (ADAM-33), a member of zinc-dependent metalloproteases, is associated with AHR and diminished lung function in asthma (Foley et al., 2007). Expression of active chemotactic factors by ASM promotes adherence and retention of circulating T cells and mast cells to airways. Recruitment and retention of T cells and mast cells to ASM are dependent on expression of functionally active chemotactic factors. For-instance, in airways of individuals with asthma, enhanced mast cell presence within ASM layers correlates with augmented expression of $TGF\beta_1$. Among other triggers, stimulation of ASM resident protease activated receptor 2 (PAR-2) by mast cell-derived tryptase enhances $TGF\beta_1$ expression, thus potentiating a "feed forward system" leading to increased mast cell recruitment (Berger et al., 2003). In addition, as demonstrated *in vitro*, TGFβ1 facilitates transformation of epithelial cells to myofibroblasts, with likely consequences to ASM hyperplasia (Zuyderduyn et al., 2008). With inflammation, expression of mast cell resident CD44 (hyaluronate receptor) and CD51 (vitronectin receptor) to ECM defines mast cell adhesion to ASM. As compared to normal cells, such interactions are enhanced in cultures derived from asthmatic airways (Girodet et al., 2010). Likewise, cytokines differentially alter expression of co-stimulatory ligands such as CD40 and OX40 among ASM from airways of normal and asthmatic individuals, implying that disease pertinent mechanisms intrinsic to ASM mitigate enhanced leukocyte adherence in asthma (Burgess et al., 2005). Besides cell adherent factors, marked increases in soluble chemotactic mediators such as IL-33, CX3CL-1 and CXCL-10 are seen in ASM tissue within bronchial biopsies in asthma (Brightling et al.,

2005; El-Shazly et al., 2006; Prefontaine et al., 2009). While CXCL-10-mediated activation of mast cell resident CXCR-3 predicts ASM microlocalization, CXCL-10 is preferentially expressed in bronchial biopsies and *ex vivo* cells from individuals compared with those from healthy control subjects. As a promoter of Th2 immunity, TNFα-mediated IL-33 secretions are refractory to corticosteroid effects (Prefontaine et al., 2009). Further, immune histochemical (IHC) analysis of bronchial biopsies shows increased IL-33 localization within ASM bundles of subjects with mild-to-moderate asthma, implying a likely role in pathogenesis of asthma. During RV-induced asthma exacerbation, cytokine secretion such as IL-6 is transcriptionally triggered by specific innate immune responses. Interestingly, such responses are differentially regulated in ASM derived from asthmatic and normal individuals (Oliver et al., 2006). As with COPD, an increase in neutrophilic inflammation correlates with CXCL-8 secretion in airways of severe asthmatics. Mechanistic studies by John et al imply that augmented binding of NF-κB, C/EBPβ and RNA Pol II elements to CXCL-8 promoter likely mediates CXCL-8 increases within asthmatic ASM (John et al., 2009) as shown in Table 1.

2.4 ASM and disease matrix

As compared to healthy individuals, ASM cells from patients with asthma secrete increased amounts of collagen I and perlecan but reduced amounts of collagen IV, chondroitin sulfate, laminin α1 and hyaluronan (Johnson et al., 2004; Klagas et al., 2009). While TGFβ1 and connective tissue growth factor (CTGF) enhance collagen I and fibronectin production in normal and asthmatic ASM, differences in intrinsic signaling mechanisms likely alter ECM deposition in asthma (Burgess et al., 2003; Johnson et al., 2006). In asthma, mast cell localization to ASM bundles promotes mutual phenotypic changes that promote development of AHR (Kaur et al., 2010). For instance, in co-cultures IgE-independent mast cell release of β-tryptase augments α-SMA within ASM via autocrine actions of TGFβ. Despite minimal effects on mast cells, TGFβ enhances ASM-derived ECM proteins such as fibronectin which modulate mast cell activation and transition to a myofibroblast phenotype (Chan et al., 2006; Johnson et al., 2006; Lam et al., 2003; Moir et al., 2008; Peng et al., 2005; Swieter et al., 1993). This altered mast cell phenotype has the potential to evoke an ASM contractile phenotype, further propagating AHR. Rhinovirus infection differentially alters ECM components such as fibronectin and collagen 4 in asthmatic ASM, thus facilitating increased cell migration and remodeling at sites of infection (Kuo et al., 2011). Others speculate that asthma pertinent ECM dysregulation likely involves imbalances in ECM modifying MMP or their endogenous enzyme inhibitors called tissue inhibitors of matrix metalloproteinases (TIMP). Supported by studies using histopathological assessment, investigators showed increased MMP-9 and -12 within ASM layers in fatal asthma (Araujo et al., 2008). Comparative assessment of BAL fluid of patients undergoing mechanical ventilation in severe asthma and those with mild etiology shows enhanced MMP-3 and -9 levels in severe disease subtypes (Lemjabbar et al., 1999). Others propose that minor allelic single-nucleotide polymorphisms in the MMP-12 gene could affect FEV_1 among children with asthma (Hunninghake et al., 2009). Besides associating rs652438, a common gene variant of MMP-12, with disease severity in young asthmatic individuals, Mukhopadhyay et al show that pharmacologic inhibition of MMP-12 downregulates allergen-induced airway responses (Mukhopadhyay et al., 2010). In comparison to corticosteroid-treated asthmatics or healthy individuals, BAL resident TIMP-1 is increased in untreated asthma, implying that a potential MMP/TIMP imbalance could also orchestrate a pro-asthmatic phenotype (Mautino et al., 1999a; Mautino et al., 1999b).

ASM function is also modulated by (i) epithelial cell-derived mediator secretion post-viral infections or (ii) air pollutants due to loss of epithelial barrier function. (Chanez, 2005). Viral infections induce epithelial cell secretion such as IFNβ which inhibits ASM proliferation, shortening or pharmacological efficacy of anti-inflammatory agents (Banerjee et al., 2008; Tliba et al., 2008b). Similarly, destruction of the epithelium elicits altered ASM responses to environmental pollutants such as ozone, as demonstrated using co-culture (Damera et al., 2009c). Epithelium also expresses mediators such as prostanoids, leukotrienes, cytokines and nitric oxide which mitigate airway bronchomotor tone (Chitano, 2011). Furthermore, epithelium-derived enzymes such as acetylcholinesterase, N-methyltransferase, angiotensin-converting enzyme and neutral endopeptidase regulate neural transmission within airways (Knight & Holgate, 2003; Spina, 1998). Studies show that post RV infections, epithelium mediates desensitization of the β2-adrenergic receptor on ASM (Trian et al., 2010). Upon injury, bronchial epithelium modulates myocyte proliferation through MMP-9 secretions or via growth factors (Malavia et al., 2009).

2.5 Asthma and ASM: Altered cell signaling

As mainstay therapy in asthma, glucocorticoids suppress inflammation by complex interactions involving their cognate nuclear receptors, glucocorticoid receptors (GR). Although studies correlate impairment in GR expression or mutations in genes encoding these receptors to asthma, no evidence exists on the direct contributory function of these receptors to asthma (Adcock et al., 1996; Corrigan et al., 1991; Lane et al., 1994). While most pharmacological effects elicited by glucocorticoids involve GR-activation, downstream signaling divergence is illustrated by studies where glucocorticoids diminish serum-stimulated IL-6, yet fail to alter proliferative responses in cells from individuals with asthma. Despite comparable levels of GR in ASM derived from asthma patients, decreased levels of co-transcription factor C/EBPα may diminish transcription of glucocorticoid-induced anti-proliferative protein $p21^{(Waf1/Cip1)}$. Compensatory induction of C/EBPα by transfection of ASM from subjects with asthma restores antiproliferative effects of glucocorticoids (Roth et al., 2004). Similarly, Damera et al suggest that inhibiting mitogen-induced phosphorylation of retinoblastoma protein (Rb) and Chk1 proteins by calcitriol inhibits ASM growth in a corticosteroid-independent manner (Damera et al., 2009a). In ASM, TGFβ induces PI3K-mediated release of VEGF and IL-6 which in turn modulates cell proliferation and angiogenesis (Johnson et al., 2006; Shin et al., 2009). As compared to asthmatic ASM, specific inhibition of p110 β isoform of PI3K alone differentially attenuates TGFβ-mediated secretion in normal tissue, implying an altered role of PI3K isoforms in asthma (Moir et al., 2011). While mitogens induce proliferation via ERK and PI3K in normal ASM, intrinsic abnormalities in expression of the endogenous ERK inhibitor, MKP-1, promote predominance of the PI3K proliferative pathway within ASM from individuals with asthma (Burgess et al., 2008). Studies by John et al suggest that increased binding of transcription factors such as NF-κB, C/EBPβ and RNA Pol II to the CXCL-8 promoter modulates pro-inflammatory outcomes in asthmatic ASM (John et al., 2009). Multiple stimuli that modulate inflammation, proliferation and asthma also activate NF-κB transcription factors, and disruption of NF-κB activation through expression of a superrepressor form of IKBα substantially impairs proliferation (Brar et al., 2002; Clarke et al., 2009; Damera et al., 2009b). Explaining increased mitochondrial mass and oxygen consumption in asthmatic ASM, Trian et al show differences in mitochondrial biogenesis and expression of transcription factors such as peroxisome proliferator-activated receptor γ co-activator (PGC)-1α, nuclear respiratory factor-1 (NRF-1) and mitochondrial transcription factor A (mtTFA) in ASM derived from asthma, COPD and normal populations (Trian et al., 2007).

3. Summary and future directions

Although asthma pathophysiology represents the complex interactions among structural and trafficking cell populations, this summary identifies factors and signaling events within ASM that promote an asthma phenotype. Evidence supports that altered cell function in cultured ASM derived from individuals with asthma exists and supports the hypothesis that an intrinsic ASM phenotype likely occurs in asthma. With this insight, focusing on the development of new pharmacological approaches that target ASM may offer unique approaches in asthma therapy.

4. References

Adcock, I.M., Gilbey, T., Gelder, C.M., Chung, K.F. & Barnes, P.J. (1996). Glucocorticoid receptor localization in normal and asthmatic lung. *American Journal of Respiratory and Critical Care Medicine*, Vol. 154(3 Pt 1): pp. 771-782.

Amishima, M., Munakata, M., Nasuhara, Y., Sato, A., Takahashi, T., Homma, Y. & Kawakami, Y. (1998). Expression of epidermal growth factor and epidermal growth factor receptor immunoreactivity in the asthmatic human airway. *American Journal of Respiratory and Critical Care Medicine*, Vol. 157(6 Pt 1): pp. 1907-1912.

Ammit, A.J., Armour, C.L. & Black, J.L. (2000). Smooth-muscle myosin light-chain kinase content is increased in human sensitized airways. *American Journal of Respiratory and Critical Care Medicine*, Vol. 161(1): pp. 257-263.

Ammit, A.J., Hastie, A.T., Edsall, L.C., Hoffman, R.K., Amrani, Y., Krymskaya, V.P., Kane, S.A., Peters, S.P., Penn, R.B., Spiegel, S. & Panettieri, R.A., Jr. (2001). Sphingosine 1-phosphate modulates human airway smooth muscle cell functions that promote inflammation and airway remodeling in asthma. *FASEB Journal*, Vol. 15(7): pp. 1212-1214.

Ammit, A.J., Moir, L.M., Oliver, B.G., Hughes, J.M., Alkhouri, H., Ge, Q., Burgess, J.K., Black, J.L. & Roth, M. (2007). Effect of IL-6 trans-signaling on the pro-remodeling phenotype of airway smooth muscle. *American Journal of Physiology. Lung Cellular and Molecular Physiology*, Vol. 292(1): pp. L199-L206.

Amrani, Y. (2006). Airway smooth muscle modulation and airway hyper-responsiveness in asthma: new cellular and molecular paradigms. *Expert Review of Clinical Immunology*, Vol. 2(3): pp. 353-364.

Amrani, Y., Syed, F., Huang, C., Li, K., Liu, V., Jain, D., Keslacy, S., Sims, M.W., Baidouri, H., Cooper, P.R., Zhao, H., Siddiqui, S., Brightling, C.E., Griswold, D., Li, L. & Panettieri, R.A., Jr. (2010). Expression and activation of the oxytocin receptor in airway smooth muscle cells: Regulation by TNFalpha and IL-13. *Respiratory Research*, Vol. 11: pp. 104.

Antonissen, L.A., Mitchell, R.W., Kroeger, E.A., Kepron, W., Tse, K.S. & Stephens, N.L. (1979). Mechanical alterations of airway smooth muscle in a canine asthmatic model. *Journal of Applied Physiology*, Vol. 46(4): pp. 681-687.

Araujo, B.B., Dolhnikoff, M., Silva, L.F., Elliot, J., Lindeman, J.H., Ferreira, D.S., Mulder, A., Gomes, H.A., Fernezlian, S.M., James, A. & Mauad, T. (2008). Extracellular matrix components and regulators in the airway smooth muscle in asthma. *European Respiratory Journal*, Vol. 32(1): pp. 61-69.

Banerjee, A., Damera, G., Bhandare, R., Gu, S., Lopez-Boado, Y., Panettieri, R.A., Jr. & Tliba, O. (2008). Vitamin D and glucocorticoids differentially modulate chemokine expression in human airway smooth muscle cells. *British Journal of Pharmacology*, Vol. 155(1): pp. 84-92.

Bansal, G., Xie, Z., Rao, S., Nocka, K.H. & Druey, K.M. (2008). Suppression of immunoglobulin E-mediated allergic responses by regulator of G protein signaling 13. *Nature Immunology*, Vol. 9(1): pp. 73-80.

Bara, I., Ozier, A., Tunon de Lara, J.M., Marthan, R. & Berger, P. (2010). Pathophysiology of bronchial smooth muscle remodelling in asthma. *European Respiratory Journal*, Vol. 36(5): pp. 1174-1184.

Baraldo, S., Faffe, D.S., Moore, P.E., Whitehead, T., McKenna, M., Silverman, E.S., Panettieri, R.A., Jr. & Shore, S.A. (2003). Interleukin-9 influences chemokine release in airway smooth muscle: role of ERK. *American Journal of Physiology. Lung Cellular and Molecular Physiology*, Vol. 284(6): pp. L1093-L1102.

Begueret, H., Berger, P., Vernejoux, J.M., Dubuisson, L., Marthan, R. & Tunon-de-Lara, J.M. (2007). Inflammation of bronchial smooth muscle in allergic asthma. *Thorax*, Vol. 62(1): pp. 8-15.

Benayoun, L., Druilhe, A., Dombret, M.C., Aubier, M. & Pretolani, M. (2003). Airway structural alterations selectively associated with severe asthma. *American Journal of Respiratory and Critical Care Medicine*, Vol. 167(10): pp. 1360-1368.

Berger, P., Girodet, P.O., Begueret, H., Ousova, O., Perng, D.W., Marthan, R., Walls, A.F. & Tunon de Lara, J.M. (2003). Tryptase-stimulated human airway smooth muscle cells induce cytokine synthesis and mast cell chemotaxis. *FASEB Journal*, Vol. 17(14): pp. 2139-2141.

Berger, P., Girodet, P.O. & Manuel Tunon-de-Lara, J. (2005). Mast cell myositis: a new feature of allergic asthma? *Allergy*, Vol. 60(10): pp. 1238-1240.

Brar, S.S., Kennedy, T.P., Sturrock, A.B., Huecksteadt, T.P., Quinn, M.T., Murphy, T.M., Chitano, P. & Hoidal, J.R. (2002). NADPH oxidase promotes NF-kappaB activation and proliferation in human airway smooth muscle. *American Journal of Physiology. Lung Cellular and Molecular Physiology*, Vol. 282(4): pp. L782-L795.

Brewster, C.E., Howarth, P.H., Djukanovic, R., Wilson, J., Holgate, S.T. & Roche, W.R. (1990). Myofibroblasts and subepithelial fibrosis in bronchial asthma. *American Journal of Respiratory Cell and Molecular Biology*, Vol. 3(5): pp. 507-511.

Brightling, C.E., Ammit, A.J., Kaur, D., Black, J.L., Wardlaw, A.J., Hughes, J.M. & Bradding, P. (2005). The CXCL10/CXCR3 axis mediates human lung mast cell migration to asthmatic airway smooth muscle. *American Journal of Respiratory and Critical Care Medicine*, Vol. 171(10): pp. 1103-1108.

Bullimore, S.R., Siddiqui, S., Donovan, G.M., Martin, J.G., Sneyd, J., Bates, J.H. & Lauzon, A.M. (2011). Could an increase in airway smooth muscle shortening velocity cause airway hyperresponsiveness? *American Journal of Physiology. Lung Cellular and Molecular Physiology*, Vol. 300(1): pp. L121-L131.

Burgess, J.K., Blake, A.E., Boustany, S., Johnson, P.R., Armour, C.L., Black, J.L., Hunt, N.H. & Hughes, J.M. (2005). CD40 and OX40 ligand are increased on stimulated asthmatic airway smooth muscle. *Journal of Allergy and Clinical Immunology*, Vol. 115(2): pp. 302-308.

Burgess, J.K., Johnson, P.R., Ge, Q., Au, W.W., Poniris, M.H., McParland, B.E., King, G., Roth, M. & Black, J.L. (2003). Expression of connective tissue growth factor in asthmatic airway smooth muscle cells. *American Journal of Respiratory and Critical Care Medicine*, Vol. 167(1): pp. 71-77.

Burgess, J.K., Lee, J.H., Ge, Q., Ramsay, E.E., Poniris, M.H., Parmentier, J., Roth, M., Johnson, P.R., Hunt, N.H., Black, J.L. & Ammit, A.J. (2008). Dual ERK and phosphatidylinositol 3-kinase pathways control airway smooth muscle proliferation: differences in asthma. *Journal of Cellular Physiology*, Vol. 216(3): pp. 673-679.

Carroll, N., Elliot, J., Morton, A. & James, A. (1993). The structure of large and small airways in nonfatal and fatal asthma. *American Review of Respiratory Disease*, Vol. 147(2): pp. 405-410.

Chan, V., Burgess, J.K., Ratoff, J.C., O'Connor B, J., Greenough, A., Lee, T.H. & Hirst, S.J. (2006). Extracellular matrix regulates enhanced eotaxin expression in asthmatic airway smooth muscle cells. *American Journal of Respiratory and Critical Care Medicine*, Vol. 174(4): pp. 379-385.

Chanez, P. (2005). Severe asthma is an epithelial disease. *European Respiratory Journal*, Vol. 25(6): pp. 945-946.

Chanez, P., Vignola, M., Stenger, R., Vic, P., Michel, F.B. & Bousquet, J. (1995). Platelet-derived growth factor in asthma. *Allergy*, Vol. 50(11): pp. 878-883.

Chitano, P. (2011). Models to understand contractile function in the airways. *Pulmonary Pharmacology & Therapeutics*, Vol.: pp. Epub ahead of print Apr 23.

Chung, K.F. (2000). Airway smooth muscle cells: contributing to and regulating airway mucosal inflammation? *European Respiratory Journal*, Vol. 15(5): pp. 961-968.

Clarke, D., Damera, G., Sukkar, M.B. & Tliba, O. (2009). Transcriptional regulation of cytokine function in airway smooth muscle cells. *Pulmonary Pharmacology & Therapeutics*, Vol. 22(5): pp. 436-445.

Corrigan, C.J., Brown, P.H., Barnes, N.C., Szefler, S.J., Tsai, J.J., Frew, A.J. & Kay, A.B. (1991). Glucocorticoid resistance in chronic asthma. Glucocorticoid pharmacokinetics, glucocorticoid receptor characteristics, and inhibition of peripheral blood T cell proliferation by glucocorticoids in vitro. *American Review of Respiratory Disease*, Vol. 144(5): pp. 1016-1025.

Damera, G., Druey, K.M., Amrani, Y., Soberman, R.J., Brightling, C.E. & Panettieri, R.A., Jr. (2010). RGS4 modulates growth factor-induced ASM proliferation In severe asthma. *American Journal of Respiratory and Critical Care Medicine*, Vol. 181(1): pp. A2303.

Damera, G., Fogle, H.W., Lim, P., Goncharova, E.A., Zhao, H., Banerjee, A., Tliba, O., Krymskaya, V.P. & Panettieri, R.A., Jr. (2009a). Vitamin D inhibits growth of human airway smooth muscle cells through growth factor-induced phosphorylation of retinoblastoma protein and checkpoint kinase 1. *British Journal of Pharmacology*, Vol. 158(6): pp. 1429-1441.

Damera, G., Tliba, O. & Panettieri, R.A., Jr. (2009b). Airway smooth muscle as an immunomodulatory cell. *Pulmonary Pharmacology & Therapeutics*, Vol. 22(5): pp. 353-359.

Damera, G., Zhao, H., Wang, M., Smith, M., Kirby, C., Jester, W.F., Lawson, J.A. & Panettieri, R.A., Jr. (2009c). Ozone modulates IL-6 secretion in human airway epithelial and smooth muscle cells. *American Journal of Physiology. Lung Cellular and Molecular Physiology*, Vol. 296(4): pp. L674-L683.

Dekkers, B.G., Maarsingh, H., Meurs, H. & Gosens, R. (2009). Airway structural components drive airway smooth muscle remodeling in asthma. *Proceedings of the American Thoracic Society*, Vol. 6(8): pp. 683-692.

Dekkers, B.G., Schaafsma, D., Nelemans, S.A., Zaagsma, J. & Meurs, H. (2007). Extracellular matrix proteins differentially regulate airway smooth muscle phenotype and function. *American Journal of Physiology. Lung Cellular and Molecular Physiology*, Vol. 292(6): pp. L1405-L1413.

Deshpande, D.A. & Penn, R.B. (2006). Targeting G protein-coupled receptor signaling in asthma. *Cellular Signalling*, Vol. 18(12): pp. 2105-2120.

Doherty, T.A., Soroosh, P., Khorram, N., Fukuyama, S., Rosenthal, P., Cho, J.Y., Norris, P.S., Choi, H., Scheu, S., Pfeffer, K., Zuraw, B.L., Ware, C.F., Broide, D.H. & Croft, M. (2011). The tumor necrosis factor family member LIGHT is a target for asthmatic airway remodeling. *Nature Medicine*, Vol. 17(5): pp. 596-603.

Dunnill, M.S., Massarella, G.R. & Anderson, J.A. (1969). A comparison of the quantitative anatomy of the bronchi in normal subjects, in status asthmaticus, in chronic bronchitis, and in emphysema. *Thorax*, Vol. 24(2): pp. 176-179.

Duplaa, C., Couffinhal, T., Dufourcq, P., Llanas, B., Moreau, C. & Bonnet, J. (1997). The integrin very late antigen-4 is expressed in human smooth muscle cell. Involvement of alpha 4 and vascular cell adhesion molecule-1 during smooth muscle cell differentiation. *Circulation Research*, Vol. 80(2): pp. 159-169.

Ebina, M., Takahashi, T., Chiba, T. & Motomiya, M. (1993). Cellular hypertrophy and hyperplasia of airway smooth muscles underlying bronchial asthma. A 3-D morphometric study. *American Review of Respiratory Disease*, Vol. 148(3): pp. 720-726.

El-Shazly, A., Berger, P., Girodet, P.O., Ousova, O., Fayon, M., Vernejoux, J.M., Marthan, R. & Tunon-de-Lara, J.M. (2006). Fraktalkine produced by airway smooth muscle cells contributes to mast cell recruitment in asthma. *Journal of Immunology*, Vol. 176(3): pp. 1860-1868.

Faffe, D.S., Flynt, L., Mellema, M., Moore, P.E., Silverman, E.S., Subramaniam, V., Jones, M.R., Mizgerd, J.P., Whitehead, T., Imrich, A., Panettieri, R.A., Jr. & Shore, S.A. (2005a). Oncostatin M causes eotaxin-1 release from airway smooth muscle: synergy with IL-4 and IL-13. *Journal of Allergy and Clinical Immunology*, Vol. 115(3): pp. 514-520.

Faffe, D.S., Flynt, L., Mellema, M., Whitehead, T.R., Bourgeois, K., Panettieri, R.A., Jr., Silverman, E.S. & Shore, S.A. (2005b). Oncostatin M causes VEGF release from human airway smooth muscle: synergy with IL-1beta. *American Journal of Physiology. Lung Cellular and Molecular Physiology*, Vol. 288(6): pp. L1040-L1048.

Fanat, A.I., Thomson, J.V., Radford, K., Nair, P. & Sehmi, R. (2009). Human airway smooth muscle promotes eosinophil differentiation. *Clinical and Experimental Allergy*, Vol. 39(7): pp. 1009-1017.

Foley, S.C., Mogas, A.K., Olivenstein, R., Fiset, P.O., Chakir, J., Bourbeau, J., Ernst, P., Lemiere, C., Martin, J.G. & Hamid, Q. (2007). Increased expression of ADAM33 and ADAM8 with disease progression in asthma. *Journal of Allergy and Clinical Immunology*, Vol. 119(4): pp. 863-871.

Gally, F., Hartney, J.M., Janssen, W.J. & Perraud, A.L. (2009). CD38 plays a dual role in allergen-induced airway hyperresponsiveness. *American Journal of Respiratory Cell and Molecular Biology*, Vol. 40(4): pp. 433-442.

Girodet, P.O., Ozier, A., Trian, T., Begueret, H., Ousova, O., Vernejoux, J.M., Chanez, P., Marthan, R., Berger, P. & Tunon de Lara, J.M. (2010). Mast cell adhesion to bronchial smooth muscle in asthma specifically depends on CD51 and CD44 variant 6. *Allergy*, Vol. 65(8): pp. 1004-1012.

Gizycki, M.J., Adelroth, E., Rogers, A.V., O'Byrne, P.M. & Jeffery, P.K. (1997). Myofibroblast involvement in the allergen-induced late response in mild atopic asthma. *American Journal of Respiratory Cell and Molecular Biology*, Vol. 16(6): pp. 664-673.

Govindaraju, V., Michoud, M.C., Al-Chalabi, M., Ferraro, P., Powell, W.S. & Martin, J.G. (2006). Interleukin-8: novel roles in human airway smooth muscle cell contraction and migration. *American Journal of Physiology. Cell Physiology*, Vol. 291(5): pp. C957-C965.

Govindaraju, V., Michoud, M.C., Ferraro, P., Arkinson, J., Safka, K., Valderrama-Carvajal, H. & Martin, J.G. (2008). The effects of interleukin-8 on airway smooth muscle contraction in cystic fibrosis. *Respiratory Research*, Vol. 9: pp. 76.

Grunstein, M.M., Hakonarson, H., Whelan, R., Yu, Z., Grunstein, J.S. & Chuang, S. (2001). Rhinovirus elicits proasthmatic changes in airway responsiveness independently of viral infection. *Journal of Allergy and Clinical Immunology*, Vol. 108(6): pp. 997-1004.

Guedes, A.G., Jude, J.A., Paulin, J., Kita, H., Lund, F.E. & Kannan, M.S. (2008). Role of CD38 in TNF-alpha-induced airway hyperresponsiveness. *American Journal of Physiology. Lung Cellular and Molecular Physiology*, Vol. 294(2): pp. L290-L299.

Guedes, A.G., Paulin, J., Rivero-Nava, L., Kita, H., Lund, F.E. & Kannan, M.S. (2006). CD38-deficient mice have reduced airway hyperresponsiveness following IL-13 challenge. *American Journal of Physiology. Lung Cellular and Molecular Physiology*, Vol. 291(6): pp. L1286-L1293.

Hakonarson, H., Kim, C., Whelan, R., Campbell, D. & Grunstein, M.M. (2001). Bi-directional activation between human airway smooth muscle cells and T lymphocytes: role in induction of altered airway responsiveness. *Journal of Immunology*, Vol. 166(1): pp. 293-303.

Halayko, A.J., Tran, T. & Gosens, R. (2008). Phenotype and functional plasticity of airway smooth muscle: role of caveolae and caveolins. *Proceedings of the American Thoracic Society*, Vol. 5(1): pp. 80-88.

Halayko, A.J., Tran, T., Ji, S.Y., Yamasaki, A. & Gosens, R. (2006). Airway smooth muscle phenotype and function: interactions with current asthma therapies. *Current Drug Targets*, Vol. 7(5): pp. 525-540.

Hirota, J.A., Nguyen, T.T., Schaafsma, D., Sharma, P. & Tran, T. (2009). Airway smooth muscle in asthma: phenotype plasticity and function. *Pulmonary Pharmacology & Therapeutics*, Vol. 22(5): pp. 370-378.

Hirst, S.J., Hallsworth, M.P., Peng, Q. & Lee, T.H. (2002). Selective induction of eotaxin release by interleukin-13 or interleukin-4 in human airway smooth muscle cells is synergistic with interleukin-1beta and is mediated by the interleukin-4 receptor alpha-chain. *American Journal of Respiratory and Critical Care Medicine*, Vol. 165(8): pp. 1161-1171.

Hirst, S.J., Martin, J.G., Bonacci, J.V., Chan, V., Fixman, E.D., Hamid, Q.A., Herszberg, B., Lavoie, J.P., McVicker, C.G., Moir, L.M., Nguyen, T.T., Peng, Q., Ramos-Barbon, D.

& Stewart, A.G. (2004). Proliferative aspects of airway smooth muscle. *Journal of Allergy and Clinical Immunology*, Vol. 114(2 Suppl): pp. S2-S17.

Hossain, S. & Heard, B.E. (1970). Hyperplasia of bronchial muscle in chronic bronchitis. *Journal of Pathology*, Vol. 101(2): pp. 171-184.

Hughes, J.M., Arthur, C.A., Baracho, S., Carlin, S.M., Hawker, K.M., Johnson, P.R. & Armour, C.L. (2000). Human eosinophil-airway smooth muscle cell interactions. *Mediators of Inflammation*, Vol. 9(2): pp. 93-99.

Hunninghake, G.M., Cho, M.H., Tesfaigzi, Y., Soto-Quiros, M.E., Avila, L., Lasky-Su, J., Stidley, C., Melen, E., Soderhall, C., Hallberg, J., Kull, I., Kere, J., Svartengren, M., Pershagen, G., Wickman, M., Lange, C., Demeo, D.L., Hersh, C.P., Klanderman, B.J., Raby, B.A., Sparrow, D., Shapiro, S.D., Silverman, E.K., Litonjua, A.A., Weiss, S.T. & Celedon, J.C. (2009). MMP12, lung function, and COPD in high-risk populations. *New England Journal of Medicine*, Vol. 361(27): pp. 2599-2608.

Ingram, J.L. & Bonner, J.C. (2006). EGF and PDGF receptor tyrosine kinases as therapeutic targets for chronic lung diseases. *Current Molecular Medicine*, Vol. 6(4): pp. 409-421.

Ito, I., Fixman, E.D., Asai, K., Yoshida, M., Gounni, A.S., Martin, J.G. & Hamid, Q. (2009). Platelet-derived growth factor and transforming growth factor-beta modulate the expression of matrix metalloproteinases and migratory function of human airway smooth muscle cells. *Clinical and Experimental Allergy*, Vol. 39(9): pp. 1370-1380.

Iwata, S., Ito, S., Iwaki, M., Kondo, M., Sashio, T., Takeda, N., Sokabe, M., Hasegawa, Y. & Kume, H. (2009). Regulation of endothelin-1-induced interleukin-6 production by Ca2+ influx in human airway smooth muscle cells. *European Journal of Pharmacology*, Vol. 605(1-3): pp. 15-22.

Jackson, A.C., Murphy, M.M., Rassulo, J., Celli, B.R. & Ingram, R.H., Jr. (2004). Deep breath reversal and exponential return of methacholine-induced obstruction in asthmatic and nonasthmatic subjects. *Journal of Applied Physiology*, Vol. 96(1): pp. 137-142.

Janssen, L.J. (1998). Calcium handling in airway smooth muscle: mechanisms and therapeutic implications. *Canadian Respiratory Journal*, Vol. 5(6): pp. 491-498.

Jensen, A., Atileh, H., Suki, B., Ingenito, E.P. & Lutchen, K.R. (2001). Selected contribution: airway caliber in healthy and asthmatic subjects: effects of bronchial challenge and deep inspirations. *Journal of Applied Physiology*, Vol. 91(1): pp. 506-515; discussion 504-505.

John, A.E., Zhu, Y.M., Brightling, C.E., Pang, L. & Knox, A.J. (2009). Human airway smooth muscle cells from asthmatic individuals have CXCL8 hypersecretion due to increased NF-kappa B p65, C/EBP beta, and RNA polymerase II binding to the CXCL8 promoter. *Journal of Immunology*, Vol. 183(7): pp. 4682-4692.

Johnson, P.R., Burgess, J.K., Ge, Q., Poniris, M., Boustany, S., Twigg, S.M. & Black, J.L. (2006). Connective tissue growth factor induces extracellular matrix in asthmatic airway smooth muscle. *American Journal of Respiratory and Critical Care Medicine*, Vol. 173(1): pp. 32-41.

Johnson, P.R., Burgess, J.K., Underwood, P.A., Au, W., Poniris, M.H., Tamm, M., Ge, Q., Roth, M. & Black, J.L. (2004). Extracellular matrix proteins modulate asthmatic airway smooth muscle cell proliferation via an autocrine mechanism. *Journal of Allergy Clinical Immunology*, Vol. 113(4): pp. 690-696.

Joubert, P. & Hamid, Q. (2005). Role of airway smooth muscle in airway remodeling. *Journal of Allergy and Clinical Immunology*, Vol. 116(3): pp. 713-716.

Jude, J.A., Solway, J., Panettieri, R.A., Jr., Walseth, T.F. & Kannan, M.S. (2010). Differential induction of CD38 expression by TNF-{alpha} in asthmatic airway smooth muscle cells. *American Journal of Physiology. Lung Cellular and Molecular Physiology*, Vol. 299(6): pp. L879-L890.

Jude, J.A., Wylam, M.E., Walseth, T.F. & Kannan, M.S. (2008). Calcium signaling in airway smooth muscle. *Proceedings of the American Thoracic Society*, Vol. 5(1): pp. 15-22.

Kaur, D., Saunders, R., Hollins, F., Woodman, L., Doe, C., Siddiqui, S., Bradding, P. & Brightling, C. (2010). Mast cell fibroblastoid differentiation mediated by airway smooth muscle in asthma. *Journal of Immunology*, Vol. 185(10): pp. 6105-6114.

Kelly, M., Hwang, J.M. & Kubes, P. (2007). Modulating leukocyte recruitment in inflammation. *Journal of Allergy and Clinical Immunology*, Vol. 120(1): pp. 3-10.

Klagas, I., Goulet, S., Karakiulakis, G., Zhong, J., Baraket, M., Black, J.L., Papakonstantinou, E. & Roth, M. (2009). Decreased hyaluronan in airway smooth muscle cells from patients with asthma and COPD. *European Respiratory Journal*, Vol. 34(3): pp. 616-628.

Knight, D.A. & Holgate, S.T. (2003). The airway epithelium: structural and functional properties in health and disease. *Respirology*, Vol. 8(4): pp. 432-446.

Knobloch, J., Peters, H., Jungck, D., Muller, K., Strauch, J. & Koch, A. (2009). TNFalpha-induced GM-CSF release from human airway smooth muscle cells depends on activation of an ET-1 autoregulatory positive feedback mechanism. *Thorax*, Vol. 64(12): pp. 1044-1052.

Krymskaya, V.P., Orsini, M.J., Eszterhas, A.J., Brodbeck, K.C., Benovic, J.L., Panettieri, R.A., Jr. & Penn, R.B. (2000). Mechanisms of proliferation synergy by receptor tyrosine kinase and G protein-coupled receptor activation in human airway smooth muscle. *American Journal of Respiratory Cell and Molecular Biology*, Vol. 23(4): pp. 546-554.

Kuo, C., Lim, S., King, N.J., Johnston, S.L., Burgess, J.K., Black, J.L. & Oliver, B.G. (2011). Rhinovirus infection induces extracellular matrix protein deposition in asthmatic and non-asthmatic airway smooth muscle cells. *American Journal of Physiology. Lung Cellular and Molecular Physiology*, Vol.: pp. Epub ahead of print Apr 5.

Lam, V., Kalesnikoff, J., Lee, C.W., Hernandez-Hansen, V., Wilson, B.S., Oliver, J.M. & Krystal, G. (2003). IgE alone stimulates mast cell adhesion to fibronectin via pathways similar to those used by IgE + antigen but distinct from those used by Steel factor. *Blood*, Vol. 102(4): pp. 1405-1413.

Lane, S.J., Arm, J.P., Staynov, D.Z. & Lee, T.H. (1994). Chemical mutational analysis of the human glucocorticoid receptor cDNA in glucocorticoid-resistant bronchial asthma. *American Journal of Respiratory Cell and Molecular Biology*, Vol. 11(1): pp. 42-48.

Lazaar, A.L., Albelda, S.M., Pilewski, J.M., Brennan, B., Pure, E. & Panettieri, R.A., Jr. (1994). T lymphocytes adhere to airway smooth muscle cells via integrins and CD44 and induce smooth muscle cell DNA synthesis. *Journal of Experimental Medicine*, Vol. 180(3): pp. 807-816.

Lazaar, A.L., Amrani, Y., Hsu, J., Panettieri, R.A., Jr., Fanslow, W.C., Albelda, S.M. & Pure, E. (1998). CD40-mediated signal transduction in human airway smooth muscle. *Journal of Immunology*, Vol. 161(6): pp. 3120-3127.

Lazaar, A.L. & Panettieri, R.A., Jr. (2005). Airway smooth muscle: a modulator of airway remodeling in asthma. *Journal of Allergy and Clinical Immunology*, Vol. 116(3): pp. 488-495; quiz 496.

Le Cras, T.D., Acciani, T.H., Mushaben, E.M., Kramer, E.L., Pastura, P.A., Hardie, W.D., Korfhagen, T.R., Sivaprasad, U., Ericksen, M., Gibson, A.M., Holtzman, M.J., Whitsett, J.A. & Hershey, G.K. (2011). Epithelial EGF receptor signaling mediates airway hyperreactivity and remodeling in a mouse model of chronic asthma.

American Journal of Physiology. Lung Cellular and Molecular Physiology, Vol. 300(3): pp. L414-L421.

Lemjabbar, H., Gosset, P., Lamblin, C., Tillie, I., Hartmann, D., Wallaert, B., Tonnel, A.B. & Lafuma, C. (1999). Contribution of 92 kDa gelatinase/type IV collagenase in bronchial inflammation during status asthmaticus. *American Journal of Respiratory and Critical Care Medicine*, Vol. 159(4 Pt 1): pp. 1298-1307.

Liang, G., Bansal, G., Xie, Z. & Druey, K.M. (2009). RGS16 inhibits breast cancer cell growth by mitigating phosphatidylinositol 3-kinase signaling. *Journal of Biological Chemistry*, Vol. 284(32): pp. 21719-21727.

Ma, X., Cheng, Z., Kong, H., Wang, Y., Unruh, H., Stephens, N.L. & Laviolette, M. (2002). Changes in biophysical and biochemical properties of single bronchial smooth muscle cells from asthmatic subjects. *American Journal of Physiology. Lung Cellular and Molecular Physiology*, Vol. 283(6): pp. L1181-L1189.

Malavia, N.K., Raub, C.B., Mahon, S.B., Brenner, M., Panettieri, R.A., Jr. & George, S.C. (2009). Airway epithelium stimulates smooth muscle proliferation. *American Journal of Respiratory Cell and Molecular Biology*, Vol. 41(3): pp. 297-304.

Marwick, J.A., Chung, K.F. & Adcock, I.M. (2010). Phosphatidylinositol 3-kinase isoforms as targets in respiratory disease. *Therapeutic Advances in Respiratory Disease*, Vol. 4(1): pp. 19-34.

Mautino, G., Henriquet, C., Gougat, C., Le Cam, A., Dayer, J.M., Bousquet, J. & Capony, F. (1999a). Increased expression of tissue inhibitor of metalloproteinase-1 and loss of correlation with matrix metalloproteinase-9 by macrophages in asthma. *Laboratory Investigation*, Vol. 79(1): pp. 39-47.

Mautino, G., Henriquet, C., Jaffuel, D., Bousquet, J. & Capony, F. (1999b). Tissue inhibitor of metalloproteinase-1 levels in bronchoalveolar lavage fluid from asthmatic subjects. *American Journal of Respiratory and Critical Care Medicine*, Vol. 160(1): pp. 324-330.

McKay, S. & Sharma, H.S. (2002). Autocrine regulation of asthmatic airway inflammation: role of airway smooth muscle. *Respiratory Research*, Vol. 3: pp. 11.

Mitchell, R.W., Ndukwu, I.M., Arbetter, K., Solway, J. & Leff, A.R. (1993). Effect of airway inflammation on smooth muscle shortening and contractility in guinea pig trachealis. *American Journal of Physiology. Lung Cellular and Molecular Physiology*, Vol. 265(6 Pt 1): pp. L549-L554.

Moir, L.M., Burgess, J.K. & Black, J.L. (2008). Transforming growth factor beta 1 increases fibronectin deposition through integrin receptor alpha 5 beta 1 on human airway smooth muscle. *Journal of Allergy and Clinical Immunology*, Vol. 121(4): pp. 1034-1039.

Moir, L.M., Trian, T., Ge, Q., Shepherd, P.R., Burgess, J.K., Oliver, B.G. & Black, J.L. (2011). Phosphatidylinositol 3-Kinase Isoform-Specific Effects in Airway Mesenchymal Cell Function. *Journal of Pharmacology and Experimental Therapeutics*, Vol. 337(2): pp. 557-566.

Mukhina, S., Stepanova, V., Traktouev, D., Poliakov, A., Beabealashvilly, R., Gursky, Y., Minashkin, M., Shevelev, A. & Tkachuk, V. (2000). The chemotactic action of urokinase on smooth muscle cells is dependent on its kringle domain. Characterization of interactions and contribution to chemotaxis. *Journal of Biological Chemistry*, Vol. 275(22): pp. 16450-16458.

Mukhopadhyay, S., Sypek, J., Tavendale, R., Gartner, U., Winter, J., Li, W., Page, K., Fleming, M., Brady, J., O'Toole, M., Macgregor, D.F., Goldman, S., Tam, S., Abraham, W., Williams, C., Miller, D.K. & Palmer, C.N. (2010). Matrix metalloproteinase-12 is a therapeutic target for asthma in children and young adults. *Journal of Allergy and Clinical Immunology*, Vol. 126(1): pp. 70-76.

Naureckas, E.T., Ndukwu, I.M., Halayko, A.J., Maxwell, C., Hershenson, M.B. & Solway, J. (1999). Bronchoalveolar lavage fluid from asthmatic subjects is mitogenic for human airway smooth muscle. *American Journal of Respiratory and Critical Care Medicine*, Vol. 160(6): pp. 2062-2066.

Oliver, B.G., Johnston, S.L., Baraket, M., Burgess, J.K., King, N.J., Roth, M., Lim, S. & Black, J.L. (2006). Increased proinflammatory responses from asthmatic human airway smooth muscle cells in response to rhinovirus infection. *Respiratory Research*, Vol. 7: pp. 71.

Oltmanns, U., Chung, K.F., Walters, M., John, M. & Mitchell, J.A. (2005). Cigarette smoke induces IL-8, but inhibits eotaxin and RANTES release from airway smooth muscle. *Respiratory Research*, Vol. 6: pp. 74.

Parameswaran, K., Janssen, L.J. & O'Byrne, P.M. (2002). Airway hyperresponsiveness and calcium handling by smooth muscle: a "deeper look". *Chest*, Vol. 121(2): pp. 621-624.

Pegorier, S., Arouche, N., Dombret, M.C., Aubier, M. & Pretolani, M. (2007). Augmented epithelial endothelin-1 expression in refractory asthma. *Journal of Allergy and Clinical Immunology*, Vol. 120(6): pp. 1301-1307.

Pellegrino, R., Wilson, O., Jenouri, G. & Rodarte, J.R. (1996). Lung mechanics during induced bronchoconstriction. *Journal of Applied Physiology*, Vol. 81(2): pp. 964-975.

Peng, Q., Lai, D., Nguyen, T.T., Chan, V., Matsuda, T. & Hirst, S.J. (2005). Multiple beta 1 integrins mediate enhancement of human airway smooth muscle cytokine secretion by fibronectin and type I collagen. *Journal of Immunology*, Vol. 174(4): pp. 2258-2264.

Peng, Q., Matsuda, T. & Hirst, S.J. (2004). Signaling pathways regulating interleukin-13-stimulated chemokine release from airway smooth muscle. *American Journal of Respiratory and Critical Care Medicine*, Vol. 169(5): pp. 596-603.

Perkett, E.A. (1995). Role of growth factors in lung repair and diseases. *Current Opinion in Pediatrics*, Vol. 7(3): pp. 242-249.

Polosa, R., Puddicombe, S.M., Krishna, M.T., Tuck, A.B., Howarth, P.H., Holgate, S.T. & Davies, D.E. (2002). Expression of c-erbB receptors and ligands in the bronchial epithelium of asthmatic subjects. *Journal of Allergy and Clinical Immunology*, Vol. 109(1): pp. 75-81.

Prefontaine, D., Lajoie-Kadoch, S., Foley, S., Audusseau, S., Olivenstein, R., Halayko, A.J., Lemiere, C., Martin, J.G. & Hamid, Q. (2009). Increased expression of IL-33 in severe asthma: evidence of expression by airway smooth muscle cells. *Journal of Immunology*, Vol. 183(8): pp. 5094-5103.

Puddicombe, S.M., Polosa, R., Richter, A., Krishna, M.T., Howarth, P.H., Holgate, S.T. & Davies, D.E. (2000). Involvement of the epidermal growth factor receptor in epithelial repair in asthma. *FASEB Journal*, Vol. 14(10): pp. 1362-1374.

Ramos-Barbon, D., Presley, J.F., Hamid, Q.A., Fixman, E.D. & Martin, J.G. (2005). Antigen-specific CD4+ T cells drive airway smooth muscle remodeling in experimental asthma. *Journal of Clinical Investigation*, Vol. 115(6): pp. 1580-1589.

Roscioni, S.S., Prins, A.G., Elzinga, C.R., Menzen, M.H., Dekkers, B.G., Halayko, A.J., Meurs, H., Maarsingh, H. & Schmidt, M. (2011). Functional roles of Epac and PKA in human airway smooth muscle phenotype plasticity. *British Journal of Pharmacology*, Vol.: pp. Epub ahead of print Mar 23.

Roth, M., Johnson, P.R., Borger, P., Bihl, M.P., Rudiger, J.J., King, G.G., Ge, Q., Hostettler, K., Burgess, J.K., Black, J.L. & Tamm, M. (2004). Dysfunctional interaction of

C/EBPalpha and the glucocorticoid receptor in asthmatic bronchial smooth-muscle cells. *New England Journal of Medicine*, Vol. 351(6): pp. 560-574.

Saetta, M., Di Stefano, A., Rosina, C., Thiene, G. & Fabbri, L.M. (1991). Quantitative structural analysis of peripheral airways and arteries in sudden fatal asthma. *American Review of Respiratory Disease*, Vol. 143(1): pp. 138-143.

Scott, P.H., Belham, C.M., al-Hafidh, J., Chilvers, E.R., Peacock, A.J., Gould, G.W. & Plevin, R. (1996). A regulatory role for cAMP in phosphatidylinositol 3-kinase/p70 ribosomal S6 kinase-mediated DNA synthesis in platelet-derived-growth-factor-stimulated bovine airway smooth-muscle cells. *Biochemical Journal*, Vol. 318 (Pt 3): pp. 965-971.

Seow, C.Y., Schellenberg, R.R. & Pare, P.D. (1998). Structural and functional changes in the airway smooth muscle of asthmatic subjects. *American Journal of Respiratory and Critical Care Medicine*, Vol. 158(5 Pt 3): pp. S179-S186.

Shan, L., Redhu, N.S., Saleh, A., Halayko, A.J., Chakir, J. & Gounni, A.S. (2010). Thymic stromal lymphopoietin receptor-mediated IL-6 and CC/CXC chemokines expression in human airway smooth muscle cells: role of MAPKs (ERK1/2, p38, and JNK) and STAT3 pathways. *Journal of Immunology*, Vol. 184(12): pp. 7134-7143.

Sharma, P., Tran, T., Stelmack, G.L., McNeill, K., Gosens, R., Mutawe, M.M., Unruh, H., Gerthoffer, W.T. & Halayko, A.J. (2008). Expression of the dystrophin-glycoprotein complex is a marker for human airway smooth muscle phenotype maturation. *American Journal of Physiology. Lung Cellular and Molecular Physiology*, Vol. 294(1): pp. L57-L68.

Shin, J.H., Shim, J.W., Kim, D.S. & Shim, J.Y. (2009). TGF-beta effects on airway smooth muscle cell proliferation, VEGF release and signal transduction pathways. *Respirology*, Vol. 14(3): pp. 347-353.

Solway, J. & Fredberg, J.J. (1997). Perhaps airway smooth muscle dysfunction contributes to asthmatic bronchial hyperresponsiveness after all. *American Journal of Respiratory Cell and Molecular Biology*, Vol. 17(2): pp. 144-146.

Spina, D. (1998). Epithelium smooth muscle regulation and interactions. *American Journal of Respiratory and Critical Care Medicine*, Vol. 158(5 Pt 3): pp. S141-S145.

Swieter, M., Hamawy, M.M., Siraganian, R.P. & Mergenhagen, S.E. (1993). Mast cells and their microenvironment: the influence of fibronectin and fibroblasts on the functional repertoire of rat basophilic leukemia cells. *Journal of Periodontology*, Vol. 64(5 Suppl): pp. 492-496.

Tao, F.C., Tolloczko, B., Eidelman, D.H. & Martin, J.G. (1999). Enhanced Ca(2+) mobilization in airway smooth muscle contributes to airway hyperresponsiveness in an inbred strain of rat. *American Journal of Respiratory and Critical Care Medicine*, Vol. 160(2): pp. 446-453.

Thomson, R.J. & Schellenberg, R.R. (1998). Increased amount of airway smooth muscle does not account for excessive bronchoconstriction in asthma. *Canadian Respiratory Journal*, Vol. 5(1): pp. 61-62.

Tliba, O., Amrani, Y. & Panettieri, R.A., Jr. (2008a). Is airway smooth muscle the "missing link" modulating airway inflammation in asthma? *Chest*, Vol. 133(1): pp. 236-342.

Tliba, O., Damera, G., Banerjee, A., Gu, S., Baidouri, H., Keslacy, S. & Amrani, Y. (2008b). Cytokines induce an early steroid resistance in airway smooth muscle cells: novel role of interferon regulatory factor-1. *American Journal of Respiratory Cell and Molecular Biology*, Vol. 38(4): pp. 463-472.

Tliba, O. & Panettieri, R.A., Jr. (2008). Regulation of inflammation by airway smooth muscle. *Current Allergy and Asthma Reports*, Vol. 8(3): pp. 262-268.

Tliba, O. & Panettieri, R.A., Jr. (2009). Noncontractile functions of airway smooth muscle cells in asthma. *Annual Review of Physiology*, Vol. 71: pp. 509-535.

Tliba, O., Tliba, S., Da Huang, C., Hoffman, R.K., DeLong, P., Panettieri, R.A., Jr. & Amrani, Y. (2003). Tumor necrosis factor alpha modulates airway smooth muscle function via the autocrine action of interferon beta. *Journal of Biological Chemistry*, Vol. 278(50): pp. 50615-50623.

Trian, T., Benard, G., Begueret, H., Rossignol, R., Girodet, P.O., Ghosh, D., Ousova, O., Vernejoux, J.M., Marthan, R., Tunon-de-Lara, J.M. & Berger, P. (2007). Bronchial smooth muscle remodeling involves calcium-dependent enhanced mitochondrial biogenesis in asthma. *Journal of Experimental Medicine*, Vol. 204(13): pp. 3173-3181.

Trian, T., Moir, L.M., Ge, Q., Burgess, J.K., Kuo, C., King, N.J., Reddel, H.K., Black, J.L., Oliver, B.G. & McParland, B.E. (2010). Rhinovirus-induced exacerbations of asthma: How is the {beta}2-adrenoceptor implicated? *American Journal of Respiratory Cell and Molecular Biology*, Vol. 43(2): pp. 227-233.

Wenzel, S.E., Schwartz, L.B., Langmack, E.L., Halliday, J.L., Trudeau, J.B., Gibbs, R.L. & Chu, H.W. (1999). Evidence that severe asthma can be divided pathologically into two inflammatory subtypes with distinct physiologic and clinical characteristics. *American Journal of Respiratory and Critical Care Medicine*, Vol. 160(3): pp. 1001-1018.

Woodruff, P.G., Dolganov, G.M., Ferrando, R.E., Donnelly, S., Hays, S.R., Solberg, O.D., Carter, R., Wong, H.H., Cadbury, P.S. & Fahy, J.V. (2004). Hyperplasia of smooth muscle in mild to moderate asthma without changes in cell size or gene expression. *American Journal of Respiratory and Critical Care Medicine*, Vol. 169(9): pp. 1001-1006.

Yamanaka, Y., Hayashi, K., Komurasaki, T., Morimoto, S., Ogihara, T. & Sobue, K. (2001). EGF family ligand-dependent phenotypic modulation of smooth muscle cells through EGF receptor. *Biochemical and Biophysical Research Communications*, Vol. 281(2): pp. 373-377.

Yamasaki, A., Saleh, A., Koussih, L., Muro, S., Halayko, A.J. & Gounni, A.S. (2010). IL-9 induces CCL11 expression via STAT3 signalling in human airway smooth muscle cells. *PLoS One*, Vol. 5(2): pp. e9178.

Yang, W., Kaur, D., Okayama, Y., Ito, A., Wardlaw, A.J., Brightling, C.E. & Bradding, P. (2006). Human lung mast cells adhere to human airway smooth muscle, in part, via tumor suppressor in lung cancer-1. *Journal of Immunology*, Vol. 176(2): pp. 1238-1243.

Zuberi, R.I., Hsu, D.K., Kalayci, O., Chen, H.Y., Sheldon, H.K., Yu, L., Apgar, J.R., Kawakami, T., Lilly, C.M. & Liu, F.T. (2004). Critical role for galectin-3 in airway inflammation and bronchial hyperresponsiveness in a murine model of asthma. *American Journal of Pathology*, Vol. 165(6): pp. 2045-2053.

Zuyderduyn, S., Sukkar, M.B., Fust, A., Dhaliwal, S. & Burgess, J.K. (2008). Treating asthma means treating airway smooth muscle cells. *European Respiratory Journal*, Vol. 32(2): pp. 265-374.

7

Fluoride and Bronchial Smooth Muscle

Fedoua Gandia[1], Sonia Rouatbi[1],
Badreddine Sriha[2] and Zouhair Tabka[1]
[1]*Laboratory of Physiology and Functional Explorations,
Faculty of Medicine Sousse, University of Sousse,*
[2]*Laboratory of Pathological Anatomy and Cytology,
Faculty of Medicine Sousse, University of Sousse,
Tunisia*

1. Introduction

Fluoride is an inhibitor of enolase, an enzyme in glycolysis leading to phosphoenolpyruvate (Mayes, 1987). Inhibition of this enzyme would be expected to reduce glycolytic ATP production and impair smooth muscle contraction. It has also been reported that fluoride has contractile effect on vascular and airway smooth muscle mediated by the activation of guanine nucleotide binding proteins (G proteins) (Himpens et al., 1991; Kawase & Van Breemen, 1992; Leurs et al., 1991).

Fluoride (NaF) may thus induce either contraction or relaxation of smooth muscle depending on the particular conditions. NaF is less potent than aluminium fluoride ($Al\ F^-_4$) in the activation of G proteins, $Al\ F^-_4$ mimics the action of GTP at micro molar concentrations by inducing dissociation of the α subunit of G protein followed by the calcium channel modulation (Stadel & Crooke, 1988).

A close relationship between fluoride exposure and asthmatic symptoms was confirmed by several studies (Taiwo et al., 2006; Viragh et al., 2006; Fritchi et al., 2003; Soyseth et al., 1994) but little is know about its potential bronchorelaxant effect. In this chapter we will explore the effect of fluoride on respiratory status, its mechanism of action, its toxicity and factors that could influence its effects.

2. Fluoride intake

Fluoride is the ionic form of fluorine, a halogen and the most electronegative of the elements of the periodic table. It's a natural component of the biosphere and the 13th most abundant element in the crust of the earth.

Sources of fluoride include natural fluoride in food stuffs and water, i.e., fluoridated water (usually at 1.0 mg/l), fluoride supplements (such as fluoride tablets), fluoride dentifrices (containing on average 100 mg/kg), and professionally applied fluoride gel (containing on average 5000 mg/kg). The main source of fluoride for humans is the intake of groundwater contaminated by geological sources (maximum concentrations reaching 30-50 mg/l). The level of fluoride contamination is dependent on the nature of rocks and the occurrence of fluoride-bearing minerals in groundwater. Fluoride concentrations in water are limited by fluorite solubility, so that in the absence of dissolved calcium, higher fluoride solubility should be expected in the groundwater of areas where fluoride-bearing minerals are common and vice versa (Barbier et al., 2010).

Fluorides accumulate in the body lead to numerous metabolic disorders even at a low concentration but with long time exposure. Chronic long-term exposure to high levels of fluoride leads to fluorosis, a serious health problem in many parts of the world, where drinking water contains more than 1-1.5 ppm of fluoride (World Health Organization, 1984). However, the exposure of humans to fluorine is also connected with its presence in the air and food.

3. Fluoride metabolism

Fluoride is very electronegative, which means that it has a strong tendency to acquire a negative charge forms fluoride ions in solution. In aqueous solutions of fluoride in acidic conditions such as those of the stomach, fluoride is converted into HF (weak acid with pK_a of 3.4) (Whitford, 1994). There is a considerable body of evidence showing that several of the transmembrane migration of the ion occurs in the form of HF in response to differences in the acidity of adjacent body fluid compartments (Whitford, 1996).

Most commonly, fluoride is absorbed and enters the body fluids by way of the lungs or the gastrointestinal tract. In the absence of high certain cations, such as calcium and aluminium, that form insoluble compounds with fluoride, about 80-90% of the ingested amount is absorbed from gastrointestinal tract (Whitford, 1994; Whitford, 1996). Most of the fluoride that escapes absorption from the stomach will be absorbed from the proximal small intestine. Roughly 50% of an absorbed amount will be excreted in the urine during the following 24h while most of the remainder will be associated with calcified tissue. 99% of the fluoride in the body is associated with calcified tissues.

There are two general forms of fluoride in human plasma. One fraction is called ionic fluoride (also called inorganic or free fluoride). This form of fluoride is the one of significance in dentistry, medicine and public health. It is detectable in plasma by the fluoride electrode and is not bound to plasma proteins. The other fraction is nonionic fluoride (also called organic of bound fluoride). Together, the ionic and nonionic fractions constitute what is commonly called 'total' plasma fluoride (whitford, 1994, 1996). The concentration of fluoride in plasma varies according to the level of intake and several physiological factors (whitford, 1996). In general, the numerical value of the fasting plasma concentration of healthy adults is equal to that in the drinking water. Then, the fasting plasma concentration of a person whose water contains 1.0ppm would be about 1.0 µmol/L. If the water contained 2.0ppm, the plasma concentration would be about 2.0µmol/L. The variations of these values would be due largely to individual differences in the rates of removal of fluoride by the kidneys and skeleton.

4. Fluoride and asthma

The relationship between exposure to fluoride and bronchial responsiveness was investigated since 1936; scientists have observed that workers exposed to airborne fluorides suffer from an elevated rate of respiratory disorders.

(Taiwo et al., 2006) in a study conducted to evaluate the respiratory risks from fluoride inhalation, showed hat there was a significant statistical relationship between the incidence of asthma and the mean gaseous fluoride exposure in the study population whereas the relationship between asthma incidence and the other contaminants was less significant.

In a 7 years study conducted by (Viragh et al., 2006) to evaluate the respiratory effects of fluorine compounds on exposed workers in a small-scale enamel enterprise found, that fluorine exposure may be responsible for the high incidence of chronic irritative respiratory diseases, especially for chronic bronchitis in exposed workers.

(Fritchi et al., 2003) had demonstrated that the relevant causative agents for respiratory symptoms in aluminum smelters are fluoride and inspirable dust.

A close relationship between the levels of fluoride exposure and work-related asthmatic symptoms has been observed by many studies (Kongerud et al., 1994; Soyseth et al., 1994; Soyseth & Kongerud, 1992; Kongerud, 1992; Tatsumi et al., 1991).The risk to respiratory function from fluoride exposure is independent of the risk from smoking, but the combination of fluoride exposure and smoking presents a risk greater than either factor by itself. In fact in a study conducted by (Kongerud & Samuelsen, 1991), they conclude that current total fluoride exposure and smoking are the major risk factors for development of dyspnea and wheezing in aluminium potroom workers.

Animal experiments studies converge of respiratory damage caused by fluoride, inflammation, emphysema and pulmonary cellular alterations (Mullenix, 2005; Yamamoto et al., 2001).

4.1 Fluoride effects on bronchial smooth muscle

The contractile effect of fluoride (NaF) was well documented. Previous studies confirms that NaF contracts several muscles such as, sheep pulmonary arterial rings (Uzun et al., 2002), rat intestinal smooth muscle (Murthy et al., 1992) isolated rat aorta and mesenteric artery (Hattori et al., 2000), and guinea-pig airway smooth muscle (Leurs et al., 1991). Several mechanisms have been proposed to explain NaF-induced contraction. In these studies, NaF was used as source of fluoride (F^-), and the effect obtained were owing to fluoride not to Na.

Flouride is a well-known G-protein activator. Activation of heterotrimetric GTP-binding proteins by F requires trace amounts of aluminum (Al^{3+}) or beryllium (Be^{2+}) ions (Li, 2003). F^- is a potent stimulator of G_s, G_i, G_p and transducin . NaF-induced vascular contractions have been proposed to be attributable to fluoride complexing with aluminum, which can come from contamination of glassware, to form fluoroaluminates (Al^{F4-}), which are activators of G proteins (Hattori et al., 2000). AlF^{4-} has a structure similar to phosphate ($PO_4{}^{3-}$) and is able to interact with the guanosine 5` -diphosphate (GDP) situated on the α-subunit of the G-proteins, resulting in activation by mimicking GTP at its binding site (Bigay et al., 1985; Wang et al., 2001).

Furthermore, it has been reported that NaF has a contractile effect on airway smooth muscle mediated by both G protein-dependent and -independent pathways (Murthy & Makhlouf,

1994). Activation of G proteins by fluoride in smooth muscle cells can initiate a series of events, such as Ca^{2+} mobilization and phospholipase C (PLC) and protein kinase C (PKC) activation (Weber et al., 1996). In vascular endothelium, NaF activates a pertussis toxin-insensitive GTP-binding protein, which leads to increases in phosphoinositide hydrolysis, Ca^{2+}mobilization from intracellular stores, arachidonate release, and prostacyclin synthesis (Garcia et al., 1991).

Fluoride has the capacity to both contract and dilate smooth muscle. These effects are closely related to the dose. NaF has been reported by (Stadel & Crooke, 1988; Cushing et al, 1990) to stimulate adenylate cyclase activity on smooth muscles and induced No synthesis which would relax bronchi. The better known bronchodilator mechanism of NaF is induced by inhibition of glycolytic enzyme, enolase, which converts 2-phosphoglycerate to phosphoenolpyruvate according to (Zhao W & Guenard H, 1997). The inhibition of glycolysis induced by NaF is illustrated by the sharp decrease in lactate production in its presence (Zhao W et al, 2002). Inhibition of this enzyme would be expected to reduce glycolytic ATP production and impair smooth muscle contraction.

This bronchodilator effect of NaF is thus far poorly documented. Inconsequence, its use as therapeutic agent for asthma disease is very limited despite its bronchodilator effect demonstrated at well defined dose both in vitro and in vivo by recent and previous studies (Gandia F et al, 2010; Rouatbi S et al, 2010; Zhao W & Guenard H, 1997; Zhao et al 2002).

4.2 Effect of fluoride dose on bronchial smooth muscle

Fluoride at a micromole level is considered an effective anabolic agent because it promotes cell proliferation whereas millimolar concentrations inhibit several enzymes, including phosphatases, both in vivo and in vitro (Barbier et al, 2010).

At toxicological concentrations, i.e. in the mM range, many effects of fluoride on respiratory status have been described which depend on three factors, the fluoride concentration, the length of exposure and the associated cation. For example, 5 mM NaF has a modest effect on the IL-6 and IL-8 secretion by of a human epithelial cell 24h after addition, which was strongly enhanced by addition of Al^{3+} (Refsnes et al, 1999). Another study showed that 0.5 mM NaF enhances IL-1 beta mRNA expression from lung lavage cells (Hirano et al, 1999). NaF, between 0.5 and 10 mM, induce a concentration-dependent contraction in bovine bronchial smooth muscle (Zhao et al, 1997). NaF at 0.5mM induce a bronchorelaxation effect by decrease of bronchial resistances in rats precontracted by acetylmethylcholine analogs and serum concentration of fluoride was within the usual range in blood samples obtained from rats receiving this drug (Gandia et al., 2010). Inhibitory effect of NaF on glycolytic enzyme enolase can be observed in the 10μM range (Curran et al, 1994) on bacteria, which could be of interest in certain lung diseases.

5. Fluoride toxicity

Fluoride toxicity is characterized by a variety of signs and symptoms poisoning most commonly occurs following ingestion (accidental or intentional) of fluoride-containing products. Symptom onset usually occurs within minutes of exposure. Fluoride has several mechanisms of toxicity. Ingested fluoride initially acts locally on the intestinal mucosa. It can form hydrofluoric acid in the stomach, which leads to G1 irritation or corrosive effects. Following ingestion, the G1 tract is the earliest and most commonly affected organ system.

Once absorbed, fluoride binds calcium ions and may lead to hypocalcaemia. Fluoride has direct cytotoxic effects and interferes with a number of enzyme systems; it disrupts oxidative phosphorylation, glycolysis, coagulation, and neurotransmission (by binding calcium). Fluoride inhibits Na^{+}/ K^{+} -ATPase, which may be partly responsible for hyper salivation, vomiting, and diarrhea (cholinergic signs). Seizures may result from both hypomagnesaemia and hypocalcaemia (Barbier et al, 2010; Whitford, 1996).

Severe fluoride toxicity will result in multiorgan failure. Central vasomotor depression as well as direct cardio toxicity also may occur. Death usually results from respiratory paralysis, dysrhythmia or cardiac failure.

The minimal risk level for daily oral fluoride uptake was determinates to be 0.05 mg/kg/day (Whitford, 1996), based on non observable adverse effect level (NOAEL) of 0.15 mg fluoride/kg/day for an increased fracture rate. Estimations of human lethal fluoride doses showed a wide range of values, from 16 to 64 mg /kg in adults and 3 to 16 kg in children (Withford, 1996).

6. Conclusion

Fluorides are known to exert a variety of effects in different cell types. Fluoride has the capacity to both contract and dilate smooth muscle. The mechanisms of the relaxant and contractile effects appear to be divers. The former being related to the inhibition of glycolysis and the latter to the calcium channel modulation. While the relationship of fluoride and asthmatic symptoms was widely studied, little is know about its potential therapeutic uses in asthma. The effects induced by fluoride are closely related to dose and concentration. However, it's important to highlight that fluoride is a strong, hard anion and a cumulative toxic agent. Then, serum fluoride determination should be carefully monitored. Further toxicological investigations are needed to conclusively determine the indications for fluoride use and dose.

7. References

Barbier, O. Mendoza, L A. & DelRazo, L M. (2010). Molecular mechanisms of fluoride toxicity. *CHEM-BIOL INTERACT.* Vol. 188, pp. (319-333).

Bigay, J.; Deterre, P.; Pfister, C. & Chadre, M. (1985). Fluoroaluminates activate transducin-GDP by mimicking the gamma-phosphate of GTP in its binding site. *FEBS Lett.* Vol. 191, pp.(181-185).

Curran, TM.; Buckley, DH.; & Marquis, RE. (1994). Quasi irreversible inhibition of enolase of Streptococcus mutans by fluoride. *FEMS Microbiol.Lett.* Vol. 119, pp.(283-288).

Cushing, DJ.; Sabouni, MH.; Brown, GL. & Mustafa, SJ. (1990). Fluoride produces endothelium-dependent relaxation and endothelium-independent contraction in coronary artery. *J. Pharm. Exp. Ther.* Vol. 254, pp.(28-32).

Fritchi L, et al. (2003). Respiratory symptoms and lung-function changes with exposure to five substances in aluminium smelters. *INT ARCH OCC ENV HEA.* Vol. 76, No.2, pp.(103-110).

Gandia, F.; Rouatbi, S.; Latiri, I.; Guenard, H. & Tabka, Z.(2010). Inhaled fluoride reverse bronchospasma. *J.Smooth Muscle Res.* Vol.46, No.3, pp.(157-165).

Garcia, JGN.; Dominguez, J. & English, D. (1991). Sodium fluoride induces phosphoinositide hydrolysis, Ca2+ mobilization, and prostacyclin synthesis in cultured human endothelium: Further evidence for regulation by a pertussis toxin-insensitive guanine nucleotide-binding protein. *Am. J. Respir. Cell. Mol. Biol.* Vol. 5, pp.(113-124).

Hattori, Y.; Matsuda, N.; Sato, A.; Watanuki, S.; Tomioka, H.; Kawasaki, H. & Kanno, M. (2000). Predominant contribution of the G protein-mediated mechanism to NaF-induced vascular contractions in diabetic rats: association with an increased level of Gq? expression. *J. Pharmacol. Exp. Ther.* Vol. 292, No.2, pp.(761-768).

Himpens, B.; Missiaen, L.; Droogmans, G. & Casteels, R. (1991). AlF^{-}_4 induces Ca^{2+} oscillations in guinea-pig ileal smooth muscle. *Pflugers Arch-Eur. J. Physiol.* Vol. 417, pp. (645-650).

Hirano, S.; Ando, M. & Kanno, S. (1999). Inflammatory responses of rat alveolar macrophages following exposure to fluoride. *Arch. Toxicol.* 73, pp. (310-315).

Kawase, T. & Van Breemen, C. (1992). Aluminium fluoride induces a reversible Ca^{2+} sensitisation in alpha-toxin-permeabilized vascular smooth muscle. *Eur. J. Pharmacol.* Vol. 214, pp. (39-44).

Kongerud, J. et al. (1994). Aluminum potroom asthma: the Norweigian experience. *EUR RESPIR J.* Vol. 7, No.1, pp.(165-172). ISSN 0903 - 1936

Kongerud, J.& Samuelsen, SO. (1991). A longitudinal study of respiratory symptoms in aluminum potroom workers. *AM REV RESPIR DIS.* Vol. 144, pp.(10-16).

Kongerud, J. (1992). Respiratory disorders in aluminium potroom workers. *Med Lav.* Vol. 83, No.5, pp.(414-417).

Leurs, R.; Bast, A. & Timmerman, H. (1991). Fluoride is a contractile agent of guinea pig airway smooth muscle. *Gen. Pharmacol.* Vol. 22, pp.(631-636).

Li, L. (2003). The biochemistry and physiology of metallic fluoride: action, mechanism, and implications. *Cr Biol. Med.* Vol.14, No. 2, pp.(100-114).

Mayes, P A. (1987). Bioenergetics and Metabolism of Suger and Lipids, In: *Glycolysis and oxidation of pyruvate,* W.W. (Eds), 177-184, Lange Medical, ISBN, San Mateo.

Mullenix, PJ. (2005). Fluoride poisoning: a puzzle with hidden pieces. *Int J Occup Environ Health.* Vol. 11, No.4, pp.(404-414).

Murthy, KS. & Makhlouf, GM. (1994). Fluoride activates G protein dependent and -independent pathways in dispersed intestinal smooth muscle cells. *Biochem. Biophys. Res. Commun.* Vol. 202, pp.(1681-1687).

Murthy, KS.; Grider, JR. & Makhlouf, M. (1992). Receptor-coupled G proteins mediate contraction in isolated intestinal muscle cells. *J. Pharmacol. Exp. Ther.* Vol. 260, pp.(98-97).

Refnes, M.; Becher, R.; Lag, M.; Skuland, T. & Scwaze, PE. (1999). Fluoride-induced interleukine-6 and interleukine-8 synthesis in human epithelial cells. *Hum. Exp. Toxicol.* Vol. 18, pp.(645-652).

Rouatbi, S.; Guandia, F.; Laatiri, I.; Tabka, Z. & Guenard, H. (2010). Inhaled fluoride, magnesium salt and L-arginine reverse bronchospasma. *Drug Test. Analysis.* Vol. 2, (February 2010), pp.(51-54).

Soyseth, V.; Kongerud, J.; Ekstrand, J. & Boe, J. (1994). Relation between exposure to fluoride and bronchial responsiveness in aluminium potroom workers with work-related asthma-like symptoms. *Thorax.* Vol. 49, No.10, pp.(984-989).

Soyseth, V. & Kongerud, J. (1992). Prevalence of respiratory disorders among aluminum potroom workers in relation to exposure to fluoride. *BRIT J IND MED* .Vol. 49, pp.(125-130).

Stadal, JM. & Crook, ST. (1988). Differential effects of fluoride on adenylate cyclase activity and guanine nucleotide regulation of agonist high affinity receptor binding. *Biochem. J.* Vol. 254, pp.(15-20).

Taiwo OA, et al. (2006). Incidence of asthma among aluminium workers. *J OCCUP ENVIRON MED* . Vol.48, No.3, pp.(275-282).

Tatsumi M et al. (1991). Healthy Survey of Workers of an Aluminum Plant in China. Respiratory symptoms and ventilatory functions. *Fluoride.* Vol. 24, No.3, pp.(90-94).

Uzun, O., Demiryurek, AT & Kanzik, I. (2002). Role of G(s) proteins in hypoxic constriction of sheep pulmonary artery rings. *Pharmacology.* Vol. 64, No.4, pp.(214-216).

Viragh E, et al. (2006). Health effects of occupational exposure to fluorine and its compound in a small-scale enterprise. *Industrial Health.* Vol. 44, No.1, pp.(64-68).

Wang, P.; Verin, AD.; Birukova, A.; Gilbert-McClain, L.; Jacobs, K. & Garcia, JGN.(2001). Mechanism of sodium fluoride-induced endothelial cell barrier dysfunction: role of MLC phosphorylation. *Am. J. Physiol.* Vol. 281, No.6, (L1472-L1483).

Weber, LP.; Chow, WL.; Abebe, W. & MacLeod, KM. (1996). Enhanced contractile responses of arteries from streptozotocin diabetic rats to sodium fluoride. *Br. J. Pharmacol.* Vol. 118, pp.(115-122).

Whitford, GM. (1994). Intake and metabolism of fluoride. *Adv Dent Res.* Vol.8, No. 1, pp.(5-14).

Whitford, GM.(1996). *The Metabolism and Toxicity of Fluoride.*(2nd, revised edition), Krager, Paris.

Yamamoto S et al. (2001). Suppression of pulmonary antibacterial defenses mechanisms and lung damage in mice exposed to fluoride aerosol.. *J TOXICOL ENV HEALTH* . Vol. 62, No.6, pp.(485-494).

Zhao, W. & Guenard, H. (1997). The inhibitory effect of fluoride on carbachol-induced bovine bronchial contraction. *RESP PHYSIOL.* Vol. 108, pp.(171-179).

Zhao, W. ; Rouatbi, S. ; Tabka, Z. & Guenard, H. (2002). Inhaled sodium fluoride decreases airway responsiveness to acetylcholine analogs in vivo. *RESP PHYSIOL NEUROBI.* Vol. 131, pp.(245-253).

Part 3

The Management of Asthma – Emerging Treatment Strategies

8

Management of Asthma in Children

Abdulrahman Al Frayh
College of Medicine, King Saud University, Riyadh
Pediatric Allergy and Pulmonology, King Khalid University Hospital, Riyadh
Kingdom of Saudi Arabia

1. Introduction

Asthma is defined as a chronic inflammatory disorder of the lower airways resulting in an obstruction of airflow, which may be completely or partially reversed with or without specific therapy. The inflammation is an interaction between various cells and cytokines. Asthmatic patients have recurrent or persistent bronchospasm, which causes symptoms e.g. wheezing, breathlessness, chest tightness, and cough, particularly at night or after exercise.

Chronic airway inflammation causes bronchial hyperresponsiveness (BHR), which is defined as the inherent tendency of the airways to narrow in response to various stimuli (eg, environmental allergens and irritants).[1]

2. Epidemiology

The prevalence of childhood asthma is 10 times higher in developed countries (UK, US, Australia and New Zealand) than in developing countries. Low income population in urban areas have higher prevalence rate than other groups (ISAAC).[2-6]

Asthma in children accounts for more school absences and more hospitalizations than any other chronic illness and is the most common diagnosis at admission.[7]

300 million individuals worldwide have asthma. Prevalence of asthma is increasing, especially in children. WHO has estimated that 15 million disability-adjusted life-years are lost and 250,000 asthma deaths are reported worldwide.[8]

3. Pathophysiology

The interplay between environment and genetic factors lead to airway inflammation, which result in functional and structural changes in the airways in the form of bronchospasm, mucosal edema, and mucus plugs, which increases resistance to airflow and decreases expiratory flow rates. Although over-distention helps maintain airway patency, and improves expiratory flow; it also alters pulmonary mechanics and increases the work of breathing, resulting ultimately in alveolar hypoventilation.[9]

Changes in airflow resistance, uneven distribution of air, and alterations in circulation (mainly vasoconstriction from increased intra-alveolar pressure due to hyperinflation) lead to ventilation-perfusion mismatch. [10-13]

Patients with acute asthma exacerbations in the **early stages**, have hypoxemia in the absence of carbon dioxide retention, as increases in alveolar ventilation prevents hypercarbia. [14]

If obstruction continues and ventilation-perfusion mismatch worsens, carbon dioxide retention and respiratory alkalosis occur. **Later**, the increased work of breathing, increased oxygen consumption, and increased cardiac output lead to metabolic acidosis. Respiratory failure leads to respiratory acidosis. [15-16]

4. Inflammation of the airways

The inflammatory process in the airways causes increased BHR, which leads to bronchospasm and typical symptoms of wheezing, shortness of breath, and coughing after exposure to allergens, environmental irritants, viruses such as RSV, Rhinovirus a.o., cold air, or exercise. [17]

Lymphocytes play a central role in the pathogenesis of asthma. Airway inflammation may represent a mis-balance between two "opposing" populations of T helper (Th) lymphocytes. Two types of Th lymphocytes have been characterized: Th1 and Th2. Th1 cells produce interleukin (IL)-2 and interferon-a (IFN-a), which are critical in cellular defense mechanisms in response to infection. Th2, in contrast, generates a family of cytokines (interleukin-4 [IL-4], IL-5, ILL6, IL-9, and IL-13) that can mediate allergic inflammation.[18-22]

Cytokines play a key role in orchestrating the chronic inflammation of asthma and other obstructive airways disease recruiting, activating, and promoting the survival of multiple inflammatory cells in the respiratory tract. Cytokines are classified into lymphokines (cytokines that are secreted by T cells and regulate immune responses), proinflammatory cytokines (cytokines that amplify and perpetuate the inflammatory process), growth factors (cytokines that promote cell survival and result in structural changes in the airways), chemokines (cytokines that negatively modulate the inflammatory response).23
Epithelial cells in the airways play an important role in orchestrating the inflammation of asthma through the release of multiple cytokines. Th2 cells orchestrate the inflammatory response in asthma through the release of IL-4 and IL-13 (which stimulate B cells to synthesize IgE), IL-5 (which is necessary for eosinophilic inflammation), and IL-9 (which stimulates mast cell proliferation). Mast celles are thus orchestrated by several interacting cytokines and play an important role in asthma through the release of the bronchoconstrictor mediator histamine, cysteinyl-leukotrienes (Cys-LTs), and PGD2)
Bronchial biopsies from asthmatics show infiltration with eosinophils, activated mast cells, and T cells that are predominantly Th2 cells. There are characteristic structural changes, with collagen deposition under the epithelium (also described as basement membrane thickening) and increased airway smooth muscle as a result of hyperplasia hypertrophy. There is also an increase in the number of blood vessels angiogenesis) as well as mucus hyperplasia.24
In patients with asthma, there is an increase in the number of CD4+ Th cells in the airways, which are predominantly of the Th2 subtype. Th2 cells are characterized by secretion of IL-4, IL-5, IL-9, and IL-13. The transcription factor GATA-binding protein 3(GATA3) is crucial for the differentiation of uncommitted naïve T cells into Th2 cells and regulates the secretion of Th2 cytokines. There is an increase in the number of GATA3+ T cells in the airways of stable asthmatic subjects. Nuclear factor of activated Tcells (NFAT) is a T-cell-specific transcription factor and enhances the transcriptional activation of the IL4 promoter by GATA3. Finally, IL-33, a member of the IL-1 family of cytokines, promotes differentiation of Th2 cells by translocating to the nucleus and regulating transcription through an effect on chromatin structure, but it also acts as a selective chemoattractant of Th2 cells.25
IL-4 plays a critical role in differentiation of Th2 cells from uncommitted Th0 cells and may be important in initial sensitization to allergens. It is also important for isotype switching of B cells from producers of IgG to producers of IgE. IL-12 mimics IL-4 in inducing IgE secretion and causing structural changes in the airways but does not play a role in promoting Th2 cell differentiation.
IL-5 plays a key role in inflammation mediated by eosinophils, since it is critically involved in the differentiation of eosinophils from bone marrow precursor cells and also prolongs eosinophils survival. Systemic and local administration of IL-5 to asthmatic patients results in an increase in circulating eosinophils and CD34+ eosinophil precursors.
The transcription factor T-bet is crucial for the Th1 cell differentiation and secretion of the Th1-type cytokine IFN-γ. Consistent with the prominent role of Th2 cells in asthma, T-bet expression is reduced in T cells from the airways of asthmatic patients compared with airway T cells from nonasthmatic patients.

Type 1 IFNs (IFN-α and IFN-β) and type III IFNs (IFN-λ) play an important role in innate immunity against viral infections, but IFN-β and IFN-λ show reduced expression in epithelial cells of asthmatic patients and are associated with increased rhinovirus replication, which may predispose these patients to viral exacerbations of asthma.

IL-12 plays an important role in differentiating the activating Th1 cells and is produced by activated macrophages, DCs, and airway epithelial cells. IL-12 induces T cells to release IFN-γ, which regulates the expression of IL-12Rβ2 and so maintains the differentiation of Th1 cells, whereas IL-4 suppresses IL-12Rβ2 expression and thus antagonizes Th1 cell differentiation.26

Thymic stromal lymphopoietin. Thymic stromal lymphopoietin (TSLP) is a cytokine belonging to the IL-7 family that shows a marked increase in expression in airway epithelium and mast cells of asthmatic patients. TSLP is released from airway epithelial cells, and its synergistic interaction with IL-1β and TNF-α results in the release of Th2 cytokines from mast cells independently of T cells. TSLP also plays a key role in programming airway DCs to release the Th2 chemoattractants CCL17 and CCL2 and thus is important in recruiting Th2 cells to the airways.

GM-CSF plays role in the differentiation and survival of neutrophils, eosinophils, and macrophages and has been implicated in asthma. Its receptor comprises and α-chain that is specific for the receptor for GM-CSF and a β-chain that is also part of the receptors for IL-3 and IL-5. GM-CSF is secreted predominantly by macrophages, epithelial cells, and T cells in response to inflammatory stimuli. Airway epithelial cells of asthmatic patients strongly express GM-CSF, which may condition DCs to direct Th2 immunity and to prolong the survival of eosinophils.27

Neutrophins are cytokines that play an important role in the function, proliferation, and survival of autonomic nerves. In sensory nerves, neutrophins increase responsiveness and expression of tachykinins. Nerve growth factor (NGF) may be produced by mast cells, lymphocytes, macrophages, and eosinophils as well as structural cells, such as epithelial cells, fibroblasts, and airwy smooth muscle cells.

In recent years more focus on **"the hygiene hypothesis"**, which is in a simplified way, a cytokine imbalance resulting in a dramatic increase in asthma prevalence in Westernized countries. This hypothesis is based on the concept that the immune system of the newborn is skewed toward Th2 cytokine generation (mediators of allergic inflammation). Environmental stimuli such as infections activate Th1 responses and bring the Th1/Th2 relationship to an appropriate balance.[28-30]

A series of epidemiological studies in Europe, Canada, and Australia showed reduced prevalence of asthma and allergy among farmers' children compared to non-farmers' children. Stable visits early in life and consumption or raw cow's milk were suggested as the main factors of the farming environment conferring protection against atopic diseases. These results have been seen as an extension of the 'hygiene hypothesis', since a farm environment provides an enormous habitat for microorganisms.

Pattern-recognition receptors (RPR) of the innate immune system, such as toll-like receptors (TLR) or CD14, recognize LPS (lipopolysaccharide), a component of the outer membrane of gram-negative bacteria, and other nonviable environmental compounds. Activation of PRR signaling pathways initiates regulatory mechanisms which in turn modulate the adaptive immune response. Interestingly, recently it has been shown that farmers' children express higher levels of PRR than children from non-farming families suggesting that innate immune mechanisms are involved in the allergy-protective effect of the farming environment.

For various genetic loci, i.a. the CD14 an association with the occurrence of atopic diseases have been described. However, studies investigating the same genetic variants in other populations often failed to reproduce the original results.

Gene environment interactions have been found for several genetic polymorphisms in PRR genes.

Several studies indicated higher gene expression of CD14,TLR 2, and TLR4 in farmers' children compared to non-farmers' children. Mainly prenatal factors accounted for these differences. Expression of CD14, TLR2, TLR4 with the number of farm animal species the mother had contact with during pregnancy, which probably serves as proxy for an increasing variation in microbial exposure. Children of mothers who worked on the farm during pregnancy were less sensitized at school age to common inhalant and food allergens than children of unexposed mothers. However development of clinical symptoms of atopic disease seemed to depend on exposures that occurred postnatally.[33]

Evidence suggests that the prevalence of asthma is less in children who experience:

- Less frequent use of antibiotics
- Exposure to other children (eg, presence of older siblings and early enrollment in childcare)
- Rural living
- Certain infections (Mycobacterium tuberculosis, measles, or hepatitis A)

On the contrary, the absence of these lifestyle events is associated with the persistence of a Th2 cytokine pattern (Allergy).

The genetic background of a child, with a cytokine imbalance toward Th2, sets the stage to promote the production of immunoglobulin E (lgE) antibody to key environmental antigens (e.g., cockroaches, dust mites, cats and alternaria). Therefore, a gene-by-environment interaction occurs in which the susceptible host is exposed to environmental factors that are capable of generating IgE, and sensitization.[34]

Allergic inflammation may be the result of an excessive expression of Th2 cytokines. Recent studies have suggested the possibility that the loss of normal immune balance arises from a cytokine dysregulation in which Th1 activity in asthma is diminished .

5. Genetic factors and asthma

Recent research studies have identified phenotypes (clusters) of genes which could predispose individuals to asthma. Cluster 1 patients have early-onset atopic asthma and preserved lung function but increased medication requirements (29% on three or more medications) and health care utilization. [35]

Genetic Factors

Genome-wide linkage studies and case-control studies have identified 18 genomic regions and more than 100 genes associated with allergy and asthma in 11 different populations. A recent genome-wide association study identified a new gene, ORMDL3, that exhibited a highly significantly association with asthma ($p < 10\text{-}12$) (for single nucleotide polymorphism rs8067378, odds ratio 1.84, 95% confidence interval 1.43-2.42) a finding that has now been replicated in several populations.

Several studies identified candidate genes in a pathway that initiates type 2 helper T-cell (Th2) inflammation in response to epithelial damage and points to other candidate genes that may act in a pathway that down-regulates airway inflammation and remodeling. Our study also shows that asthma is heterogeneous: later-onset cases are influenced more by the MHC (major histocompatibility complex) than are childhood-onset cases. There is a strong and specific effect of the chromosome 17q locus on childhood-onset disease.[37]

SNPs at the chromosome 17q21 locus associated with asthma are also strongly associated with variation in the expression of ORMDL3 and GSDMB.

There is an association between SNPs flanking IL33 on chromosome 9 and atopic asthma. [38]

The locus chromosome at 2, implicating 1L1RL1 and IL 18R1 is also associated with asthma. The effect at this locus has been attributed to IL 1RL1 (encoding the receptor for interleukin) [6] and synergizes with IL 12 to induce the production of interferon-y and to promote Th1 responses. The expression of IL 18R1 is also concentrated within the respiratory epithelium.[39]

SMAD3 is a transcriptional modulator activated by transforming growth factor β, a polypeptide that controls proliferation, differentiation, and other functions in many cell types, including regulatory T cells. [40]

HLA-DQ was the first identified asthma susceptibility locus. Extended haplotypes encompassing HLA-DQ and HLA-DR have been studied for their effects on specific allergen sensitization and on the formation of tumor necrosis factor and related gene products.

Two other genes, SLC22A5 and RORA. SLC22A5 encodes a carnitine transporter and, like ORMDL3/GSDMB and IL18R1/IL1RL1.[41]

Cluster 2 comprises mostly older obese women with late-onset non-atopic asthma, moderate reductions in pulmonary function, and frequent oral corticosteroid use to manage exacerbations. Cluster 3 and cluster 4 patients have severe airflow obstruction with bronchodilator responsiveness but differ in to their ability to attain normal lung function, age of asthma onset, atopic status, and use of oral corticosteroids. [36]

6. Specific and non-specific triggers

Specific immune-response to triggers entails 2 types of bronchoconstrictor responses to allergens: early and late. [42]

Early asthmatic responses occur via IgE-induced mediator release from mast cells within minutes of exposure and last for 20-30 minutes. [43-45]

William et al found an increase rates of sensitization to indoor and outdoor aeroallergens throughout childhood. He also found different aeroallergens to be prominent at different ages. For example, dogs and cats were the most likely sensitizers in children younger than 4, whereas dust mites and trees were the most prominent in older children and adolescents.[46]
There was a relatively high rate of tree sensitization in the children less than 4 years of age.
The same study found that 57.2% of the referred patients who under SPT were sensitized to at least 1 of the studied aeroallergens, 51.3% of patients were sensitized to at least 1 indoor aeroallergen, and 38% were sensitized to at least 1 outdoor aeroallergen.[47-49]
Cat, dogs, and dust mites are the predominant sensitizers in younger children, whereas trees and dust mites are the most prevalent sensitizers in older children and adolescents. In contrast to grass and ragweed tree sensitization is much more common than expected in very young children.[50]

Late asthmatic responses occur 4-12 hours after antigen exposure and result in more severe symptoms that can last for hours and contribute to the duration and severity of the disease. Inflammatory cell infiltration and inflammatory mediators play a role in the late asthmatic response. Allergens can be foods, household inhalants (eg, animal allergens, molds, fungi, cockroach allergens, dust mites), or seasonal outdoor allergens (eg, mold spores, pollens, grass, trees).

Non-specific response e.g. tobacco smoke, cold air, chemicals, perfumes, paint odors, hair sprays, air pollutants, and ozone can initiate BHR by inducing inflammation. [9]

Sudden changes in ambient temperature, barometric pressure, and the quality of air (eg, humidity, allergen and irritant content) can also induce asthma exacerbations.[10]

Exercise can trigger an early asthmatic response. Different mechanisms are hypothesized to play a role. Heat and water loss from the airways can increase the osillolarity of the fluid lining the airways and result in mediator release. Cooling of the airways results in congestion and dilatation of bronchial vessels. During the rewarming phase after exercise, the changes are magnified because the ambient air breathed during recovery is warm rather than cool.

Emotional factors are sometimes incriminate to trigger asthma exacerbation (stress, emotional upsets a.o.)

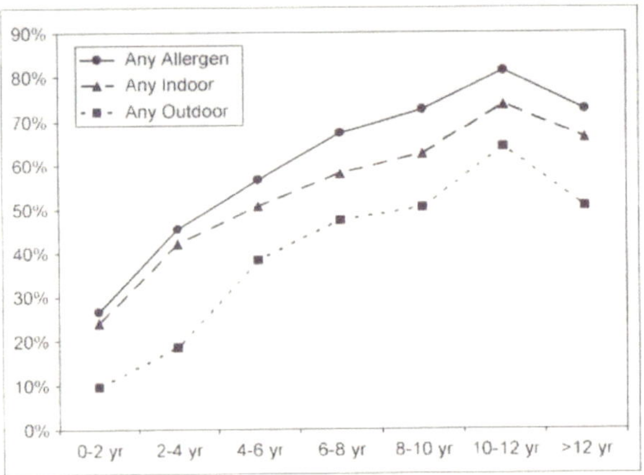

Figure 1. Age-specific prevalence of sensitization[a]
▲, Sensitization to at least 1 of the aeroallergens studied; •, sensitization to at least 1 of the indoor aeroallergens (cats, dogs, dust mites, mice, cockroaches); ■, sensitization to at least 1 of the outdoor aeroallergens (trees, grass, ragweed).

Table 2. Prevalence of Positive Skin Prick Test for Each Allergen (All Ages)[a]

	Indoor Allergens					Outdoor Allergens		
Age (years)	Mice	Roaches	Dogs	Cats	Mites	Trees	Grass	Weeds
0-2	3.2 (93)	3.6 (138)	15.5 (174)	9.2 (174)	8.2 (195)	7.8 (103)	1.0 (98)	1.0 (97)
2-4	8.1 (235)	10.9 (239)	21.0 (271)	22.5 (267)	22.3 (287)	17.1 (252)	2.8 (246)	5.7 (245)
4-6	8.3 (206)	8.8 (205)	25.0 (216)	33.3 (222)	37.2 (231)	35.3 (221)	9.3 (215)	17.9 (218)
6-8	10.9 (184)	14.2 (183)	31.1 (190)	37.0 (189)	41.9 (191)	46.6 (191)	10.1 (189)	20.9 (187)
8-10	5.6 (142)	15.8 (139)	28.4 (148)	41.1 (146)	47.9 (140)	46.6 (148)	19.6 (143)	23.6 (144)
10-12	13.5 (111)	19.8 (111)	26.5 (113)	48.2 (110)	53.1 (113)	56.4 (110)	28.8 (111)	34.2 (111)
>12	10.4 (182)	22.2 (180)	23.0 (187)	38.5 (187)	56.8 (185)	45.2 (188)	21.7 (184)	24.3 (185)
Total	8.8 (1153)	13.3 (1195)	24.0 (1299)	31.3 (1295)	35.6 (1342)	35.8 (1213)	12.4 (1186)	17.7 (1187)

7. Gastroesophageal reflux

The presence of acid in the distal esophagus, mediated via vagal or other neural reflexes, can significantly increase airway resistance and airway reactivity.

8. Upper respiratory tract: conditions

Inflammatory conditions of the upper airways (eg, allergic rhinitis, sinusitis, or chronic and persistent infections) must be treated before asthmatic symptoms can be completely controlled.

9. Circadian rhythm

Circadian variation in lung function and inflammatory mediator release in the circulation and airways (including parenchyma) have been demonstrated to explain nocturnal asthma. Other factors, such as allergen exposure and posture-related irritation of airways (eg, gastroesophageal reflux, sinusitis), can also play a role. In some cases, abnormalities in CNS control of the respiratory drive may be present, particularly in patients with a defective hypoxic drive and obstructive sleep apnea. [51]

It is well known that there is a circadian variation in asthma severity and exacerbation.
Wheezing, cough and dyspnea are worse during the late night and early morning hours[3]. Most dyspneic episodes occurring nocturnally, with a 50-fold increase in the number of attacks between 4 am and 5 am compared with the number of attacks between 4 pm and 5 pm.[4] Objective indicators of disease severity correlate closely with subjective dyspnea PEFR begins declining rapidly at midnight, and at 4 am is between 8% and 40% below its mean 24-hour value at 9 am. The PEFR then increases sharply and reaches its mean 24 hour value at 8 am.[5] Normal subjects also show circadian changes in airflow, with mild nocturnal bronchoconstriction, although the variation is far less pronounced than that seen in asthmatic subjects.[52]
The pathophysiology of nocturnal asthma exacerbation is not completely understood and appears to be multifactorial. Plasma cortisol levels vary markedly, reaching a nadir at midnight and peaking at 8 am. Serum histamine levels peak dramatically at about 4 am, dropping to baseline levels by 8 am. Plasma cyclic AMP(cAMP) levels reaches a nadir at 4 am, as do the density and responsiveness of beta-adrenergic receptors located on circulating leukocytes. A nocturnal increase in vagal tone has been described. All of these factors appear to play a role in destabilizing the inflammatory environment of the airways at night. Additionally, sleep-induced oxygen dessaturation, gastroesophageal reflux, and body temperature decline during sleep may all predispose to nocturnal airway hyperresponsiveness.[55-53]
The circadian nature of asthma has led to the argument that nocturnal presentation of asthma is marker of more severe disease, warranting more aggressive therapy and lower threshold for hospitalization than for other asthmatic patients. Data demonstrating increased asthma mortality between midnight and 4 am, although limited to inpatient settings, appear to support this argument. However, some studies of asthmatic patients in the emergency department failed to validate this hypothesis. Several studies however demonstrate no significant disease severity between asthmatic patients who presented during late night/early-morning hours.[58-56]

10. Asthma outcome

Children with mild asthma who are asymptomatic between attacks are likely to improve and be symptom-free later in life.

Children with asthma appear to have less severe symptoms as they enter adolescence, but half of these children continue to have asthma. Asthma has a tendency to remit during puberty, with a somewhat earlier remission in girls. However, compared with men, women have more BHR. [59]

Of infants who wheeze with URTIs, 60% are asymptomatic by age 6 years. However, children who have asthma (recurrent symptoms continuing at age 6 years) have airway reactivity later in childhood. Some findings suggest a poor prognosis if asthma develops in children younger than 3 years, unless it occurs solely in association with viral infections. [60-62]

Individuals who have asthma during childhood have significantly lower forced expiratory volume in 1 second (FEV1), higher airway reactivity, and more persistent bronchospastic symptoms than those with infection-associated wheezing.

11. Patient education

11.1 Pediatrician and/or asthma educator should instruct

Patient and parent on how to use medications and devices (eg, spacers, nebulizers, metered-dose inhalers [MDls]). The patient's MOl technique should be assessed on every visit.[63]

Instruction should also includes the use of medications, precautions with drug and/or device usage, monitoring symptoms and their severity (peak flow meter reading), and identifying potential adverse effects and necessary actions. [64]

Parents should understand that asthma is a chronic disorder with acute exacerbations; hence, continuity of management with active participation by the patient and/or parents and interaction with asthma care medical personnel is important. Adherence to treatment is the key to full control of symptoms including nocturnal and exercise-induced symptoms. Emphasize the importance of adherence to treatment.[65]

Parents caregiver and teachers should expect the child to participate in recreational activities and sports and to attend school as usual. [66]

12. Differential diagnoses

12.1 Problems to be considered include the following

- Vascular ring
- Vocal cord dysfunction
- Tracheobronchomalacia
- Pulmonary edema
- Gastroesophageal Reflux
- Bronchopulmonary Dysplasia
- Bronchiectasis
- Aspiration Syndromes
- Airway Foreign Body
- Allergic Rhinitis
- Aspergillosis
- Cystic Fibrosis
- Primary Ciliary Dyskinesia [67]

13. Clinical presentation

13.1 History is very important in asthma the clinician should confirm

- Airflow obstruction or symptoms are at least partially reversible
- Episodic symptoms of airflow obstruction are present
- Alternative diagnoses are excluded

Obtaining a good patient history is crucial when diagnosing asthma and excluding other causes, symptoms, aggravating factors and co-existing conditions should be asked.

- Shortness of breath
- Cough
- Wheezing
- Cough at night or with exercise
- Chest tightness
- Sputum production
- Onset and duration
- Perennial, seasonal, or both
- Daytime or nighttime

- Continuous or intermittent
- Exercise
- Viral infections
- Irritants (eg, smoke exposure, chemicals, vapors, dust)
- Environmental allergens
- Changes in weather
- Emotions
- Stress
- Foods
- Home environment (eg, carpets, pets, mold)
- Drugs (eg, aspirin, beta blockers)
- Rhinitis
- Sinusitis
- Gastroesophageal reflux disease (GERD)
- Thyroid disease

Vascular rings are unusual congenital anomalies that occur early in the development of the aortic arch and great vessels. The primary symptomatology associated with vascular rings relates to the structure that are encircled by the ring, chiefly the trachea, large airways and esophagus.

PERINATAL AND FAMILY HISTORY	POSSIBLE DIAGNOSIS
Symptoms present from birth or perinatal lung problem	Cystic fibrosis; chronic lung disease of prematurity; ciliary dyskinesia; developmental anomal
Family history of unusual chest disease	Cystic fibrosis; neuromuscular disorder
Severe upper respiratory tract disease	Defect of host defence; ciliary dyskinesia
Symptoms and signs	
Persistent moist cough	Cystic fibrosis; bronchiectasis; protracted bronchitis; recurrent aspiration; host defence disorder; ciliary dyskinesia
Excessive vomiting	Gastroesophageal reflux (+-aspiration)
Dysphagia	Swallowing problems (+- aspiration)
Breathlessness with light-headedness and peripheral tingling	Hyperventilation/panic attacks
Inspiratory stridor	Tracheal or laryngeal disorder
Abnormal voice or cry	Laryngeal problem
Focal signs in chest	Developmental anomaly; post-infective syndrome; bronchiectasis; tuberculosis
Finger clubbing	Cystic fibrosis; bronchiectasis
Failure to thrive	Cystic fibrosis; host defense disorder; gastroesophageal
Other conditions	
Transient infant wheezing	Onset in infancy; no associated atopy associated with parental smoking
Inhaled foreign body	Suddent onset

Differential Diagnosis of Asthma in Children 5 years and younger
Infections: • Recurrent Respiratory tract infections • Chronic rhino-sinusitis • Tuberculosis. Congenital problems: • Tracheomalacia • Cystic Fibrosis • Bronchopulmonary dysplasia • Congenital malformation causing narrowing of the intratoracic airways. • Primary ciliary dyskinesia syndrome • Immune deficiency • Congenital heart disease Mechanical Problems • Foreign body aspiration • Gastroesophageal reflux *Adopted from GINA Guide 2011*

The family history should include any history of asthma, allergy, sinusitis, rhinitis, eczema, or nasal polyps in close relatives, and the social history should cover factors that may contribute to non adherence of asthma medications, as well as any illicit drug use.[68-72]

Physical findings vary with the absence or presence of an acute episode and its severity.

A patient with mild asthma may have normal findings on physical examination. Patients with more severe asthma are likely to have signs of chronic respiratory distress and chronic hyperinflation.

Signs of atopy or allergic rhinitis, such as conjunctival congestion and inflammation, allergic shiners, a transverse crease on the nose due to constant rubbing associated with allergic rhinitis, and pale nasal mucosa covered with transparent mucus due to allergic rhinitis, may be present.

The anteroposterior diameter of the chest may be increased because of hyperinflation. Hyperinflation may also cause an abdominal breathing pattern.

Lung examination may reveal prolonged expiratory phase, expiratory wheezing, coarse crackles, or unequal breath sounds.

Clubbing of the fingers is not a usual feature of asthma and indicates a need for more extensive evaluation and work-up to exclude other conditions, such as cystic fibrosis. [73-77]

A child with an acute episode may reveal different findings in mild, moderately severe, and severe episodes and in status asthmaticus with imminent respiratory arrest.

13.2 Mild episode asthma reveals

- Accessory muscles of respiration are not used
- Increased respiratory rate

- The heart rate is less than 100 beats per minute
- Auscultation of chest reveals moderate wheezing, which is often end expiratory
- Pulsus paradoxus is not present
- Oxyhemoglobin saturation with room air is greater than 95%

13.3 Moderately severe asthma include the following

- Increased respiratory rate
- Accessory muscles of respiration typically are used
- Suprasternal retractions are present
- The heart rate is 100-120 beats per minute
- Loud expiratory wheezing can be heard
- Pulsus paradoxus may be present (10-20 mm Hg)
- Oxyhemoglobin saturation with room air is 91-95%

13.4 Severe asthma include the following:

- The respiratory rate is often greater than 30 breaths per minute
- Accessory muscles of respiration are usually used
- Suprasternal retractions are commonly present
- The heart rate is greater than 120 beats per minute
- Loud biphasic (expiratory and inspiratory) wheezing can be heard
- Pulsus paradoxus is often present (20-40 mm Hg)
- Oxyhemoglobin saturation with room air is less than 91 %.

13.5 Status asthmaticus may include the following

- Paradoxical thoracoabaominal movement
- Wheezing may be absent (in patients with the most severe airway obstruction)
- Severe hypoxemia may manifest as bradycardia
- Pulsus paradoxus may disappear; this finding suggests respiratory muscle fatigue

14. Workup

Spirometry is indicated in children >6 years, as younger children < 6 years are unable to perform spirometry, unless modern techniques such as measurement of airway resistance using oscillometry is applied.

In a typical case, an obstructive defect is present in the form of normal forced vital capacity (FVC), reduced forced expiratory volume in 1 second (FEV1), and reduced forced expiratory flow more than 25-75% of the FVC (FEF 25-75). The flow-volume loop can be concave. Documentation of reversibility of airway obstruction after bronchodilator therapy is essential to the definition of asthma. FEF 25-75 is a sensitive indicator of obstruction and may be the only abnormality in a child with mild disease.

In an outpatient or office setting, measurement of the peak flow rate by using a peak flow meter can provide useful information about obstruction in the large airways.

	Daytime symptoms between exacerbations	Night-time symptoms between exacerbations	Exacerbations	PEF or FEV1*	PEF variability**
Infrequent intermittent	Nil	Nil	Brief Mild Occur less than every 4-6 weeks	More than 80% predicted	Less than 20%
Frequent intermittent	Nil	Nil	More than 2 per month	At least 80% predicted	Less than 20%
Mild persistent	More than once per week but not every day	More than twice per month but not every week	May affect activity and sleep	At least 80% predicted	20%-30%
Moderate persistent	Daily	More than once per week	At least twice per week Restricts activity or affects sleep	60%-80% predicted	More than 30%
Severe presistent	Continual	Frequent	Frequent restricts activity	60% predicted or less	More than 30%
ADAPTED GINA 2008					

An individual's asthma pattern (infrequent intermittent, frequent intermittent, mild persistent, moderate persistent or severe persistent) is determined by the level of the table that corresponds to the most severe feature present. Other features associated with that pattern need not be present.
*Predicted values are based on age, sex, and height.
*Difference between morning and evening values.
FEV_1: Forced expiratory volume in 1 second: PEF: Peak expiratory flow.

15. Plethysmography

Patients with chronic persistent asthma may have hyperinflation, as evidenced by an increased total lung capacity (TLC) at plethysmography. Increased residual volume (RV) and functional residual capacity (FRC) with normal TLC suggests air trapping. Airway resistance is increased when significant obstruction is present.

16. Bronchial provocation tests

Bronchial provocation tests may be performed to diagnose bronchial hyper-responsiveness (BHR). These tests are performed in specialized laboratories by specially trained personnel to document airway hyper-responsiveness to substances (eg, methacholine, histamine). Increasing doses of provocation agents are given, and FEV1 is measured. The endpoint is a 20% decrease in FEV1 (PD20).[90-92]

17. Exercise challenge

In a patient with a history of exercise-induced symptoms (eg, cough, wheeze, chest tightness or pain), the diagnosis of asthma can be confirmed with the exercise challenge. In children >6 years old, the procedure involves baseline spirometry followed by exercise on a treadmill or bicycle to a heart rate greater than 60% of the predicted maximum, with monitoring of the electrocardiogram and oxyhemoglobin saturation.93

Spirographic findings and the peak expiratory flow (PEF) rate (PEFR) are determined immediately after the exercise period and at 3 minutes, 5 minutes, 10 minutes, 15 minutes, and 20 minutes after the first measurement. The maximal decrease in lung function is calculated by using the lowest post-exercise and highest pre -exercise values. The reversibility of airway obstruction can be assessed by administering aerosolized bronchodilators.94-95

18. Chest X-ray

Chest X-ray is indicated in the initial work-up of asthmatic patients. Typical findings are hyperinflation and increased bronchial markings, a chest radiograph may reveal evidence of parenchymal disease, atelectasis, pneumonia, congenital anomaly, or a foreign body.

In a patient with an acute asthmatic episode that responds poorly to therapy, a chest radiograph helps in the diagnosis of complications such as pneumothorax or pneumomediastinum.

19. Paranasal sinus and CT scanning

Consider sinus radiography and CT scanning to rule out sinusitis, co-existing with allergic rhinitis and asthma.

20. Blood testing

CBC, Eosinophil counts, total IgE and RAST may be useful when allergic factors are suspected.

21. Skin prick test

Allergy testing can be used to identify allergic factors that may significantly contribute to the asthma. Once identified, environmental factors (eg, dust mites, cockroaches, molds, animal dander) and outdoor factors (eg, pollen, grass, trees, molds) may be controlled or avoided to reduce asthmatic symptoms.

Allergens for skin testing are selected on the basis of suspected or known allergens identified from a detailed environmental history. Antihistamines can suppress the skin test results and should be discontinued for an appropriate period (according to the particular agent's duration of action) before allergy testing. Topical or systemic corticosteroids do not affect the skin reaction.

22. Fraction of Exhaled Nitric Oxide testing

Measuring the fraction of exhaled nitric oxide (FeNO) has proved useful as a non-invasive marker of airway inflammation, in order to guide adjustment of the dose of inhaled corticosteroids. [96-98]

23. Histologic findings

Asthma is an inflammatory disease characterized by inflammatory cells, vascular congestion, increased vascular permeability, increased tissue volume, and the presence of an exudate.

Eosinophilic infiltration, a universal finding, is considered a major marker of the inflammatory activity of the disease.

Histologic evaluations of the airways in a typical patient reveal infiltration with inflammatory cells, narrowing of airway lumina, bronchial and bronchiolar epithelial denudation, and mucus plugs. [99-104]

Additionally, a patient with severe asthma may have a markedly thickened basement membrane and airway remodeling in the form of subepithelial fibrosis and smooth muscle hypertrophy or hyperplasia.

24. Management

24.1 Goal for therapy

- Control asthma by reducing impairment through prevention of chronic and troublesome symptoms (eg, coughing or breathlessness in the daytime, in the night, or after exertion)
- Maintain near-normal pulmonary function
- Maintain normal activity levels (including exercise and other physical activity and attendance at work or school)
- Reduce the need for a short-acting beta2-agonist (SABA) for quick relief of symptoms (not including prevention of exercise-induced bronchospasm)
- Satisfy patients' and families' expectations for asthma care105

Reduction in risk can be achieved by preventing recurrent exacerbations of asthma and minimizing the need for emergency room visits and hospitalizations, and preventing progressive loss of lung growth and function providing optimal pharmacotherapy with minimal or no adverse effects is important.

24.2 Pharmacologic treatment

Pharmacologic management includes the use of agents for control and agents for relief. Control agents include inhaled corticosteroids, inhaled cromolyn or nedocromil, long acting bronchodilators, theophylline, leukotriene modifiers, and more recent strategies such as the use of anti-immunoglobulin E (lgE) antibodies (omalizumab). Relief medications include short-acting bronchodilators, systemic corticosteroids, and ipratropium.[106-107]

For all but the most severely affected patients, the ultimate goal is to prevent symptoms, minimize morbidity from acute episodes, and prevent functional and psychological morbidity to provide a healthy (or near healthy) lifestyle appropriate to the age of child. 108

A stepwise approach to pharmacologic therapy is recommended to gain and maintain control of asthma in both the impairment and risk domains. The type, amount, and scheduling of medication is dictated by asthma severity (for initiating therapy) and the level of asthma control (for adjusting therapy). Step-down therapy is essential to identify the minimum medication necessary to maintain control. See table below.

For pharmacotherapy, children with asthma are divided into 3 groups based on age: 0-4 y, 5-11 y, 12 Y and older.[109]

For all patients, quick-relief medications include rapid-acting beta2-agonists as needed for symptoms. The intensity of treatment depends on the severity of symptoms. If rapid acting beta2-agonists are used more than 2 days a week for symptom relief (not including use of rapid-acting beta2-agonists for prevention of exercise induce symptoms), stepping up treatment may be considered. See the stepwise approach to asthma medications in Table 1, below.

	Intermittent Asthma	**Persistent Asthma: Daily Medication**				
Age	Step 1	Step 2	Step 3	Step 4	Step 5	Step 6
< 5 y	Rapid-acting beta2-agonist prn	Low-dose inhaled corticosteroid (ICS) Alternate regimen: cromolyn or montelukast	Medium-dose ICS	Medium-dose ICS plus either long-acting beta2-agonist (LABA) or montelukast	High-dose ICS plus either LABA or montelukast	High-dose ICS plus either LABA or montelukast; Oral systemic corticosteroid
5-11 y	Rapid-acting beta2-agonist prn	Low-dose ICS Alternate regimen: cromolyn, leukotriene receptor antagonist (LTRA), or theophylline	Either low-dose ICS plus either LABA, LTRA, or theophylline OR Medium-dose	Medium-dose ICS plus LABA Alternate regimen: medium-dose ICS plus either LTRA or theophylline	High-dose ICS plus LABA Alternate regimen: high-dose ICS plus either LABA or theophylline	High-dose ICS plus LABA plus oral systemic corticosteroid Alternate regimen: high-dose ICS plus LRTA or theophylline plus systemic corticosteroid
12 y or older	Rapid-acting beta2-agonist as needed	Low-dose ICS Alternate regimen: cromolyn, LTRA, or theophylline	Low-dose ICS plus LABA OR Medium-dose ICS Alternate regimen: low-dose ICS plus either LTRA, theophylline, or zileuton	Medium-dose ICS plus LABA Alternate regimen: medium-dose ICS plus either LTRA, theophylline, or zileuton	High-dose ICS plus LABA (and consider omalizumab for patients with allergies)	High-dose ICS plus either LABA plus oral corticosteroid (and consider omalizumab for patients with allergies)

Table 1. Stepwise Approach to Asthma Medications

In the Salmeterol Multicenter Asthma Research Trial (SMART), salmeterol use in asthma patients, particularly African Americans, was associated with a small but significantly increased risk of serious asthma-related events. This trial was a large, double-blind, randomized, placebo-controlled, safety trial in which salmeterol 42 mcg twice daily or placebo was added to usual asthma therapy for 28 weeks. [110]

The study was halted following interim analysis of 26,355 participants because patients exposed to salmeterol (n = 13,176) were found to experience a higher rate of fatal asthma events compared with individuals receiving placebo (n = 13,179); the rates were 0.1 % and 0.02%, respectively. This resulted in an estimated 8 excess deaths per 10,000 patients treated with salmeterol. 111

In the post-hoc subgroup analysis, the relative risks of asthma-related deaths were similar among whites and blacks, although the corresponding estimated excess deaths per 10,000 patients exposed to salmeterol were higher among blacks than whites.

A meta-analysis by Salpeter et al found that LABAs increased the risk for asthma related intubations and deaths by 2-fold, even when used in a controlled fashion with concomitant inhaled corticosteroids. However, the absolute number of adverse events remained small. The large pooled trial included 36,588 patients, most of them adults. 112

The US Food and Drug Administration (FDA) has reviewed the data and the issues and has determined that the benefits of LABAs in improving asthma symptoms outweigh the potential risks when LABAs are used appropriately with an asthma controller medication in patients who need the addition of LABAs. The FDA recommends the following measures for improving the safe use of these drugs :

- LABAs should be used long-term only in patients whose asthma cannot be adequately controlled on inhaled steroids 113
- LABAs should be used for the shortest duration of time required to achieve control of asthma symptoms and discontinued, if possible, once asthma control is achieved; patients should then be switched to an asthma controller medication
- Pediatric and adolescent patients who require the addition of a LABA to an inhaled corticosteroid should use a combination product containing both an inhaled corticosteroid and a LABA to ensure compliance with both medications

Concerns about the safety of long-acting beta2-agonists and resultant drug safety communications create a question as to the course of treatment if asthma is not controlled by inhaled corticosteroidsY4] A study by Lemanske et al addressed this question and concluded that addition of long-acting beta2-agonist was more likely to provide the best response than either inhaled corticosteroids or leukotriene-receptor antagonists. Asthma therapy should be regularly monitored and adjusted accordingly.

A systematic review of 18 placebo-controlled clinical trials evaluating monotherapy with inhaled corticosteroids supports their safety and efficacy in children with asthma. In addition, the data provide new evidence linking inhaled corticosteroids use in children with asthma to improved asthma control. A recent study to assess the effectiveness of an inhaled corticosteroid used as rescue treatment recommends that children with mild persistent asthma should not be treated with rescue albuterol alone and the most effective treatment to prevent exacerbations is daily inhaled corticosteroids. This study suggests that inhaled corticosteroids as rescue medication with albuterol might be an effective step down strategy, for children as it is more effective at reducing exacerbations than is use of rescue albuterol alone. A recent Cochrane review concluded that more research is needed to assess the effectiveness of increased inhaled corticosteroid doses at the onset of asthma exacerbation]

In children, long-term use of high-dose steroids (systemic or inhaled) may lead to adverse effects, including growth failure. Recent data from the Childhood Asthma Management Program (CAMP) study and results of the long-term use of inhaled steroids (budesonide) suggest that the long-term use of inhaled steroids has no sustained adverse effect on growth in children. 114-116

Low Daily Doses of Inhaled Glucocorticosteroids for Children 5 years and younger	
Drug	Low Daily Dose (µg)
Beclomethasone dipropianate	100
Budesonide MDI+spacer	200
Budesonide nebulized	500
Fluticasone propionate	100

GINA Guidelines

Omalizumab is a recombinant humanized IgG1 monoclonal anti-IgE antibody that binds to the IgE molecule at the same epitope on the Fc region that binds to FcεRL, Omalizumab binds to circulating IgE regardless of allergen specificity, forming small, biologically inert IgE-anti-IgE complexes without activating the complement cascade. An 89 to 99 percent reduction in free serum IgE (i.e., IgE not bound to Omalizumab) occurs soon after the administration of omalizumab and low levels persist throughout treatment with appropriate doses. Proof-of-concept studies have shown that Omalizumab reduces both early-and late –phase asthmatic responses after allergen inhalation challenge, has a marked effect on late-phase as compared with early-phase skin responses, decreases eosinophil numbers in sputum and submucosal bronchial specimens and also down-regulates FcεRI on basophils, mast cells, and dendritic cells. A reduction in the expression of FcεRI on basophils and mast cells decreases the binding of circulating IgE, thus, preventing the release of inflammatory mediators. A reduction in the expression of FcεRI on dendritic cells may decrease allergen processing.

Several randomized, double-blind clinical trials compared omalizumab, administered subcutaneously, with placebo.

These trials demonstrated a clinical benefit from Omalizumab, although the specific findings varied. Three of the trials evaluated patients with moderate-t0-severe persistent asthma (requiring doses of inhaled bleclomethasone, or its equivalent, ranging from 168-1200 µg per day). Two of these tree trials included adolescents and adults, and one was a study of children 6-12 years of age. Treatment with Omalizumab as compared with placebo was associated with significantly fewer exacerbations of asthma per patient, and a significantly lower percentage of patients had an exacerbation, the dose of inhaled corticosteroids required to control symptoms was significantly less among patients treated with Omalizumab than among those who received placebo.

A review by Rodrigo et al looked at 8 studies of omalizumab in children with moderateeto-severe asthma and elevated IgE levels. Children treated with omalizumab were more significantly able to reduce their use of rescue inhalers and their inhaled and/or oral steroid dose than patients in the placebo group. Although no significant differences in pulmonary function were observed, patients receiving omalizumab had fewer exacerbations than the children receiving placebo. These studies lasted a year or less and did not reveal any significant adverse effects of the omalizumab.

Clinical Use

The role of Omalizumab in the management of asthma has not yet been precisely defined. Patients with persistent asthma (defined as asthma with symptoms that occur more than two days a week or nocturnal symptoms that occur more than twice a month) have several treatment options in addition to the use of inhaled β-adrenergic agonist. These include environmental control (i.e., the elimination or minimization of exposure to aeroallergens), pharmacologic control (i.e., the use of inhaled corticosteroids, leukotriene modifiers, or both), and possibly, immunologic control (i.e., immunotherapy for relevant antigens). In addition, evaluation for coexisting conditions such as allergic rhinitis, sinusitis, and gastroesophageal reflux disease may prove beneficial.

Patients who are particularly likely to benefit from the use of Omalizumab include those with evidence of sensitization to perennial aeroallergens who require high doses of inhaled corticosteroids that have a potential for adverse side effects, those with frequent exacerbations of asthma associated with unstable disease and possibly, those with severe symptoms related in part to poor adherence to daily medication. Analysis of pooled data from published clinical trials have indicated that patients who had a response to Omalizumab had a ration of observed to expected forced expiratory volume in one second (FEV1) of less than 65 percent, were taking doses of inhaled corticosteroids equivalent to more than 800 μg of beclomethasone dipropionate per day, and had at least one visit to the emergency department in the past year. Patients requiring daily oral corticosteroids to control their stamina may be less likely to have response to Omalizumab.

A total serum IgE level should be measured in all patients who are being considered for treatment with Omalizumab, because the dose of Omalizumab is determined on the basis of the IgE level and body weight. The recommended dose is 0.016 mg per kilogram of body weight per international unit of IgE every four weeks, administered subcutaneously at either two-week or four-week intervals. This dose is based on the estimated amount of drug that is required to reduce circulating free IgE levels to less than 10 IU per milliliter.

Monitoring of total serum IgE levels during the course of therapy with Omalizumab is not indicated, because these levels will be elevated as a result of the presence of circulating IgE-anti-IgE complexes. No other laboratory tests seems to be necessary, since there have been no clinically significant laboratory abnormalities noted during treatment.

Cost

Omalizumab is considerably more expensive than conventional asthma therapy, with an average of approximately $12,000 per year. This compares with approximate cosets per year of $1,289 for montelukast, $2,160 for the combination of fluticasone dipropionate and salmeterol, $680 for extended-release theophylline.

A randomized trial of omalizumab for asthma in inner-city children showed improved asthma control, elimination of seasonal peaks in asthmatic exacerbations, and reduced need for other medications for asthma control.

25. Delivery devices and best route of administration

In pediatric asthma, inhaled treatment is the cornerstone of asthma management. Inhaler devices currently used to deliver inhaled corticosteroids (ICSs) fall into the following 4 categories:64

- Pressurized metered dose inhaler (pMDI) - Propellant used to dispense steroid when canister is pressed manually
- Dry powder inhaler (DPI) - Does not require hand-breath coordination to operate
- Breath-actuated pMDI - Propellant used to dispense steroid when patient inhales
- Nebulized solution devices

Go to Use of Metered Dose Inhalers, Spacers, and Nebulizers for complete information on this topic.

In pediatric patients, the inhaler device must be chosen on the basis of age, cost, safety, convenience, and efficacy of drug delivery

Based on current research, the preferred device for children younger than 4 years is a pMDI with a valved holding chamber and age-appropriate mask. Children aged 4-6 years should use a pMDI plus a valved holding chamber. Lastly, children older than 6 years can use either a pMDl, a DPI, or a breath-actuated pMDI. For all 3 groups, a nebulizer with a valved holding chamber (and mask in children younger than 4 y) is recommended as alternate therapy.

Valved holding chambers are important. The addition of a valved holding chamber can increase the amount of drug reaching the lungs to 20%. The use of a valved holding chamber helps reduce the amount of drug particles deposited in the oropharynx, thereby helping to reduce systemic and local effects from oral and gastrointestinal absorption.

A Cochrane review on the use of valved holding chambers versus nebulizers for inhaled steroids found no evidence that nebulizers are better than valved holding chamber. Nebulizers are expensive, inconvenient to use, require longer time for administration, require maintenance, and have been shown to have imprecise dosing.

Newer devices such as…. have been associated with a greater efficacy (as evidenced by…). For MDls, chlorofluorocarbon (CFC) propellants (implicated in ozone depletion) have been phased out in favor of the hydrofluoroalkane-134a (HFA) propellant. Surprisingly, the HFA component is more environmentally friendly and has proven to be more effective, due to its smaller aerosol particle size, which results in better drug delivery. MDls with HFA propellant have better deposition of drug in the small airways and greater efficacy at equivalent doses compared with CFC-MDls.[117]

26. Long-term monitoring

Regular follow-up visits are essential to ensure control and appropriate therapeutic adjustments. In general, patients should be assessed every 1-6 months. At every visit, adherence, environmental control, and comorbid conditions should be checked.

If patients have good control of their asthma for at least 3 months, treatment can be stepped down. However, the patient should be reassessed in 2-4 weeks to make sure that control is maintained with the new regimen. If patients require step 2 asthma medications or higher, consultation with an asthma specialist should be considered.

27. Outpatient visits should include the following

- Interval history of asthmatic complaints, including history of acute episodes (eg, severity, measures and treatment taken, response to therapy)
- History of nocturnal symptoms
- History of symptoms with exercise, and exercise tolerance
- Review of medications, including use of rescue medications
- Review of home-monitoring data (eg, symptom diary, peak flow meter readings, daily treatments)

28. Patient evaluation should include the following

- Assessment for signs of bronchospasm and complications
- Evaluation of associated conditions (eg, allergic rhinitis)
- Pulmonary function testing (in appropriate age group)

Address issues of treatment adherence and avoidance of environmental triggers and irritants.

Long-term asthma care pathways that incorporate the aforementioned factors can serve as roadmaps for ambulatory asthma care and help streamline outpatient care by different providers.

In the author's asthma clinic, a member of the asthma care team sits with each patient to review the written asthma care plan and to write and discuss in detail a rescue plan for acute episodes, which includes instructions about identifying signs of an acute episode, using rescue medications, monitoring, and contacting the asthma care team. These items are reviewed at each visit.

One study using directly observed administration of daily preventive asthma medications by a school nurse showed significantly improved symptoms among urban children with persistent asthma.

29. Control of environmental factors and comorbid conditions

As mentioned above, environmental exposures and irritants can play a strong role in symptom exacerbations. Therefore, in patients who have persistent asthma, the use of skin testing or in vitro testing to assess sensitivity to perennial indoor allergens is important. Once the offending allergens are identified, counsel patients on avoidance from these exposures. In addition, education to avoid tobacco smoke (both first-hand and second-hand exposure) is important for patients with asthma. 118

Lastly, comorbid conditions that may affect asthma must be appropriately managed. These include the following:

- Bronchopulmonary aspergillosis
- Gastroesophageal reflux disease (GERD)

- Obesity
- Obstructive sleep apnea
- Rhinitis
- Sinusitis
- Depression
- Stress

Inactivated influenza vaccine may be helpful in those who are older than 6 months.

30. Education

Patient education continues to be important in all areas of medicine and is particularly important in asthma. Self-management education should focus on teaching patients the importance of recognizing their own their level of control and signs of progressively worsening asthma symptoms.

Both peak flow monitoring and symptom monitoring have been shown to be equally effective; however, peak flow monitoring may be more helpful in cases in which patients have a history of difficulty in perceiving symptoms, a history of severe exacerbations, or moderate-to-severe asthma.

Educational strategies should also focus on environmental control and avoidance strategies and medication use and adherence (eg, correct inhaler techniques and use of other devices).

Using a variety of methods to reinforce educational messages is crucial in patient understanding. Providing written asthma action plans in partnership with the patient (making sure to review the differences between long-term control and quick-relief medications), education through the involvement of other members of the healthcare team (eg, nurses, pharmacists, physicians), and education at all points of care (eg, clinics, hospitals, schools) are examples of various educational tools that are available and valuable for good patient adherence and understanding.

31. Status asthmaticus

Treatment goals for acute severe asthmatic episodes (status asthmaticus) are as follows:

> Acute exacerbation of asthma induces the release of inflammatory mediators prime adhesion molecules in the airway epithelium and capillary endothelium, which then allows inflammatory cells, such as eosinophils neutrophils, and basophils, to attach to the epithelium and endothelium and subsequently migrate into the tissues of the airway. Eosinophils release eosinophilic cationic protein (ECP) and major basic protein (MBP). Both ECP and MBP induce deqsquamation of the airway epithelium and expose nerve endings. This interaction promotes further airway hyperresponsiveness in asthma. This inflammatory component may even occur in individuals with mild asthma exacerbation.

- Correction of significant hypoxemia with supplemental oxygen; in severe cases, alveolar hypoventilation requires mechanically assisted ventilation

- Rapid reversal of airflow obstruction with repeated or continuous administration of an inhaled beta2-agonist; early administration of systemic corticosteroids (eg, oral prednisone or intravenous methylprednisolone) is suggested in children with asthma that fails to respond promptly and completely to inhaled beta2-agonists

1. Yes, See British Guidelines on Management of Asthma (revised 2009).
   : second line treatment of acute asthma in children aged over 2 years.
2. Indications for admission to intensive care or high-dependency units include patients requiring ventilator support and those with severe acute or life threatening asthma who are failing to respond to therapy, as evidenced by:
   - Deteriorating PEF
   - Persisting or worsening hypoxia
   - Hypercapnea
   - Arterial blood gas analysis showing fall in pH or rising H+ concentration
   - Exhaustion, feeble respiration
   - Drowsiness, confusion, altered conscious state
   - Respiratory arrest.

Not all patients admitted to the Intensive Care Unit (ICU) need ventilation, but those with worsening hypixia or hypercapnea, drowsiness or uncousciousness and those who have had a respiratory arrest require intermittent positive pressure ventilation, intubation in such patients is very difficult and should ideally be performed by an anaesthetist or ICU consultant.

- Reduction in the likelihood of recurrence of severe airflow obstruction by intensifying therapy: Often, a short course of systemic corticosteroids is helpful 119-120

Achieving these goals requires close monitoring by means of serial clinical assessment and measurement of lung function (in patients of appropriate ages) to quantify the severity of airflow obstruction and its response to treatment. Improvement in FEV1 after 30 minutes of treatment is significantly correlated with a broad range of indices of the severity of asthmatic exacerbations, and repeated measurement of airflow in the emergency department can help reduce unnecessary admissions.

The use of the peak flow rate or FEV1 values, patient's history, current symptoms, and physical findings to guide treatment decisions is helpful in achieving the aforementioned goals. When using the peak expiratory flow (PEF) expressed as a percentage of the patient's best value, the effect of irreversible airflow obstruction should be considered. For example, in a patient whose best peak flow rate is 160 L/min, a decrease of 40% represents severe and potentially life-threatening obstruction.

An Australian study by Vuillermin et al found that asthma severity decreased in school aged children when parents initiated a short course of prednisolone for acute asthma. Children who received parent-initiated prednisolone for episodes of asthma had lower daytime and nighttime asthma scores, reduced risk of health resource use, and reduced school absenteeism compared with children who received placebo.

32. Prevention of asthma

The goal of long-term therapy is to prevent acute exacerbations. The patient should avoid exposure to environmental allergens and irritants that are identified during the evaluation.

Recurrent acute exacerbation of asthma cause the following histoopathological change in the airways. The airways becomes blocked by viscous, tenacious mucus distended lung parenchyma are composed of eosinophils and epithelial cells. There is an increase in smooth airway muscle with hyperplasia and hypertrophy in the major airways. Shedding of the cilated bronchial wall cells, mainly eosinophils. Apart from the bronchial infiltration of eosinophils there is dilatation of the capillary blood cells. The connective tissue in which these vessels lie consists of strands of widely separated collagen.

Numerous vasoactive agents have been found in broncoalveolar lavage of ___ with recurrent acute exacerbation of asthma including cell-derived mediators, such as histamine, the cysteinyl leukotriene, LTC4, LTD4 and LTE4, and PAF, and also neural-derived mediators, e.g. substance P(SP), neurokinin A and B (NKA, NKB), and calcitonin gene-related peptide (CGRP), PAF is a phospholipid that induces neutropenia, bronchocosntriction, and abnormal airway microvascular leakage, possibly through postcapillary venoconstriction in the tracheobroncial circulation. Thus microvascular leakage of plasma is an inflammatory hallmark of paramount relevance n asthma, generally referred to as abnormally increased vascular permeability. A substantially increased number of PAF receptors are reported in the lungs of asthmatic individuals.

33. Dietary adjustments

When a patient has major allergies to dietary products, avoidance of particular foods may help. In the absence of specific food allergies, dietary changes are not necessary. Unless compelling evidence for a specific allergy exists, milk products do not have to be avoided.

34. Consultations

Any patient with high-risk asthma should be referred to a specialist. The following may suggest high risk:

- History of sudden severe exacerbations
- History of prior intubation for asthma
- Admission to an ICU because of asthma
- Two or more hospitalizations for asthma in the past year
- Three or more emergency department visits for asthma in the past year
- Hospitalization or an emergency department visit for asthma within the past month
- Use of 2 or more canisters of inhaled short-acting beta2-agonists per month
- Current use of systemic corticosteroids or recent withdrawal from systemic corticosteroids

Referral to an asthma specialist for consultation or co-management of the patient is also recommended if additional education is needed to improve adherence or if the patient requires step 4 care or higher (step 3 care or higher for children aged 0-4 y). Consider referral if a patient requires step 3 care (step 2 care for children aged 0-4 y) or if additional testing for the role of allergy is indicated.

The choice between a pediatric pulmonologist and an allergist may depend on local availability and practices. A patient with frequent ICU admissions, previous intubation, and a history of complicating factors or comorbidity (eg, cystic fibrosis) should be referred to a pediatric pulmonologist. When allergies are thought to significantly contribute to the morbidity, an allergist may be helpful.

Consider consultation with an ear, nose, and throat (ENT) specialist for help in managing chronic rhinosinusitis. Consider consultation with a gastroenterologist for help in excluding and/or treating gastroesophageal reflux.

35. Appendix: Specific pharmacologic treatment

35.1 Bronchodilators, Beta2-Agonists

These agents are used to treat bronchospasm in acute asthmatic episodes, and used to prevent bronchospasm associated with exercise-induced asthma or nocturnal asthma. Recent studies have suggested that short-acting beta2-agonists may produce adverse outcomes (eg, decreased peak flow or increased risk of exacerbations) in patients homozygous for arginine (Arg/Arg) at the 16th amino acid position of beta-adrenergic receptor gene compared with patients homozygous for glycine (Gly-Gly). Similar findings are reported for long-acting beta2-agonists, such as salmeterol. 121-122

35.2 Salbutamol sulfate (Proventil HFA, Ventolin HFA, ProAir HFA)

This beta2-agonist is the most commonly used bronchodilator that is available in multiple forms (eg, solution for nebulization, MOl, PO solution, butalin, ventolin, asthalin, salamol, a.o.). This is most commonly used in rescue therapy for acute asthmatic symptoms. Used as needed. Prolonged use: may be associated with tachyphylaxis due to beta2-receptor down regulation and receptor hyposensitivity.

Some MD is/are available as a breath-actuated inhalers. The ease of administration with the breath-actuated devices make it an attractive choice in the treatment of acute symptoms in younger children who otherwise cannot use an ordinary MDl. The Autohaler delivers 200 mcg per actuation.

Terbutalin, a partial beta-2-agonist is short-acting bronchodilator. The inhaled form of terbutalin starts working within 15 minutes and can last for up to 6 hours.

This nonracemic form of beta-2-agonist (albuterol) offers a significant reduction in the adverse effects associated with racemic albuterol (eg, muscle tremors, tachycardia, hyperglycemia, hypokalemia).

The noncarcemic form of albuterol Levabuterol offers a significant reduction in the adverse effects associated with racemic albuterol (eg, muscle tremors, tachycardia, hyperglycemia, Hypokalemia.
The dose may be doubled in acute severe episodes when even a slight increase in the bronchodilator response may make a big difference in the management strategy (eg, in avoiding patient ventilation). It is available as an MDI (45 mcg per actuation) or solution for nebulized inhalation).

35.3 Xopenex

Nonracemic form of albuterol (xopenex), levalbuterol (R isomer) is effective in smaller doses and is reported to have fewer adverse effects (eg, tachycardia, hyperglycemia, hypokalemia). The dose may be doubled in acute severe episodes when even a slight increase in the bronchodilator response may make a big difference in the management strategy (eg, in avoiding patient ventilation). It is available as an MOl (45 mcg per actuation) or solution for nebulized inhalation.

35.4 Long-Acting Beta2-Agonists

Long-acting bronchodilators (LABA) are not used for the treatment of acute bronchospasm. They are used for the preventive treatment of nocturnal asthma or exercise-induced asthmatic symptoms, for example.

There are 2 LABA are available: salmeterol and formoterol. Both are available as combination products with inhaled corticosteroids.

LABA may increase the chance of severe asthma episodes and death when those episodes occur. Most cases have occurred in patients with severe and/or acutely deteriorating asthma; they have also occurred in a few patients with less severe asthma.

LABAs are not considered first-line medications to treat asthma. LABAs should not be used as isolated medications and should be added to the asthma treatment plan only if other medicines do not control asthma, including the use of low- or medium-dose corticosteroids. If used as isolated medication, LABAs should be prescribed by pulmonologist / allergist.

35.5 Salmeterol

This long-acting preparation of a beta2-agonist is used primarily to treat nocturnal or exercise-induced symptoms. It has no anti-inflammatory action and is not indicated in the treatment of acute bronchospastic episodes. It may be used as an adjunct to inhaled corticosteroids to re9uce the potential adverse effects of the steroids. The medication is delivered via a Diskus DPI.

35.6 Formoterol

Formoterol is a long-acting B2-agonist. It is marketed in dry powder inhalation, a metered-dose inhaler, an inhalation solution and oral tablet.

Formoterol relieves bronchospasm by relaxing the smooth muscles of the bronchioles in conditions associated with asthma. They are used for long-term control and prevention of symptoms, especially nocturnal symptoms.

35.7 Methylxanthines

35.7.1 Theophylline

Theophylline is available in short-acting and long-acting formulations. Because of the need to monitor serum concentrations, this agent is used infrequently. The dose and frequency depend on the particular product selected. The actions of theophylline involve:

- relaxing bronchial smooth muscle
- increasing heart muscle contractility and efficiency as a positive inotropic
- increasing heart rate positive chronotrope
- increasing blood pressure
- increasing renal blood flow
- some anti-inflammatory effects
- central nervous system stimulatory effect mainly on medullary respiratory center.123-125

Parenteral methylxanthines (aminophylline, theophylline) may circumvent the dimininshed delivery of aerosolized β-agonists in acute asthma and young children thus augmenting submaximal bronchial smooth-muscle relaxation. Molecular mechanisms specific to theophylline that may be responsible for its beneficial effect include phosphodiesterase enzyme inhibition, adenosine receptor antagonism, enhanced catecholamine secretion, and modulation of transmembrane calcium fluxes in muscle cells. The influence on calcium may be respoinsble for an increase in respiratory muscle contractility and resistance to diaphragmatic fatigue particularly advantageous in asthmatics with early respiratory failure. Methylxanthines may also assume greater importance during β-receptor desensitization where the response to β agonist drugs is attenuated but a response to aminophylline persists. Clinical trials involving submaximal bronchodialation have shown that the benefit from combinations of methylxanthines and β-agnosits are more likely additive and synergistic.

The use of theophylline is complicated by its interaction with other drugs, chiefly cimetidine and phenytoin, erythromycin, ciprofloxacin and fluoroquinolones and that it has a narrow therapeutic index. It can cause nausea, diarrhea, tachycardia, headache, insomnia

35.8 Inhaled corticosteroids

Steroids are the most potent anti-inflammatory agents. Inhaled forms are topically active, poorly absorbed and thus less likely to cause adverse effects. They are used for long-term control of asthma symptoms and airway inflammation. Inhaled forms reduce the need for systemic corticosteroids.

Inhaled steroids block late asthmatic response to allergens; reduce airway hyper responsiveness; inhibit inflammatory process e.g. cytokine production, adhesion protein activation, and inflammatory cell migration and activation; and reverse beta2-receptor downregulation and subsensitivity (in acute asthmatic episodes with LABA use). 126-127

35.8.1 Fluticasone

Fluticasone has extremely potent vasoconstrictive and anti-inflammatory activity. It has a weak hypothalamic-pituitary adrenocortical axis inhibitory potency when applied topically. It is available as an MDl aerosolized product (HFA) or DPI (Diskus).

35.8.2 Budesonide

Budesonide has extremely potent vasoconstrictive and anti-inflammatory activity. It has a weak hypothalamic-pituitary adrenocortical axis inhibitory potency when applied topically. It is available as a DPI, MDI and nebulized susp (ie, Respules).

35.8.3 Beclomethasone

Beclomethasone inhibits bronchoconstriction mechanisms; causes direct smooth muscle relaxation, decrease the number and activity of inflammatory cells, and decreases airway hyperresponsiveness. It is available as MDI.

35.8.4 Ciclesonide

Ciclesonide is an aerosol inhaled corticosteroid indicated for maintenance treatment of asthma as prophylactic therapy in adolescent patients aged 12 y and older. Not indicated for relief of acute bronchospasm.

Corticosteroids have wide range of effects on multiple cell types (eg, mast cells, eosinophils, neutrophils, macrophages, lymphocytes) and mediators (eg, histamines, eicosanoids, leukotrienes, cytokines) involved in inflammation.

Maximum benefit may not be achieved for 4 wk or longer after initiation of therapy.

After asthma stability is achieved, it is best to titrate to lowest effective dosage to reduce the possibility of adverse effects. For patients who do not adequately respond to the starting dose after 4 wk of therapy, higher doses may provide additional asthma control. It is available as MDI.[127]

35.8.5 Mometasone furoate inhalation powder (Asmanex Twisthaler)

Mometasone is a corticosteroid for inhalation. It is indicated for asthma as prophylactic therapy.

35.9 Systemic corticosteroids

Corticosteroids are the most potent anti-inflammatory used in asthma. Systemic corticosteroids (SCS) are effective in acute asthma, pulmonary function slowly improves beginning within 6-12 hours, SCS reduces to relapse rate and admission ranks. Several studies suggest duration of 3-5 days. The anti-inflammatory effects of corticosteroids are mediated to a major extent via TRANSREPRESSION, while many side-effects are due to TRANSACTIVATION. New generations of corticosteroids are being developed that preferentially induce TRANSREPRESSION with little or no TRANSACTIVATION.

These agents are used for short courses (3-10 d) to gain prompt control of inadequately controlled acute asthmatic episodes. They are also used for long-term prevention of symptoms in severe persistent asthma as well as for suppression, control, and reversal of inflammation. Frequent and repetitive use of beta2-agonists has been associated with beta2-receptor sub-sensitivity and down regulation; these processes are reversed with corticosteroids.

Higher-dose corticosteroids have no advantage in severe asthma exacerbations, and intravenous administration has no advantage over oral therapy, provided that 81 transit time or absorption is not impaired. The usual regimen is to continue frequent multiple daily dosing until the FEV1 or peak expiratory flow (PEF) is 50% of the predicted or personal best values; then, the dose is changed to twice daily. This usually occurs within 48 hours.

35.9.1 Prednisone

An immunosuppressant for the treatment of autoimmune disorders, prednisone may decrease inflammation by reversing increased capillary permeability and suppressing polymorphonuclear neutrophil (PMN) activity.

35.9.2 Methylprednisolone

Methylprednisolone may decrease inflammation by reversing increased capillary permeability and suppressing PMN activity.

35.10 Leukotriene modifiers

Knowledge that leukotrienes cause bronchospasm, increased vascular permeability, mucosal edema, and inflammatory cell infiltration has led to the concept of modifying their action by using pharmacologic agents. These are either 5-lipoxygenase inhibitors or leukotriene-receptor antagonists.

35.11 Leukotriene antagonists

These are drugs that inhibit leukotrienes and thus suppress inflammation. Leukotriene antagonists such as montelukast, zafirlukast are used in asthma to block the actions of leukotrienes, either by inhibition of the cysteinyl-leukotriene type 1 receptors. (Montelukast, Zafirlukast)

35.11.1 Zafirlukast

Zapirlukast is a selective competitive inhibitor of LTD4 and LTE4 receptors.

The leukotriene-antagonist zafirlukast (Accolate), and montelukast (Singulaire) are proving to be effective for long-term prevention of asthma, including exercise-induced asthma and aspirin (or NSAID)-induced asthma. Their anti-inflammatory actions are different from those of steroids.

Studies suggest that montelukast, wheich comes in a chewable tablet, may be particularly useful for managing asthma in small children (ages two to five) with asthma, since they have trouble with inhaled steroids. Zafirlukast may also reduce the severity of cat allergies, regardless of whether or not asthma is also present.

Of some concern are reports of Churg-Satrauss syncrome in a few people taking zafirlukast or montelukast. Churg-Strauss syndrome is very rare, but it causes blood vessel inflammation in the lungs and can be life threatening. Oral steroids quickly resolve the problem. In fact, usually the syndrome has occurred in patients who were tapering off steroids and changing over to the leukotrines-antagonist. Some experts believe that, in such cases, the steroids may simply have masked the presence of the disorder, which then developed when the steroid drugs were withdrawn. Symptoms include severe sinusitis, flu-like symptoms, rash, and numbness in the hands and feet.

35.11.2 Montelukast

The last agent introduced in its class, montelukast has the advantages that it is chewable, it has a once-a-day dosing, and it has no significant adverse effects.

35.11.3 Omalizumab

Omalizumab is a recombinant, DNA-derived, humanized IgG 1K monoclonal antibody that selectively binds to human Immunoglobulin (IgE). Omalizumab's cost is very high as compared with other drugs used for asthma, and hence is mainly prescribed for patients with severe persistent asthma, which can not be controlled even with high doses of corticosteroids like other protein drugs, omalizumab may cause anaphylaxis in 1 to 2 patients per 1000.

35.12 Combination inhaled steroids/Long-Acting Beta2-Agonists

These combinations may de\crease asthma exacerbations when inhaled short-acting beta2-agonists and corticosteroids have failed. Refer to previous discussion in the LABAs section regarding increased risk of severe asthma episodes and death with LABAs. In a recent study, use of combination therapy using fluticasone propionate and salmeterol prolonged time to first severe asthma exacerbation.

Budesonide is an inhaled corticosteroid that alters level of inflammation in airways by inhibiting multiple types of inflammatory cells and decreasing production of cytokines and other mediators involved in the asthmatic response. Available as MDl in 2 strengths; each actuation delivers formoterol 4.5 mcg with either 80 mcg or 160 mcg.

35.12.1 Budesonide and formoterol

Formoterol relieves bronchospasm by relaxing the smooth muscles of the bronchioles in conditions associated with asthma. Budesonide is an inhaled corticosteroid that alters the level of inflammation in airways by inhibiting multiple types of inflammatory cells and decreasing production of cytokines and other mediators involved in the asthmatic response. This combination is available as an MOl in 2 strengths; each actuation delivers formoterol 4.5-mcg with either 80-mcg or 160-mcg of budesonide.

35.12.2 Mometasone and formoterol

This is a combination corticosteroid and LABA metered-dose inhaler. Mometasone elicits local anti-inflammatory effects in the respiratory tract with minimal systemic absorption. Formoterol elicits bronchial smooth muscle relaxation.

This combination is indicated for prevention and maintenance of asthma symptoms in patients inadequately controlled with other asthma controller medications (eg, low-dose to medium-dose inhaled corticosteroids) or whose disease severity clearly warrants initiation of treatment with 2 maintenance therapies, including a LABA. Available in 2 strengths; each actuation delivers mometasone/formoterol 100 mcg/5 mcg or 200 mcg/5 mcg.

35.12.3 Fluticasone and salmeterol

This is a combination corticosteroid and LABA metered-dose inhaler. Fluticasone inhibits bronchoconstriction mechanisms, produces direct smooth muscle relaxation, and may decrease number and activity of inflammatory cells, in turn decreasing airway hyper-responsiveness. It also has vasoconstrictive activity. Salmeterol relaxes the smooth muscles of the bronchioles in conditions associated with bronchitis, emphysema, asthma, or bronchiectasis and can relieve bronchospasms. Its effect may also facilitate expectoration. Adverse effects are more likely to occur when administered at high or more frequent doses than recommended. Two delivery mechanisms are available (ie, powder for inhalation [Diskus], metered-dose inhaler [MDl]). Diskus is available as a combination of salmeterol 50 mcg with fluticasone 100 mcg, 250 mcg, or 500 mcg. The MDl is available as 21 mcg salmeterol with fluticasone 45 mcg, 115 mcg, or 230 mcg.

35.13 Anticholinergic drugs

Anticholinergic drugs are group of bronchodilators that block the neurotransmitter acetylcholine on the muscarinic receptor on bronchial smooth muscle.

35.13.1 Ipratropium bromide

Chemically related to atropine, protropium has antisecretory properties and, when applied locally, inhibits secretions from serous and seromucous glands lining the nasal mucosa. The MDl delivers 17 mcg/actuation. Solution for inhalation contains 500 mcg/2.5 mL (ie, 0.02% solution for nebulization).

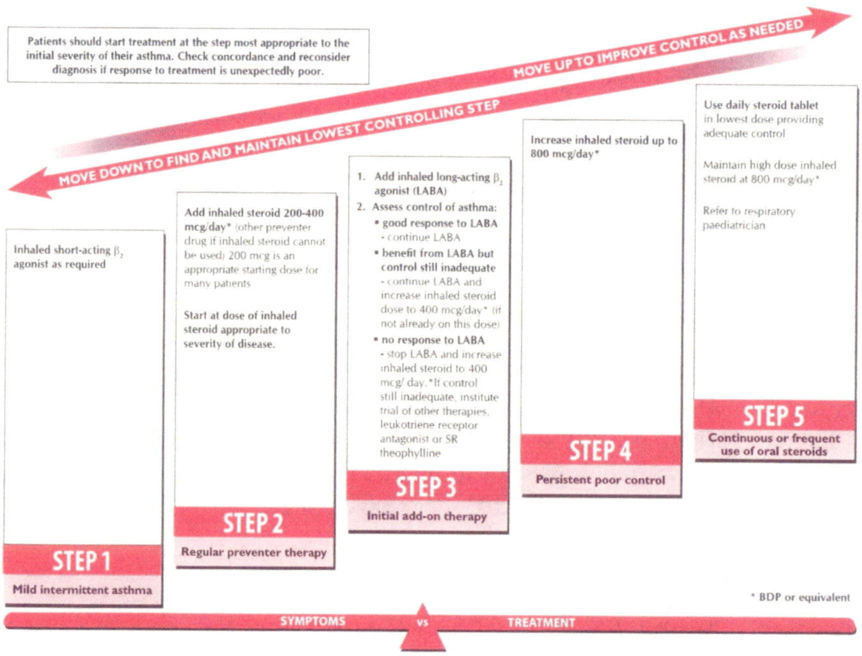

Figure 5. Summary of stepwise management in children aged 5-12 years

ITISH GUIDELINE ON THE MANAGEMENT OF ASTHMA

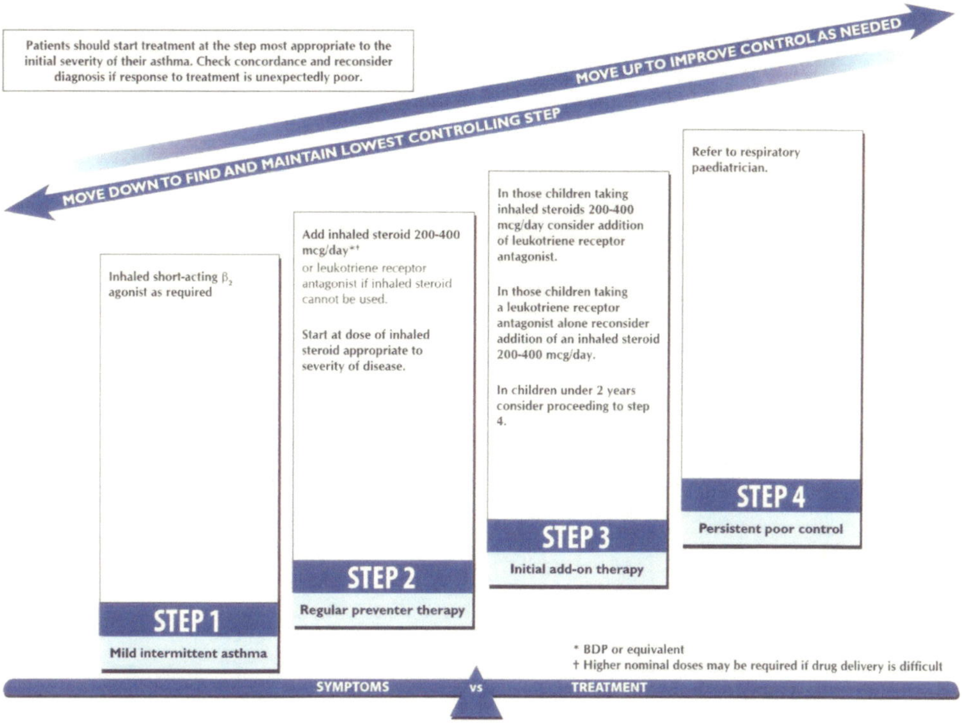

Figure 6: Summary of stepwise management in children less than 5 years

Steroid Therapy

Give prednisolone or prednisone early in the treatment of acute asthma attacks.	A
Use a dose of prednisolone or prednisone 1-2mg/kg/day. A maximum dose of 40mg per day is usually sufficient but up to 60mg may be used.	☑
Repeat the dose of prednisolone/ prednisone in children who vomit within an hour of the dose, and consider IV steroids hydrocortisone 4mg/kg/dose six hourly	☑
Treatment with systemic steroids for up to three days is usually sufficient, but tailor length of course to the number of days necessary to bring about recovery. Tapering of short courses (up to 7-14 days) of steroids is not necessary.	☑

Inhaled corticosteroids (ICS)

There is insufficient evidence to support the use of ICS as alternative or additional treatment to steroid tablets for acute asthma. There is no evidence that increasing the dose of ICS is effective in treating acute symptoms, but it is good practice for children already receiving ICS to continue with their usual maintenance doses.

Do not initiate inhaled corticosteroids in preference to steroid tablets to treat acute childhood asthma.	☑
There is no evidence that increasing the dose of inhaled corticosteroid is beneficial in acute attacks of asthma.	☑
Betamethasone (Betnesol) and Dexamethasone are not recommended for use with asthma.	☑

)ne MANAGEMENT OF CHRONIC ASTHMA

)CESS OF REVIEW IN THE MANAGEMENT OF PERSISTENT ASTHMA.

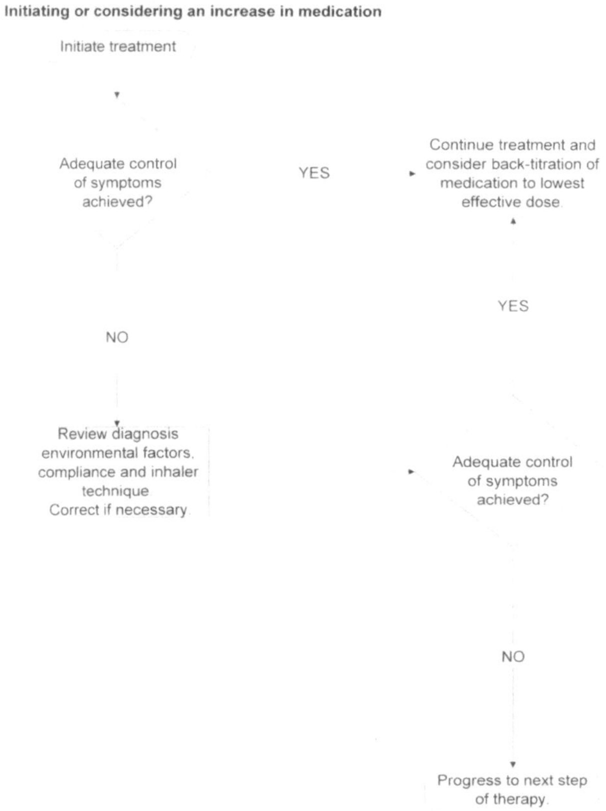

Management of Acute Asthma

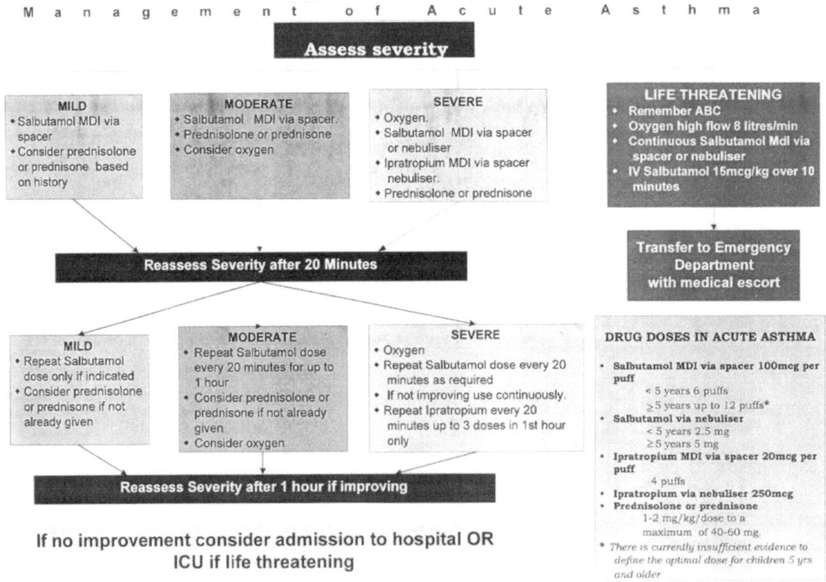

Summary of Stepwise Pharmacological Management in Children Aged 5-15 Years.

STEP 1: MILD INTERMITTENT ASTHMA

Inhaled short acting β_2 agonist as required

↕

STEP 2: REGULAR PREVENTER THERAPY

Add inhaled steroid 200-400mcg/day BDP or BUD, or 100-200 mcg/day FP

- use the higher dose for greater severity,

(cromoglycate, nedocromil or montelukast[a] if inhaled steroid cannot be used)

↕

STEP 3: ADD ON THERAPY

1. **Add inhaled long acting ß2 agonist (LABA)[b]**
2. **Assess response to LABA:**

- **good response to LABA** --- continue LABA

some benefit from LABA in maximum dose[c] but control still inadequate, increase inhaled steroid to 400mcg/day BDP or BUD, **or** 200 mcg/day FP (if not already on this dose)

- **no response to LABA** - Stop LABA consider trial of montelukast[a] **or** SR theophylline

↕

STEP 4: PERSISTENT POOR CONTROL

Increase inhaled steroid to 600-800 mcg/day BDP or BUD, or 300-400 mcg/day FP[d]

Continue to review add on therapy

Refer to paediatrician if not improving

↕

STEP 5: CONTINUED POOR CONTROL

Refer to paediatrician

Maintain high dose inhaled steroid

Consider steroid tablet in lowest dose providing adequate control.

[a] The only New Zealand Registered Leukotriene Receptor Antagonist, montelukast, is not currently on the Pharmaceutical Schedule

[b] The current Special Authority criteria of the Pharmaceutical schedule allows LABA to be introduced at the higher threshold of 400mcg/day BDP or BUD, or 200mcg/day

[c] Maximum recommended dose of eformoterol is 12mcg bd, and salmeterol 50mcg bd

[d] These levels of ICS are greater than usually required to achieve optimal control (See Dose Response Curve pg 21) and do not hesitate to seek advice from a paediatrician.

ALTERNATIVE DIAGNOSES IN WHEEZY CHILDREN

Clinical clue*	Possible diagnosis*
Perinatal and family history	
• symptoms present from birth or perinatal lung problem	• cystic fibrosis, chronic lung disease of prematurity, ciliary dyskinesia, developmental anomaly
• family history of unusual chest disease	• cystic fibrosis, developmental anomaly, neuromuscular disorder
• persistent sinusitis	• defect of host defence
Symptoms and Signs	
• persistent wet cough	• cystic fibrosis, recurrent aspiration, bronchiectasis, host defence disorder
• excessive vomiting or spilling	• reflux (± aspiration)
• dysphagia	• swallowing problems (± aspiration)
• abnormal voice or cry	• laryngeal problem
• focal signs in the chest	• developmental anomaly, post adenoviral pneumonia, bronchiectasis, tuberculosis
• inspiratory stridor as well as wheeze	• central airway or laryngeal disorder • inhaled foreign body
• failure to thrive	• cystic fibrosis, host defence disorder, gastroesophageal reflux
• clubbing	• bronchiectasis, cystic fibrosis
Chest Xray	
• focal radiological changes	• developmental anomaly, inhaled foreign body, bronchiectasis, tuberculosis, segmental or lobar collapse
• persistent radiological changes	• recurrent aspiration, bronchiectasis,cystic fibrosis

*List not comprehensive

Note: Recurrent cough in the absence of wheeze is unlikely to be due to asthma

ALTERNATIVE DIAGNOSES IN COUGHING CHILDREN

Clinical clue*	Possible diagnosis*
History	
• day care	• recurrent bronchitis
• unimmunised	• pertussis
• symptoms present from birth or perinatal lung problem	• cystic fibrosis, ciliary dyskinesia, developmental anomaly
• family history of unusual chest disease	• cystic fibrosis, developmental anomaly, neuromuscular disorder
• persistent upper respiratory tract disease	• defect of host defence
Symptoms and Signs	
• recurrent cough, asymptomatic between episodes	• recurrent bronchitis, tracheomalacia, mild airway compression
• paroxysmal cough	• pertussis
• persistent wet cough	• cystic fibrosis, recurrent aspiration, bronchiectasis; host defence disorder
• excessive vomiting or spilling	• reflux (± aspiration)
• dysphagia	• swallowing problems (± aspiration)
• abnormal voice or cry	• laryngeal problem
• focal signs in the chest	• developmental anomaly, post adenoviral pneumonia, bronchiectasis, tuberculosis
• inspiratory stridor as well as wheeze	• central airway or laryngeal disorder
• failure to thrive	• cystic fibrosis, host defence disorder; gastroesophageal reflux
• older child	• psychogenic cough, tobacco smoking
• clubbing	• bronchiectasis, cystic fibrosis
Chest Xray	
• focal radiological changes	• developmental anomaly, inhaled foreign body, bronchiectasis, tuberculosis, segmental or lobar collapse
• persistent radiological changes	• recurrent aspiration, bronchiectasis, cystic fibrosis

*List not comprehensive

Source: Management of Asthma in Children aged 1-15 years (Ped. Society of New Zealand)

36. References

[1] Bousquet J, Jeffrey P-/, Busse WW, Johnson M, Vignola AM. Asthma. From Bronchoconstriction to airways inflammation and remodeling. Am J Respir Crit Care Med. May 2000; 161 (5):1720-45 (Medline)

[2] Nagel G, Buchele G. Weinmayr G, Bjorksten B, Chen Y-Z, Wang H, Nystad W, Saraclar Y, B Batlles-Garrido J, Garcia-Hernandez G, Weiland SK, and the ISAAC Phase Two Study Group. Effective Breastfeeding on Asthma, Lung function, and Bronchial Hyperreactivity in ISAAC-Phase-Two. Eur 33:993-1002;Epub 2009 Jan 22.

[3] Genuneit J, Cantelmo JL., Weinmayr G, Wong GWK, Cooper PJ, Riikjarv MA, Gotua M, Kabe Mutius E, Forastiere F, Crane J, Nystad W, El Sharif N, Battles-Garrido J, Garcia-Marcos L, Garci G, Morales Suarez-Varela MM, Nillsson L, Braback L, Saraclar Y, Weiland SK, Cookson WOC, S Moffatt M, ISAAC Phase Two Study Group. A multi-centre study of candidate genes for wheez. The International Study of Asthma and Allergies in Childhood Phase Two. Clin Exp Allergy 2009 I 1875-1888

[4] Bjorksten B, Clayton T, Ellwood P, Stewart A, Strachan D, and the ISAAC Phase Three Study Group. Worldwide trends for symptoms of rhinitis: Phase III of the Internaional Asthma and Allergies in Childhood Pediatr Allergy Immunol 2008; 19(2) 110-24.

[5] Ait-Khaled N, Pearce N, Anderson HR, Ellwood P, Montefort S, Shah J, and the ISAAC Phase Group. Global map of the prevalence of symptoms of rhinoconjunctivitis in children: The International Asthma and Allergies in Childhood (ISAAC). Phase Three Allergy 2009;64:123-148.

[6] Lai CKW, Beasley R, Crane J, Foliaki S, Shah J, Weiland S, and the ISAAC Phase Three Study viariation in the prevalence of severity of asthma symptoms: Phase Three of the international Study and Allergies in Childhood (ISAAC). Thorax 2009;64:476-483. Epub Feb 2009.

[7] Odhiambo J, Williams H, Clayton T, Robertson C, Asher MI, and ISAAC Phase Three Study Group. Global variations in prevalenc of eczema symptoms in children for ISAAC Phase Three. Immunol. Dec 2009:124 (6):1251-8.

[8] Ellwood P, Asher MI, Stewart AW and the ISAAC Phase III Study Group The impact of the me on response rates in the ISAAC time trends study. Int J Tuberc Lung Dis. 2010 Aug; 14 (8(: 1059-65.

[9] [Best Evidence] Salpeter SR, Wall AJ, Buckley NS. Long-acting beta-agonists with and without inhaled corticosteroids and catastrophic asthma events. Am J Med. Apr 2010; 123(4):322-8.e2. [Medline].

[10] Wechsler ME, Lehman E, Lazarus SC, Lemanske RF Jr, Boushey HA, Deykin A, et al. beta-Adrenergic receptor polymorph isms and response to salmeterol. Am J Respir Crit Care Med. Mar 1 2006; 173(5):519-26. [Medline]. [Full Text].

[11] Robertson D, Kerigan AT, Hargreave FE, Chalmers R, Dolovich J. late asthmatic responses induced by ragweed pollen allergen. J Allergy Clin Immunol 1974; 54:244-254.

[12] D Ho I.C., Pai S. Y. 2007. GATA-3-not just for Th2 cells anymore. Cell Mol Immunol 4:15-29. Boulet LP, Robers RS, Dolovich J, Hargreave FE. Prediction of late sthmatic rsponses to inhaled allergen. Clin Allergy 1984;14:379-385.

[13] Lipworth BJ, White PS: Allergic inflammation in the unified airway: start with the nose. Thorax 55:878-881, 2000.
[14] Minoguchi H, Minoguchi K, Tanaka A, Matsou H, Kihara N, Adachi M: Cough receptor sensitivity to capsaicin does not change after allergen bronchoprovocation in allergic asthma. Thorax 58: 19-22, 2003.
[15] De Magalhaes Simoes S, dos Santos MA, da Silva Oliveira M, Fontes ES, Fernezlian S, Garippo AL, Castro I, Castro FF, de Arruda Martins M, Saldiva PH, Mauad T, and Dolhnikoff M. Inflammatory cell mapping of ther espoiratory tract in fatal asthma. Clin Exp Allergy 35:602-611, 2005.
[16] Homma T, Bates JH, and Irvin CG. Airway hyperresponsiveness induced by cationic proteins in vivo: site of action. Am J Physiol Lung Cell Mol Physiol 289:L413-L418, 2005.
[17] Boulet LP, Robers RS, Dolovich J, Hargreave FE. Prediction of late sthmatic rsponses to inhaled allergen. Clin Allergy 1984;14:379-385.
[18] Zhou Y., McLane, M., Levitt, R.C. 2001. Interleukin-9 as a therapeutic target for asthma. Respir Res 2:80-84.
[19] Steenwinckel V, et al 2007. IL-13 mediates in vivo IL-9 activities on lung epithelial cells but not on hematopoietic cells. J Immunol 178:3244-3251.
[20] Szabo S.J., et al. 2002. Distinct effects of T-bet in TH1 lineage commitment and IFN-gamma production in CD4 and CD8 T cells. Science 295:338-342. View this article via:
[21] Wark P.A., et al 2005. Asthmatic bronchial epithelial cells have a deficient innate immune response to infection with rhinovirus. J Exp Med 201:937-947.
[22] Cooper A.M., Khader S.A. 2007. IL-12p40: an inherently agonistic cytokine. Trends Immunol 28:33-38.
[23] Manel N, Unutmaz D, Littman D.R. 2008. The differentiation of human T(H)-17 cells requires transforming growth factor-beta and induction of the nuclear receptor RORgammat. Nat Immunol 9:641-649.
[24] Pene J, et al 2008. Chronically inflamed human tissues are infiltrated by highly differentiated th17 lymphocytes. J Immunol 180:7423-7430.
[25] Ballantyne S.J. et al. 2007. Blocking IL-25 prevents airway hyperresponsiveness in allergic asthma. J Allergy Clin Immunol 120:1324-1331.
[26] Erin E.M., et al. 2008. Rapid anti-inflammatory effect of inhaled ciclesonide in asthma: a randomized, placebo-controlled study. Chest. Online publication ahead of print.doi: View this article via: CrossRef
[27] Gauvreau G.M. et al 2008. Antisense therapy against CCR3 and the common beta chain attenuates allergen-induced eosinophilic responses. Am J Respir Crit Care Med 177:952-958.
[28] Strachan DP (August 2000). Family size, infection and atopy: the first decade of the "hygiene hypothesis" (http://thorax.bmj.com/cgi/pmidlookup?view=long&pmid=10943631). Thorax. 55 Suppl 1(90001):S2-10.doi: 10.1136/thorax.55.suppl_1.S2 (http://dx.doi.org/10.1136%2Fthorax.55.suppl_1.S2). PMC 1765943631).
[29] The Hyginene hypothesis for autoimmune and allergic disease: an update. Okada H, Kuhn C, Feillet H, Bach JF. INSERM U1013, Necker-Enfants Malades Hospital, Paris, France.

[30] Marra F, Lynd L, Coombes M "et al." (2006). " Does antibiotic exposure during infancy lead to development of asthma? : a systematic review and metaanalysis" Chest 129 (3):610-8. Doi:10.1378/chest. 129.3.610 (http://dx.doi.org/10.1378% Chest 129 3:610). PMD 16537858).
[31] Moffat, Miriam F. et al. Gene in Asthma: New genes and new ways, Current opinion in allergy and clinical immunology, 2008. Volume 8. Issue 5 411-417
[32] Bouzigon E, Corda E, Aschard H, et al. Effect of 17q21 variants and smoking exposure in early-onset asthma. N Engl J Med
[33] Cookson W, Liang L, Abecasis G, Moffatt M, Lathrop M. Mapping complex disease traits with global gene expression. Nat Rev Genet 2009;10:184-194.
[34] Verlaan DJ, Berlivet S, Hunninghake GM, et al. Allele-specific chromatin remodeling in the ZPBP2/GSDMB/ORMDL3 locus associated with the risk of asthma and autoimmune disease. Am J Hum Genet 2009;85:377-393,
[35] Gudbjartsson DF, Bjornsdottir US, Halapi E, et al. Sequence variants affecting eosinophil numbers associate with asthma and myocardial infarction. Nat Genet 2009;41:342-347.
[36] Moussion C, Ortega N, Girard JP. The IL-1-like cytokine IL-33 is constitutively expressed in the nucleus of endothelial cells and epithelial cells in vivo: a novel alarmin? PLoS ONE 2008;3:e3331-e3331.
[37] Fukao T, Matsuda S, Koyasu S. Synergistic effects of IL-4 and IL-18 on IL-12 dependent IFN-gamma production by dendritic cells. J Immunol 2000;164:64-71.
[38] Nouri-Aria KT, Durham SR. Regulatory T cells and allergic disease. Inflamm Allergy Drug Targets 2008;7:237-252.
[39] Moffatt MF, Cookson WO. Tumour necrosis factor haplotypes and asthma. Hum Mol Genet 1997;6:551-554.
[40] Taylor JM, Street TL, Hao L, et al. Dynamic and physical clustering of gene expression during epidermal barrier formation in differentiating keratinocytes. PLoS ONE 2009;4:e7651-e7651.
[41] Vercelli D. Advances in asthma and allergy genetics in 2007. J Allergy Clin Immunol 2008;122:267-271.
[42] William J. Sheehan, MD, et. al. Age Specific Prevalence of Outdoor and Indoor Aeroallergen Sensitization in Boston. Clinical Pediatrics 49 (6) 579-585.
[43] Guilbert TW, Morgan WJ, Zeiger RS, et al. Atopic characteristics of children with recurrent wheezing and high risk for the development of childhood asthma. J Allergy Clin Immunol. 2004;114:1282-1287.
[44] Calabria CW, Dice JP, Hagan LL. Prevalence of positive skin test responses to 53 allergens in patients with rhinitis symptoms. Allergy Asthma Proc. 2007;28:442-448.
[45] Phipatanakul W. Allergic rhinoconjunctivitis: epidemiology. Immunol Allergy Clin North Am. 2005;25:263-281,vi
[46] B ernstein IL, Li JT, Bernstein DI, et al. Allergy diagnostic testing: an updated practice parameter. Ann Allergy Asthma Immunol. 2008; 100 (3, suppl 3):A1-S148.
[47] Ogershok PR, Warner DJ, Hogan MB, Wilson NW. Prevalence of pollen sensitization in younger children who have asthma. Allergy Asthma Proc. 2007;28:654-658.
[48] LeMasters GK, Wilson K, Levin L, et al. High prevalence of aeroallergen sensitization among infants of atopic parents. J Pediatr. 2006;149:505-511.

[49] Pastorino AC, Kuschnir FC, Arruda LK, et al. Sensitization of aeroallergens in Brazilian adolescents living at the periphery of large subtropical urban centres. Allergol Immunopathol (Madr). 2008;36:-9-16.
[50] Calabria CW, dice J Aeroallergen sensitization rates in military children with rhinitis symptoms. Ann Allergy Asthma Immunol. 2007;99:161-169.
[51] Turner-Warnick M: Epidemiology of norcturnal asthma. Am J Med 1988;85 (suppl 1B):6-8.
[52] Barnes P, FitzGerald G, Brown M, et al: Nocturnal asthma and changes in circulating epinephrine, histamine, and cortisol. N Engl J Med 1980;303:263-267.
[53] Douglas NJ: Asthma at night. Clin Chest Med 1985;6;663-674
[54] Peiffer C. Marsac C. Marsac A, Lockhart A: Chronobiological study of the relationship between dyspnea and airway obstruction in symptomatic asthmatic subjects. Clin Sci 1989;77:237-244.
[55] Clark TJH, Hetzel MR: Diurnal variation of asthma. Br J Dis Chest 1977;71:87-92.
[56] Szefler SJ, Ando R, Cicutto LC, et al: Plasma histamine epinephrine, cortisol, and leukocyte b-adrenergic receptors in nocturnal asthma, Clin Pharmacol Ther 1991;49:59-68
[57] Martin RJ: Nocturnal asthma: Circadian rhythms and therapeutic interventions. Am Rev Respir Dis 1993; 147(suppl): S25-S28.
[58] David J Karras MD, et al. Is Circadian Variation in Asthma Severity Relevant in the Emergency Department?. Anals of Emergency Medicine Volume 26 1995. 558-563.
[59] Payne DN, Wilson NM, James A, Hablas H, Agrefioti C, Bush A. Evidence for different subgroups of difficult asthma in children. Thorax 2001;56:345-350.
[60] Marguet C, Dean TP, Basuyau JP, Warner JO. Eosinophil cationic protein and interleukin-8 levels in bronchial lavage fluid from children with asthma and infantile wheeze. Pediatr Allergy Immunol 2001; 12:27-33.
[61] Van Den Tooorn LM, Prins JB, Overbreak SE, Hoogstenden HC, de Jongste JC. Adolescents in clinical remission of atopic asthma have elevated exhaled nitric oxide levels and bronchial hyperresponsiveness. Am J Respair Crit Care Med 3000;162:953-957.
[62] Christie GL, Helms PJ, Godden DJ, et. al. Asthma, wheezy bronchitis, and atopy across two generations. Am J Respir Crit Care Med 1999; 159:125-129.
[63] (Best Evidence) Coffman JM, Cabana MD, Yelin EH. Do school-based asthma education programs improve self-management and health outcoms? Pediatrics. Aug 2009; " 124(2):729-42 (Medline). (Full Text)
[64] (Best Evidence) Cates CJ, Bestall J, Adams N. Holding chambers versus nebulisers for inhaled steroids in chronic asthma. Cochrane Database Syst Rev. Jan 25 2006; C0001491, (Medline).
[65] Halternman JS, Szilagyi PG, Fisher SG, Fagnano M, Tremblay P, Conn KM, e al. randomized controlled trial to improve care for urban children with asthma: results of the school-based asthma therapy trial. Arch Pediatr Adolesc Med. Mar 2011; 165 (3): 262-8. (Medline)
[66] Global strategy for asthma management and prevention. Global initiative for asthma (GINA) 2006. Available at http://ginasthma.org.

[67] (Gudeline) Expert Panel Report 3 (EPR-3): Guidelines for the diagnosis and Management of Asthma –Summary Report 2007. J Allergy Clin Immunol. Nov 2007; 120 (5 Suppl): S94-138. (Medline).

[68] Togias AG. Systemic Immunologic and Inflammatory aspects of allergic rhinitis. J Allergy Clin Immunol. Nov 2000; 1065 (6 Suppl):s247-50.

[69] Thompson AK, Juniper E, Meltzer EO. Quality of life in patients with allergic rhinitis. Ann Allergy Asthma Immunol. Nov. 2000;85(5):338-47; quiz 347-8. (Medline).

[70] Bhattacharyya N. Incremental healthcare utilization and expenditures for allergic rhinitis in the United States. Laryngoscope. Sep 2011; 121 (9):1830-3

[71] Habera I, Corey JP. The role of leukotrienes in nasal allergy. Otolaryngol Head Neck Surg. Sep 2003;129(3):274-9. (Medline)

[72] Iwasaki M, Saito K, Takemura M, Sekikawa K, Fujii H, Yamada Y. TNF-alpha contributes to the development of allergic rhinitis in mice. J Allergy Clin Immunol. Jul 2003;112(1):134-40. (Medline)

[73] O'Malley CA (May 2009). "Infection control in cystic fibrosis: cohorting, cross contamination and the respiratory therapist" (http://rcjournal.com/contents05.09/05.09.0641.pdf). Respir 2Faarc0446. PMID 19393108.

[74] Reeves J, Wallace G. Unexplained bruising: weighing the pros and cons of possible causes.

[75] Franco LP, Camargos PA, Becker HM, Guimaraes RE (December 2009). Nasal Endoscopic evaluation of children and adolescents with cystic Fibrosis" (http://www.scielo.br/scielo.php?script=sci_arttext&pid=S1808-86942009006000006&lng=en&nrm=iso&tlng-en). Braz J Otorhinolaryngol 75 (6):806-13. PMID 2-2-9279 (http:ncbi.nlm.nih.gov/pubmed/20209279). 86942009000600006&lng=en&nrm=iso&tlng-en.

[76] Childers M, Eckel G, Himmel A, Caldwell J(2007). "A new model of cystic fibrosis pathology: Lack of transport of glutathione and its thiocyanate conjugates". Medical Hypotheses (68 (1):101-12. Doi:10.1016/j. mehy.2006.06.020 (http://dx.doi.org/10.1016%.Freudenheim, Mild (2009-12-22). "Tool in Cystic Fibrosis Fight: A Registry" (http://www.nytimes.com/2009/12/22/health/22cyst.html?8dpc=& pagewanted=all.Retrieved 2009-12-21.

[77] Quon BS, Fitzgerald JM, Lemiere C, Shahidi N, Oucharme FM. Increased versus stable doses of inhaled corticosteroids for exacerbations of chronic asthma in adults and children. Cochrane Database Syst Rev. Dec 8 2010;C0007524. [Medline].

[78] Ciprandi Giorgio;Cirillo, Ignazio (1 february 2011). "Forced expiratory flow between 25% and 75% of vital capacity may be marker of bronchial impairment in allergic rhinitis". Journal of Allergy and Clinical Immunology 127 (2):549-549.doi:10.1016/j.jaci.2010.10.053 (http://dx.doi.org/10/1016%2F.jaci.2010.1-.053.)

[79] Pellegrino,R; Viegi, G, Brusasco, V, Crabo, RO, Burgos, F, Casaburi, R, Coates, A, van der Griten, CP, Gustafsson, P, Hankinson,J, Jensen, R, Johnson, DC, Macintyer, N, McKay, R, Mller, Mr, Navajas, D, Pederson, OF, Wanger, J (2005 Nov). "Interpretative strategies for lung function tests". The European respiratory journa:official journal of he European Society for Clinical Respiratory Physioogy 26 (5):948_68.doi:20.1183/09031936.05.00035205

(http://dx.doi.org/10.1183%2F09031936.05.00035205). PMID 15264058 (http://dx.doi.org/org/10.1183%2F09031936.05.00035205). PMID 16264058 (http://www.ncbi.nlm.nih.gov/pubmed/162

[80] Stanojevic S, Wade A, Stocks J, et. al. (February 2008). "Reference Ranges for Spirometry Across All Ages: A new Approach" (http://www.pubmedcentral. Nih.gov/articlerender.fegi?tool=pmcentrez&artid=2643211). PMID 18006882 (http://www.ncbi.nlm.nih.gov/pubmed/18006882 http://www.pubmedcentral.nih.gov/articlerender.fcgi?tool=pmcentrez&artid=26 43211.

[81] MVV and MBC (http://www.biology-online.org/dictionary/Maximum_breathing_capacity)

[82] Kreider, Maryl. "Chapter 14.1 Pulmonary Function Testing" NoteID=48177&grpalias=TEX). ACP Medicine. Decker Intellectual Properties. (http://online.statref.com/Notes/ResolveNote.aspx? http://online.statref.com/Notes/ResolveNote.aspx?

[83] Nunn AJ, Gregg I (April 1989). "New regressional equaltions for predicting peek expiratory flow in adults" (http://www.pubmedcentral.nih.gov/articlerender.fegi?tool=pmcentrez &artid=1836460). BMJ 298 (6680):1068-70. Doi:1-1136/bmj.298.6680). PMC 1836460). PMD 2497892). http://www.pubmedcentra.gov/articlerender.fcgi?tool=pmcentral &artid=.1836460). PMID 2497892 (http://www.ncbi.nlm.nih.gov/pubmed/2497892 (http://.pubmedcentral.nih.gov/articlerender.fcgi?too=pmcentrez&artid=1836460. Adapted by clement Clarke for use in EU scale - see Peakflow.com = Predictive Normal Values (Nomogram, EU scale) (http://www.peakflow.com/top_nav/normal_values/index.html)

[84] MedlinePlus Encyclopedia Diffuse Lung Capacity (http://www.nlm.nih.gov/medlineplus/ency/article/003854.htm)

[85] George, Ronald B. (2005). Chest medicine: essentials of pulmonary and critical care medicine (http://books.google.com/books?id=2zJMbdgC).Lippincott Williams and Wilkins. P.96.ISBN 978-0-7817-5273-2.

[86] Sud, A.;Gupta, D.; Wanchu, A.; Jindal, S. K.; Bambery, P. (2001). "Static lung compliance as an index of early pulmonary disease in systemic sclerosis". Clinical rheumatology 20 (3): 177-180. Doi:10.1007/s100670170060 (http://dx.doi.org/10.1007%2Fs100670170060). PMID 11434468 (http://www.ncbi.nlm.nih.gov/pubmed/11434468).

[87] Rossi A, Gottfried SB, Zocchi L, et al. (May 1985). "Measurement of static failure during mechanical ventilation. The effect of intrinsic positive end-expiratory pressure". The American review of respiratory disease 131 (5):672 - 7. PMID 4003913 (http://www.ncbi,nlm.nih.gov/pubmed/4003913).

[88] Lausted, c.; Johnson, A.; Scott, W.; Johnson, M.; Coyne, K.; Coursey, D. (2006). "Maximum static inspiratory and expiratory pressure with different lung volumes" (http://www.pubmedcentral.nih.gov/articlerender.fcgi? Tool=pmcentrez&artid=1501025). Biomedical engineering online 5 (1): 29. Doi: 10.1186/1475-925X-5-29 (http:// dx.doi.org/10.1186%2F1475-925X-5-29).

[89] Borth, F. M. (1982). "The derivation of an index of ventilator function from spirometric recordings using canonical analysis" British Journal of Disease of the Chest 76:400-756. Doi:10.1016/0007-0971 (82)90077-8 (http://dx.doi.org/10.1016%2F0007-0971%288%2990077-8).

[90] Brannan, J.D., P. G.D. Subbarao, B. Ho, S. D. Anderson, H.K Chan, and A.L. Coates. 1999. Inhaled mannitol identifies metacholine responsive children with current asthma (abstract). Am. J. Respir. Crit. Care Med. 159:A911.

[91] Jensen, E. J., R. Dahl, and F. Steffensen. 1998. Bronchial reactivity to cigarette smoke in smokers: repeatability, relationship to metacholine reactivity, smoking, and atopy. Eur. Respir. J. 11:870-676.

[92] Hayes, R. D., J.R. Beach, D. M. Rutherford, and M.R. Sim. 1998. Statbility of methacholine chloride solutions under different storage conditions over a 9 month period. Eur Respir. J. 11:946- 948.

[93] Pathogenesis, prevalence, diagnosis, and management of exercise-induced bronchoconstriction: A practice parameter. Palatine, III.: The American Academy of Allergy, Asthma and Immunology and the American College of Allergy, Asthma and Immunology. http://www.aaaai.org/Aaaai/media/MediaLibrary/PDF%20Documents/ Practice%20and%20Parameters/Exercise-induced -bronchoconstriction-2011.pdf. Accessed. Accessed Sept 26, 2011.

[94] Asthma and exercise: Tips to remember. American Academy of Allergy Asthma and Immunology. http://www.aaaai.org/conditions-and-treatments/library/asthma-library/asthma-and exercise.aspx. Accessed Sept.26, 2011.

[95] Asthma action plan. National Heart, Lung, and Blood Institute. http://ww.nhlbi.nih.gov/health/publik/lung/asthma/asthma_actplan.Accessed

[96] Valkvists S, Sinding M, Skampstrup K, Bisgaard H (June 2006). "Daily home measurements of exhaled n itric oxide in asthmatic children during natural birch pollen exposure" (http://linkinghub.elsevir.com/retrieve/pii/S0091-6749 (06) 00659-2). J. aLLERGY Clin. Immunol. 117 (6)"1272-6. Doi:10.1016/j.jaci.2006.03.018 (http://www.ncbi.nlm.nih.gov/pubmed/16750986). http://linkinghub.elsevier.com/retrieve/pii/S0091-6749 (06) 00659-2.

[97] Petsky HL, Cates CJ, Li AM, Kynaston JA, Turner C, Chang AB (2008). Petsky, Helen L. ed. "Tailored interventions based on exhaled nitric oxide versus clinical symptoms for asthma in children and adults". Cochrane Data Syst Rev (2): CD006340. Doi:10.1002%2F14651858. CD006340.pub2). PMID 18425949 (http://www.ncbi.nlm.nih.gov/pubmed/18425949).

[98] Malmberg LP, Pelkonen AS. Haahtela T, Turppeinen M (June 2003). "Exhaled nitric oxide rather than lung function distringuishes preschool children probable asthma "http://thorax.bmj.com/cgi/pmidlookup? view=long&pmid=12775859). Thorax 58 (6):494-9. doi: 10.1136/thorax. 58.6.494 (http://dx.doi.org/10.1136%2Fthorax.58.6.494). PMC 1746693 (http:www.ncbi.nlm.nih.gov.pubmed/12775859 (http://www.ncbi.nlm.nih.gov/pubmed/12775859) http://thorax.bmj.com/cgi/pmidlookup?view-long&pmid=12775859.

[99] Fahy JV, Kim KW, Liu J, Boushey HA. Prominent neutrophilic inflammation in sputum from subjects with sthma exacerbations. J Allergy Clin Immunol 19995;4:843-852.

[100] Lamblin C. Gosset P, Tillie-Leblond I, et al. Bronchial neturophilia in patients with noninfectious status asthmaticus. Am J Respir Crit Care Med 1998; 157:349-402.

[101] Wenzel SE Shwartz LB, Langmack ELM, et al. Evidence that asthma can be divided pathologically into two inflammatory subtypes with distinct physiologic and clinical characteristics. Am J Respir Crit Care Med 1999; 160: 1001-1008.

[102] Di Stefano A, Capelli A, LUsuardi M, et al. Severity of airflow limitation is associated with severity of airway inflammation in smokers. Am J Respir Crit Care Med 1998; 158:1277-1285.

[103] Jeffrey PK. Comparison of the structural and inflammatory features of COPD and asthma. Chest 2000; 117: 2518 - 260S.

[104] Saetta M, Turato G, Baraldo S, et al. Goblet cell hyperplasia and epithelial inflammation in peripheral airways of smokers with both symptoms of chronic bronchitis and airflow limitation. Am J respire Crit Care Med 2000; 161: 1-16-1021.

[105] Wu AC, Tantisira K, Li L, Scuemann B, Weiss ST, Fuhlbrigge AL. Predictors of Symptoms are Different from Predictors of Severe Exacerbations from Asthma in Children. Chest. Fbe 3, 2011; (Medline).

[106] Rodrigo GJ, Neffen H, Castro-Rodriguez JA. Efficacy and safety of subcutaneious Omalizumab vs placebo as add-on therapy to corticosteroids for children and adults with asthma: a systematic review. Chest. Jan 2011; 139 (1): 28-35. (Medline).

[107] Busse WW, Morgan WJ, Gergen PJ, Mitchell, Gem JE, Liu AH, et al Randomized trial of Omalizumab (anti-IgE) for asthma in inner-city children. N Engl J Med. Mar 17 2011; 364 (11):1—5-15 (Medline).

[108] Quon BS. Fitzgerald JM, Lemiere C, Shahidi N, Ducharme FM. Increased versus stable doeses of inhaled corticosteroids for exacerbations of chronic asthma in adults and children. Cochrane Database Syst Rev. Dec 8 2010; CD007524.

[109] (Best Evidence) Rachelefsky G. Inhaled corticosteroids and asthma control in children: assessing impairment and risk. Pediatrics. Jan 2009; 123(1):353-66.

[110] Wechsler ME, Lehman E, Lazarus SC, Lemanske RF Jr, Boushey HA, Deykin A, et al. beta-adrenergic receptor polymorphisms and response to salmeterol. AM j Respir Crit Care Med. Mar 1 2006; 173(5):519.(Medline).Full Text).

[111] The Salmeterol Multicenter Astma Research Trial: A comparison of usual Phamacotherapy plus salmeterol.

[112] US Food and Drug Administration. FDA Drug Safety Communication: New Safety requirements for along-acting ialed asthma medications called Long-Acting Beta-Agonist (LABA): Human Department of Health and Human Services. Feb 18, 2010; 1-4(Full Text).

[113] Postma OS, q'Byrne PM, Pederson S. Comparison of the effect of low-dose circlesonide and fixed-dose fluticasone propionate and salmeterol combination on long-term asthma control. Chest. Feb 2011; 139(2); 311-8. (Medline).

[114] (Best Evidence) Rachelefsky G. Inhaled corticosteroids and asthma control in children: assessing impairment and risk. Pediatrics. Jan 2009; 1231 (1):353-66. (Medline).

[115] Martinex FO, Chinchilli VM, Morgan WJ, Boehmer SJ, Lenmanske RF Jr, Mauger OT, et al. Use of beclomethasone dipropionate as rescue treatment for children with mild persistent asthma (TREXA): a randomized, double-blind, placeboocontrolled trial. Lancet. Feb 19 2011;377(9766(:650-7. (Medline)

[116] Quon BS, Fitzgerald JM, Lenmiere C, Shahidi N, Ducharme FM. Increased versus stable doses of inhaled corticosteroids for exacerbations of chronic asthma in adults and children. Cochrane Database Syst Rev. Dec 8 2010; CD007524. (Medline).
[117] Agertoft L, Pedersen S. Effect of long-term treatment with inhaled budesonide on adult height in children with asthma. N Eng/JmED. Oct 12 2000;343(15): 1 064-9, (Medline).
[118] Ege MJ, Mayer M, Normand AC, Genuneit J, et al. Exposure to environmental microorganisms and childhood asthma. N Engl J Med. Feb 24 2011; 364 (8): 701-9. (Medline)
[119] Lenmanske RF, Mauger DT, Sorkness CA, et al. Step-up therapy for children with uncontrolled asthma receiving inhaled conrticosteroids. N Eng/J Med. Mar 30, 2010; 364(11):1 005-15. (Medline)
[120] Castro-Rodriguez JA, Holberg CJ, Wright AL, Martinez FD. A clinical index to define risk of asthma in young children with recurrent wheezing. Am J Respir Crit Care Med. Oct, 2000; 162 (4 Pt1): 1403-6. (Medline).
[121] Lipworth BJ, Clark DJ, Effects of airway caliber on lung delivery of nebulized salbutamol. Thorax 1997:52:1036-1039.
[122] Penna AC, Dawson KP, Manglick P, et. Al. Systemic absorption of salbutamol after nebulizer delivery in acute asthma. Acta Paediatr 1993;82:963-966.
[123] Vassallo R, Lipsky JJ. Theophylline; recent advances in the understanding of its mode of action and uses in clinical practice. Mayo Cline Proc 1998;73:346-354
[124] Fanta CH, Bossing Th, McFadden ER, Treatment of acute asthma: is combination therapy with sympathomimetics and methylxanthines indicated? Am J Med 1986;80:5-10
[125] Handslip PDJ, Dart AM Davies BH, Intravenous salbutamol and aminophylline in asthma: a search for synergy. Thorax 1981:36:741-744.
[126] Best Evidence Guilbert TW, Morgan WJ, Zeiger RS, Mauger DT, Boehmer SJ, Szfler SJ, et al. Long term inhaled corticosteroids in preschool children at high risk of asthma. N Engl J Med. May 11 2006;354 (19):1985-97 (Medline).
[127] Postma OS, q'Byrne PM, Pederson S. Comparison of the effect of low-dose circlesonide and fixed-dose fluticasone propionate and salmeterol combination on long-term asthma control. Chest. Feb 2011; 139(2); 311-8. (Medline)

9

Mechanisms of Reduced Glucocorticoid Sensitivity in Bronchial Asthma

Yasuhiro Matsumura
Akishima Hospital
Japan

1. Introduction

Although glucocorticoids (GCs) are among the most widely used compounds for treating asthma, patients with severe asthma sometimes have uncontrolled symptoms despite GC therapy. These patients have an impaired response to GCs, and may demonstrate a temporal reduction in GC reactivity when asthma deteriorates. Although it can be difficult to differentiate truly GC-resistant (GC-R) asthma (Hakonarson et al., 2005), it may correspond to severe asthma. It is defined as persistence of airway obstruction associated with an increase of less than 15% in the forced expiratory volume in 1 second (FEV1) following 2-week high-dose prednisolone administration, as evaluated mainly by reversibility of airflow obstruction (Corrigan & Loke, 2007; Woolcock, 1996). A definition referring to the inhalation route remains obscure (Hakonarson et al., 2005).

Co-administration of certain drugs, e.g. rifampicin, phenytoin and phenobarbital, which may possibly reduce steroid availability by affecting steroid metabolism through CYP3A4, should always be considered by clinicians.

Many processes involved in inflammation escape GC modulation, and resistance to the anti-inflammatory effects of these compounds is mediated via several mechanisms.

2. Actions of GCs

GCs upregulate mRNAs of molecules that suppress inflammatory cytokines and downregulate mRNAs of various inflammatory cytokines and chemokines. GCs increase gene expression of GC-induced leucine zipper (GILZ), mitogen-activated protein kinase phosphatase-1 (MKP-1), and the RNA-binding protein tristetraprolin. Expression of lipocortin-1, interleukin (IL)-10, IL-1 receptor antagonist, and inhibitor-κBα (I-κBα) is also induced. GCs suppress expression of epithelial-derived cytokines and chemoattractants that promote inflammatory cell recruitment. Cytokine expressions is inhibited through reversal of histone acetylation at sites of cytokine gene expression by direct interaction of GC receptors (GRs) with nuclear factor kappa B (NF-κB)-associated coactivators or by recruitment of histone deacetylases (HDAC) to the activated transcription complex.

Low concentrations of dexamethasone (DEX) reportedly rapidly regulate intracellular pH, Ca^{2+} and cAMP-dependent protein kinase activity, and inhibit Cl^- secretion in bronchial epithelial cells via nongenomic mechanisms (Urbach et al., 2006).

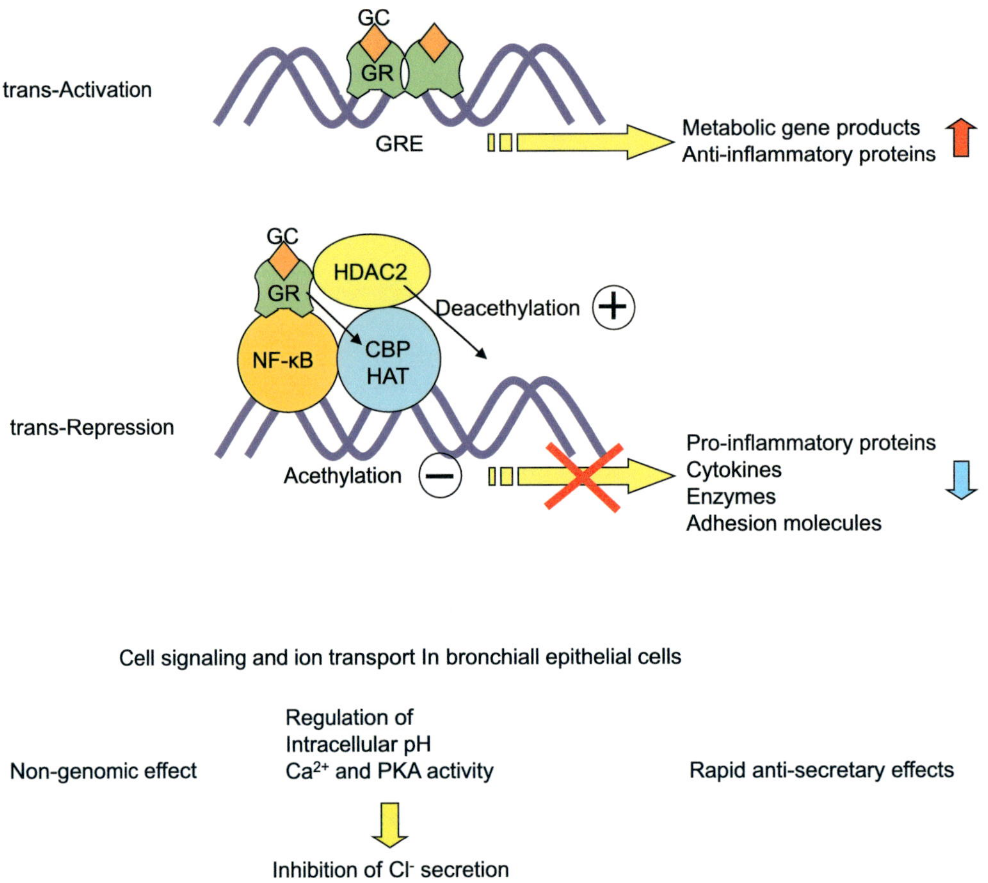

Fig. 1. **Anti-inflammatory actions of GC**
Trans-Activation: GRs bind to GREs and activate genes encoding β2-adrenergic receptors and anti-inflammatory proteins, such as secretory leukoprotease inhibitor (SLPI), MKP-1, IκB-α, and GILZ.
Trans-Repression: GRs inhibit transcription factors such as NF-κB and AP-1. GRs bind to co-activators, such as cAMP-response element-binding protein (CREB)-binding protein (CBP), and thereby inhibit HAT activity. GRs also recruit HDAC2 to the NF-κB -activated inflammatory gene complex.
Nongenomic effect: GCs rapidly regulate intracellular pH, Ca^{2+} and cAMP-dependent protein kinase (PKA) activity and inhibit Cl^- secretion in human bronchial epithelial cells, suggesting GC modulate secretion.

3. Transcription factors

Overexpression of chemokines and cytokines induces inflammatory processes in the airways of asthmatics. These mediators are downstream targets of transcription factors that antagonize steroid signaling via competition with GR-associated co-activators. This mutual transcriptional activity competition between GR and other regulators is among the mechanisms contributing to GC-R asthma.

3.1 GRs

GRs belong to the steroid/thyroid/retinoic acid nuclear receptor superfamily of transcription factor proteins.

Anti-inflammatory actions of GCs are often attenuated in inflamed tissues and differ among tissues. Ligand-dependent downregulation of GR expression via proteasomes was apparent in a respiratory epithelial cell line as compared to keratinocyte-like and hematopoietic cell lines, and was enhanced by lipopolysaccharide (LPS) via activation of p38 mitogen-activated protein kinase (MAPK), c-Jun N-terminal (JNK) and cyclin-dependent kinases (Hirasawa et al., 2009).

GRs are phosphorylated on specific serine residues after hormone binding and also by several kinases and phosphatases as a substrate. Although the precise roles of each specific phosphorylation event remain unclear, GR phosphorylation is involved in its stability, subcellular localization, interactions with coregulators, and transcriptional responses. Phosphorylation of GR on one or more residues adds increasing complexity to GC signaling and may explain how GR differentially regulates subsets of genes in various cell types. GR phosphorylation patterns via enhanced kinase activities of p38 MAPK, JNK, and GSK-3 in diseased cells contribute to different GC signaling within normal and diseased tissues (Bantel et al., 2002; Galliher-Beckley et al., 2008; Irusen et al., 2002; Itoh et al., 2002; Rogatsky et al., 1998; Szatmáry et al., 2004; Wang et al., 2004). GC-induced alterations in GR phosphorylation status are suggested to be associated with acquired GC resistance (Galliher-Beckley & Cidlowski, 2009).

Although phosphor-Ser226-GR reportedly associates with endogenous GRE-containing promoters and remains transcriptionally active, most studies suggest that Ser226 phosphorylation of GR attenuates GR signaling (Ismaili & Garabedian, 2004). Furthermore, JNK-mediated phosphorylation of GR at Serine 226 blunted hormone signaling by enhancing nuclear export of GR (Itoh et al., 2002). Activation of p38 MAPK by IL-2 and IL-4 induces GR phosphorylation and reduces ligand-binding affinity of GR in the nucleus (Irusen et al., 2002). Reduced GR ligand-binding affinity induced by IL-2/IL-4 (Kam et al., 1993; Sher et al., 1994) can be blocked with specific p38 MAPK inhibitors, suggesting that p38 MAPK inhibitors may reverse GC insensitivity (Irusen et al., 2002). IL-2/IL-4 pretreatment and p38 MAPK activation may affect the expression and/or activity of phosphatases, thereby inhibiting DEX-induced S211 phosphorylation of GR, which serves as a biomarker for activated GR in vivo, and preventing GR nuclear translocation in response to hormones (Goleva et al., 2009).

Sensitivity to GCs could reflect the degree of GC-induced GR nuclear translocation (Matthews et al., 2004). The IL-2/IL-4 combination alters GR nuclear translocation in T cells, an effect reversed by IFN-γ via inhibition of p38MAPK activation, suggesting critical role of INF-γ for maintaining GC sensitivity (Goleva et al., 2009). Combined budesonide and formoterol can stimulate GR and promote its translocation to the nucleus (Roth et al., 2002).

GRβ is an alternatively spliced form that binds to DNA but cannot be activated by GC, and reportedly antagonizes the trans-activating activity of GRα. GRβ expression is significantly increased in some patients with GC-R asthma and GRβ might be involved in GC resistance (Goleva et al., 2006; Hamid et al., 1999; Kelly et al., 2008; Pujols et al., 2001; Sousa et al.,

2000). CD38 expression upregulates the GRβ isoform, becoming insensitive to GC action thus providing a novel in vitro cellular model for ascertaining how GC resistance develops in primary cells (Tliba et al., 2006). A recent study demonstrated that GRβ promotes steroid insensitivity by controlling HDAC2 expression by inhibiting GC response elements in its promoter (Li et al., 2010). Hypoxia impairs anti-inflammatory actions of GCs by decreasing expression of GRα, but not GRβ, in A549 cells (Huang et al., 2009). However, the role of GRβ in modulating sensitivity to GCs remains controversial.

FK506-binding protein 51 (FKBP51) expression might affect clinical responsiveness to GCs (Denny at al., 2005; Reynolds et al., 1999; Vermeer et al., 2004a; Vermeer et al., 2004b). FKBP51 is an immunophilin chaperone protein residing in the cytoplasm before GC binding. GC dissociates GR from chaperone complexes, translocates GR to the nucleus, and modulates transcription. FKBP51 overexpression inhibits GR signaling by impairing nuclear translocation (Wochnik et al., 2005) and reducing GC binding (Denny et al., 2000). FKBP51 was induced by GCs (Rogatsky et al., 2003; Vermeer et al., 2003), suggesting FKBP51 to function in a negative-feedback loop limiting GR signaling. Airway epithelial cells collected from asthmatics showed high FKBP51 expression associated with a poor GC response (Woodruff et al., 2007).

3.2 Activator protein-1 (AP-1)

AP-1 expression is enhanced in asthmatic airways by Th2 cytokines (Demoly et al., 1992). GC resistance was associated with inability of GCs to deactivate JNK MAPK, as reflected by elevated phosphorylated c-Jun and c-fos gene expression in GC resistance and coinciding with decreased GR-AP-1 interaction intensity in steroid-resistant asthmatics as compared with peripheral blood mononuclear cells (PBMC) (Adcock et al., 1995; Takahashi et al., 2002), monocytes and T lymphocytes (Lane et al., 1998), immunohistochemical analysis of the tuberculin-mediated cutaneous response (Sousa et al., 1999), and bronchial biopsies (Loke et al., 2006) from GC-responsive patients.

3.3 NF-κB

NF-κB, a homo- or heterodimer consisting of subunits from the Rel family of proteins comprised of c-Rel, NF-κB1 (p50), NF-κB2 (p52), Rel A (p65), and Rel B, is activated by a broad range of inflammatory and environmental stimuli, e.g. tumor necrosis factor-α (TNF-α), IL-1β, IL-2, leukotriene B4, allergens, mitogens, LPS, viral infection, oxidative stress, and reactive oxygen exposure. The inflammation target is the prevalent heterodimer NF-κB p65-p50. p50 can increase DNA binding and p65 confers transcriptional regulation.

In patients with bronchial asthma, like other inflammatory diseases, NF-κB activity is increased. Increased activity has been reported in airway epithelial cells, submucosal cells, and sputum macrophages (Caramori et al., 2009; Hart et al., 1998; Vignola et al., 2001). Increases in activated p65, phosphorylated IκBα (p-IκBα), and IκB kinase β (IKKβ) have been documented in PBMC from subjects with severe uncontrolled asthma (Gagliardo et al., 2003). Rhinovirus infection activates NF-κB, leading to cytokine production and expression of adhesion molecules (Papi & Johnston, 1999; Zhu et al., 1996; Zhu et al., 1997), exacerbating asthma and steroid refractoriness. Excess active NF-κB in severe uncontrolled asthma, which may reflect inflammatory stimuli, may impair the anti-inflammatory actions of GCs by interacting with GR.

3.4 GATA-3

The zincfinger transcription factor GATA-3 is essential for expression of the IL-4, IL-5 and IL-13 genes (Ray & Cohn, 1999; Zhu et al., 2006). Upon activation, GATA-3 is phosphorylated by p38 MAPK and translocates from the cytoplasm to the nucleus via the nuclear import protein importin-α. GCs inhibit GATA-3 function by rapidly blocking GATA-3 nuclear translocation via preferential binding to shared importin-α and also by inhibiting p38 MAPK via MKP-1 induction (Barnes, 2008).

3.5 CCAAT enhancer-binding protein (C/EBP)

C/EBP belongs to the basic region-leucine zipper transcription factor family. C/EBP-α, which binds the zinc finger motif of single active GR molecules and translocates to the nucleus, modulates GR function allowing induction of key anti-inflammatory mediators (Roth et al., 2004). Airway smooth muscle (ASM) cells from asthmatics are deficient in C/EBP-α, seemingly due to reduced translation controlling factor eukaryotic initiation factor-4E (eIF-4E) (Borger et al., 2009), resulting in poor inhibition of smooth muscle proliferation in vitro (Borger et al., 2007; Roth & Black, 2009). Budesonide plus formoterol simultaneously activates GR and C/EBP-α, resulting in synergistic stimulatory effects on p21 promoter activity and additive inhibitory effects on serum-induced proliferation (Roth et al., 2002).

3.6 Interferon regulatory factor-1 (IRF-1)

Recent investigations demonstrated elevated IRF-1, an early response gene involved in diverse transcriptional regulatory processes, in cells exposed to multiple cytokines that reduce GC responsiveness. IRF-1 promotes GC insensitivity in human ASM cells by interfering with GR signaling (Tliba et al., 2008). Inhibition of GR function by IRF-1 involves its interaction with transcriptional co-regulator GR-interacting protein 1 (GRIP-1). Under GC-R conditions, cytokines enhance expression of IRF-1, depleting GRIP-1 from the GR complex, thereby reducing transcriptions of GR-dependent genes such as MKP-1 and promoting expressions of IRF-1-dependent pro-inflammatory genes such as CD38 (Bhandare et al., 2010). As IRF-1 expression is markedly increased after viral infections, suppressive effects of IRF-1 on GC signaling may explain the reduced GC responsiveness in asthmatics experiencing viral infections (Kröger et al., 2002; Vianna et al., 1998; Yamada et al., 2000).

4. Chromatin modification; histone acetyltransferase (HAT) and HDAC

Reduced HDAC activity and reciprocally increased HAT activity are reported to be among the mechanisms underlying reduced GC sensitivity in bronchial asthma patients (Ito et al., 2002a). Patients with severe asthma have diminished GC sensitivity of PBMC compared to those with nonsevere asthma, associated with reduced HDAC activity paralleling impaired GC sensitivity (Hew et al., 2006). HDAC2 deacetylates GR, enabling p65–NF-κB association and subsequent attenuation of pro-inflammatory gene transcription (Ito et al., 2006). Low-dose theophylline restores HDAC activity in vivo (Ito et al., 2002b).

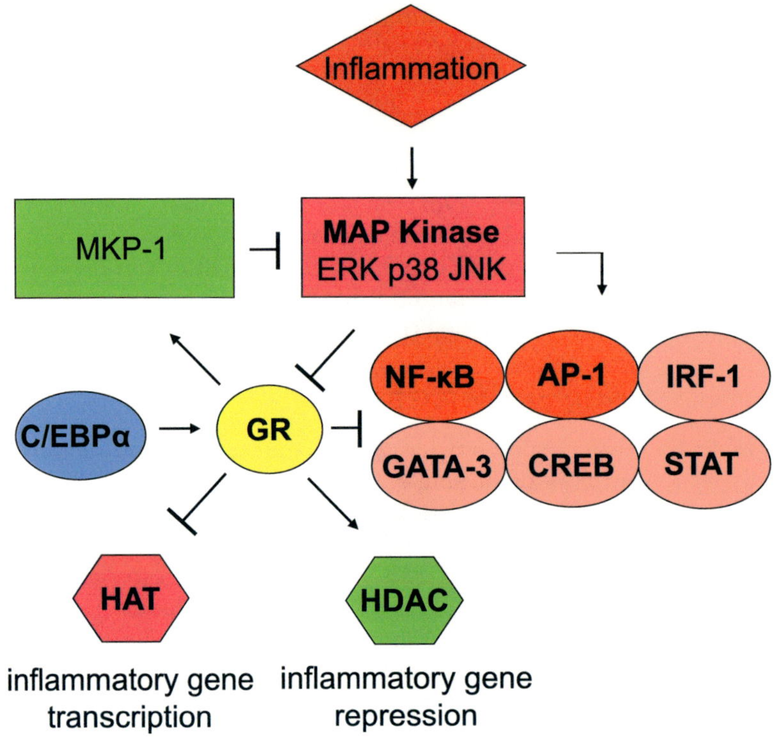

Fig. 2. **Intracellular factors and pathways of GC-R asthma.**
GC acts through switching on the expression of anti-inflammatory genes such as MKP-1 or switching off inflammatory genes through negatively regulate the activity of various other DNA-bound transcription factors, including NF-κB, AP-1 ,CREB, IRF-1, STAT, and GATA-3, via the transrepression mechanism or tethering mechanism. Inflammatory stimulation provokes activation of protein kinase pathways and transcription factors, resulting in attenuation of GR function and reduction of HDAC activity or recruitment.

5. Protein kinase signaling

Intracellular protein kinases are involved in the expression and activation of inflammatory mediators in the airways. MAPK family members, e.g. p38MAPK, JNK and extracellular signal-regulated kinase (ERK), are implicated in airway inflammation via activation of pro-inflammatory transcription factors including AP-1 and NF-κB, or via regulation of stabilization and increased translation of pro-inflammatory cytokine mRNA, dependent on conserved AU-rich elements in the 3′-UTRregion (Dean et al., 2004).

GCs not only induce MKP-1, an endogenous inhibitor of MAPK genes, but also reduce its degradation (Abraham et al., 2006; Clark, 2003). MKP-1 inhibits MAPK pathways and thereby inhibits JNK and to a lesser extent ERK.

Alveolar macrophages from patients with severe asthma show reduced inhibition of cytokine release by DEX with increased p38 MAPK activation, possibly resulting from impaired MKP-1 inducibility (Bhavsar et al., 2008), suggesting that GC insensitivity in severe asthma could be improved by p38 MAPK inhibitors (Bhavsar et al., 2010).

Moreover, GC responses of GC-R patient samples were restored by adding MAPK inhibitors (Goleva et al., 2009; Irusen et al., 2002; Li et al., 2004; Tsitoura & Rothman, 2004). Thus, MAPK-mediated inhibition of GR function appears to be key to GC resistance.

In GC-R asthma patients, increased p38 MAPK phosphorylation corresponds to reduced induction of dual-specificity phosphatases (DUSP) 1 expression (Bhavsar et al., 2008). Taken together, these observations suggest GC unresponsiveness to play central roles in MAPK dysregulation and probably also impaired DUSP1 induction.

Cytokine signaling, including type I interferon signaling, through cognate Jak/signal transduction and activators of transcription (STAT) pathways is reported to be unaffected or even stimulated by GR. Inhibition of JAK/STAT signaling may be of therapeutic benefit in GC-R airway disease (Clarke et al., 2010; Flammer et al., 2010).

PI3K plays an integral role in the immune system, for both mast cells and eosinophil function (Marwick et al., 2010), and may contribute to GC sensitivity by reducing HDAC activity (Ito et al., 2007). Therapeutic inhibition of PI3Kδ is reported to restore GC function in oxidative stress-induced GC-insensitive mice (Marwick et al., 2009).

6. Cytokine-induced GC insensitivity

Inflammatory cytokines alter GC cellular responses. Cytokines from Th2 cells are implicated in the pathogenesis of athma. IL-4 and IL-13 switch B cells to IgE synthesis, IL-5 plays a role in eosinophil maturation and survival, and IL-13 regulates airway hyper-responsiveness (AHR) and mucus hyperplasia. A study of bronchoalveolar lavage (BAL) fluid showed significantly greater numbers of cells expressing IL-2 and IL-4 mRNA in GC-R than in GC-sensitive asthmatics (Leung et al., 1995). Bronchial biopsy specimens from GC-R asthma patients revealed overexpression of IL-2, IL-4 and IL-13 and reduced GR affinity of inflammatory cells (Leung et al., 1999; Szefler & Leung, 1997).

IL-33, described as a promoter of Th2 immunity and systemic inflammation (Schmitz et al., 2005), is expressed at higher levels in ASM cells of asthmatics. DEX failed to abrogate TNF-α-induced IL-33 expression (Préfontaine et al., 2009).

TNF-α, a pro-inflammatory cytokine, is often associated with conditions that might activate innate immunity in the lung. Upregulation of the TNF-α axis in bronchial asthma with reduced sensitivity was reported (Berry et al., 2006; Howarth et al., 2005; Morjaria et al., 2008). TNF-α is produced by Th1 cells and macrophages and to a lesser extent mast cells in ASM, possibly inducing AHR. TNF-α is increased in BAL and bronchial biopsy specimens from severe asthma patients and is associated with GC-R (Howarth et al., 2005). TNF-α suppresses GC responsiveness in monocytes (Franchimont et al., 1999) and upregulates pathways involved in chronic airway remodeling and subepithelial fibrosis (Sullivan et al., 2005). TNFα upregulates the ERK1/ERK2 and p38MAPK pathways and induces expression of CXCL8, a neutrophil chemoattractant. Activation of the ERK1/ERK2 MAPK cascade is completely insensitive to actions of GCs in ASM cells and is involved in neutrophil recruitment contributing to inflammation (Robins et al., 2011).

Cytokines associated with Th1 immunity rather than allergic Th2 responses may contribute to the pathogenesis of severe GC-R asthma (Heaton et al., 2005). Th1 cells induce steroid-resistant AHR through an INF-γ/TLR4-MyD88-dependent mechanism after LPS-priming of the innate host defense system (Yang et al., 2009). Although interferon γ (IFN-γ), a Th1 cytokine, prevented airway inflammation, some studies suggest that Th1 cells, secreting IFN-γ, might cause severe airway inflammation (Cui et al., 2005; Hansen et al., 1999). Sputum IFN-γ levels were markedly increased in airway cells obtained by sputum induction in patients with moderate to severe asthma and nonallergic asthma (Truyen et al., 2006). IFN-γ is expressed by an increased percentage of cells in the airways of severe asthmatics (Shannon et al., 2008).

TNF-α and IFN-γ synergistically enhance transcriptional activation of interferon- γ -inducible protein-10 (CXCL10), a potent chemoattractant for mast cells and T lymphocytes, cells implicated in asthma pathophysiology and elevated in patients suffering viral exacerbation of asthma, in human ASM cells via STAT-1, NF-κB and the transcriptional coactivator CREB-binding protein. Abrogation of JAK2 and subsequent STAT-1 signaling was more effective than fluticasone in an in vitro model of steroid-resistant inflammation, suggesting JAK/STAT signaling inhibition to be of therapeutic benefit in GC-R (Clarke et al., 2010).

Dysregulation of INF-γ producing Th1 cells or IL-10-producing regulatory T cells can counterbalance the number of Th2 cells. IL-10, a potent anti-inflammatory and immunosuppressive cytokine, appears to correlate inversely with the incidence and/or severity of asthma (Akdis et al., 2004; Borish et al., 1996; Heaton et al., 2005; Lim et al., 1998). Induction of IL-10 synthesis may contribute to the clinical efficacy of GCs in allergy and asthma. CD4+ T cells from GC-R asthmatics show markedly reduced capacity to synthesize IL-10, which inhibits pro-inflammatory cytokine production, antigen presentation, T cell activation and mast cell and eosinophil function, following in vitro stimulation in the presence of DEX, as compared with those from GC-sensitive patients with similar disease severity (Hawrylowicz et al., 2002).

Thus, GC-R asthma is associated with an altered cytokine gene expression profile; i.e. failure to suppress production of inflammatory cytokines and to induce production of anti-inflammatory cytokines.

Dehydroepiandrosterone (DHEA) can reverse cytokine imbalances associated with asthma, possibly preventing and attenuating allergic airway inflammation. Clinically, a steroid-sparing effect is observed with DHEA. DHEA and its analogs might prove useful in reversing relative GC-insensitivity in patients with GC-R asthma (Kasperska-Zajac, 2010).

7. Inflammatory cells

In severe asthma, pathological features different from those in mild-to-moderate asthma include mixed Th2/Th1 phenotypes with possible Th17 or regulatory T cell involvement. This type of asthma is GC-refractory.

Some asthma patients have neutrophils instead of eosinophils in their sputum. In general, asthma associated with neutrophils tends to show increased airway gland secretion, AHR, tissue destruction and airway remodeling, resulting in a severe condition (Douwes et al., 2002; Wenzel et al., 1998; Wenzel, 2009). Epidermal growth factor receptor (EGFR) (Puddicombe et al., 2000), which correlates with IL-8 (Hamilton et al., 2003; Hamilton et al., 2005), could contribute to sustained neutrophilic inflammation. Subjects with neutrophilic asthma have increased activation of proteolytic enzymes, such as neutrophil elastase, indicating protease/anti-protease imbalance, as compared with other asthma phenotypes (Simpson et al., 2005). Moreover, it is characterized by a poor response to GC (Green et al., 2002; Pavord et al., 1999; Pavord, 2007). A mouse model suggested GC-R neutrophilic inflammation in acute exacerbation of asthma to be related to impaired nuclear recruitment of HDAC2, leading to ongoing enhanced expression of neutrophil chemoattractant and survival factors (Ito et al., 2008). The neutrophil infiltrates in these patients suggest activation of innate host defense pathways. This is consistent with evidence that infection and allergen exposure function synergistically in the pathogenesis of asthma exacerbations.

In a mouse model, Th17 cells, which play a central role in regulating neutrophilic inflammation during infection, were linked to GC-R AHR (McKinley et al., 2008). IL-17 is reported to be increased in the lungs, sputum, and BAL fluid of asthmatics (Bullens et al., 2006), and its expression level correlates with disease severity (Kawaguchi et al., 2009). IL-17 is especially important for neutrophil recruitment (Pène et al., 2008). Th17 cytokine responses are not sensitive to DEX. Th17 cell-mediated airway inflammation and AHR are steroid-resistant, indicating a potential role of Th17 cells in GC-R asthma. IL-17F plays a pro-inflammatory role in asthma, by activating transcription factors such as C/EBPβ, C/EBPγ and NF-κB.

8. Other novel intracellular mechanisms causing GC-R

Amphiregulin is secreted by human mast cells after exposure to antigens via aggregation of FcεRI, resulting in sputum production. Its expression is not inhibited by DEX. This may explain GC treatment being largely ineffective against sputum overproduction (Okumura et al., 2005).

Cofilin is a novel factor causing GC-R. Cofilin is known to promote actin depolymerization and filament severing. Cofilin 1, the evolutionarily conserved ADF/cofilin family, is crucial for many cellular processes, e.g. cell motility, cell division and membrane organization. The inhibitory action of cofilin on GR may have physiological relevance. Overexpressions of cofilin and actin as well as chemical cytoskeletal disruption changed the subcellular receptor distribution and upregulated c-Jun, possibly explaining the inhibitory mechanism of cofilin-1. Increased cofilin-1 expression is important for regulating GC sensitivity in peripheral blood lymphocytes of patients with severe treatment-resistant asthma (Vasavda et al., 2006).

9. Air way structure and remodeling

The effects of GC on airway remodeling are not completely understood. Airway remodeling is associated with increased deposition of extracellular matrix (ECM) proteins such as type I collagen. Immunoreactivity of type I collagen was not reduced in the submucosa of moderate to severe asthmatics after a 2-week oral GC course (Chakir et al., 2003). Overexpression of AP-1, which is known to be involved in regulating the procollagen-α II promoter by inhibiting its activity, impairs GC inhibition of collagen production by fibroblasts in asthmatics (Jacques et al., 2010).

The ratio of matrix metalloprotease (MMP)-9 to tissue inhibitor of MMP (TIMP)-1 is higher in the lungs of patients with severe asthma. MMP-9 is produced in neutrophils (Cundall et al., 2003). This is poorly inhibited by GCs. Eosinophilic asthma is characterized by active MMP-9 without free elastase (Simpson et al., 2005). DEX upregulates TIMP-1 mRNA in BAL fluid cells from patients with GC-sensitive asthma, but not in cells from those with GC-R asthma. Inability of GC to enhance TIMP-1 production shifts the MMP-9/TIMP-1 ratio in GC-R asthma, potentially promoting proteolytic activity and possibly resulting in abnormal tissue remodeling of airways (Goleva et al., 2007), leading to reduced lung function and β-agonist reversibility in these patients.

10. Environmental and behavioral factors

The classical macrophage activation and induction of LPS signaling pathways along with high endotoxin levels in BAL fluid from GC-R asthma patients suggest LPS exposure to contribute to GC-R asthma (Goleva et al., 2008).

Increased T-cell receptor vβ8+ T cells in BAL fluid of subjects with poorly controlled asthma suggests a role for microbial superantigens (Hauk et al., 1999). Microbial superantigens may contribute to GC insensitivity through induction of GR (Hauk et al., 2000). Microbial superantigens induce human T-cell resistance to GC, via the Raf-MEK-ERK1/ERK2 pathway of T-cell receptor signaling, which leads to GCRα phosphorylation and inhibition of DEX-induced GCRα nuclear translocation (Li et al., 2004). This may occur in exacerbation of asthma symptoms by bacterial infection.

Clinically, bronchial asthma patients who smoke have an impaired GC response as compared to nonsmokers (Chaudhuri et al., 2006). The sputum of asthmatic patients who smoke contains more neutrophils and CXCL8, which is closely associated with severe asthma (Thomson et al., 2004). Smoking increases NF-κB activity, resulting in increased expression of inflammatory genes such as IL-8, MMP and monocyte chemoattractant protein. Smoking can inhibit GR function by suppressing GR-associated HDAC2 activity and expression (Ito et al., 2001). It also reduces the GRα:β ratio in PBMC (Livingston et al., 2004), and GC insensitivity in smokers with asthma may be more generalized, affecting tissue sites other than the airways (Livingston et al., 2007).

In asthma patients, reduced vitamin D levels are associated with impaired lung function, increased AHR and reduced GC responsiveness (Ginde et al., 2009; Sutherland et al., 2010). Impaired induction of IL-10 by GCs in T cells from GC-R asthmatics can be reversed by vitamin D3 and IL-10 (Xystrakis et al., 2006). This may reflect IL-10 increasing GR expression by human $CD4^+$ T cells while vitamin D3 overcomes ligand-induced downregulation of GR. Vitamin D reduced human ASM expression of chemokines, including fractalkine and CX_3C chemokine (Banerjee et al., 2008; Sukkar et al., 2004). Thus, vitamin D may hold promise in treating GC-R asthma.

Asthma appears to be more severe in obese individuals (Moore et al., 2007). Obese asthma patients have increased illness severity and altered responses to conventional therapy, as well as leukotriene antagonists (Sin & Sutherland, 2008), as compared with lean asthmatics. Elevated body mass index is associated with a blunted in vitro response to DEX in asthma patients. MKP-1 induction by GC is impaired in PBMC and alveolar macrophages from obese asthmatics. Increased TNF-α in overweight and obese patients with asthma might be involved in downregulation of MKP-1 (Sutherland et al., 2008).

Extracellular factors	Reported GR-R mechanisms
Viral infection	NF-κB ↑ IRF-1 ↑
Microbial superantigens	GRα phosphorylation ↑
	GRα nuclear translocation ↓
Smoking	NF-κB ↑
	HDAC ↓
	GR α:β ratio ↓
Vitamin D ↓	GR downregulation ↑
	Chemokines ↑
Obesity	TNF-α ↑
	MKP-1 ↓

Table 1. **Extracellular factors and reported mechanisms of GC-R.**
In general, the factors exacerbate asthma symptoms occur largely at the same time the factors of GC-R. Those extracellular factors control the intensity of inflammation,which may explain the very common clinical observation that resistance is relative, and patients often respond to high doses of GCs. GC-R asthma may be attributable mostly to reduced GR function resulting from enhanced activations of AP-1 and NF-κB and upstream kinase pathways, or reduced HDAC activity.

11. Conclusions

The inflammatory processes in asthma are complex and heterogeneous (Anderson, 2008; Gibson et al., 2001). GC insensitivity may contribute to disease severity. GC-R asthma is usually an acquired condition. Variable intensity of inflammation may explain the very common clinical observation that resistance is relative. Reduced GC sensitivity in asthmatics is largely due to altered activation of GR by upstream kinase activity, enhanced activation of AP-1 and NF-κB or reduced HDAC activity, associated with inflammation. Th2 independent mechanisms tend to involve GC-R. Understanding the contributing factors and cellular and molecular mechanisms of GR-asthma is important for identifying new targets for biological intervention.

12. References

Abraham, SM., Lawrence, T., Kleiman, A., Warden, P., Medghalchi, M., Tuckermann, J., Saklatvala, J., & Clark, AR. (1896). Antiinflammatory effects of dexamethasone are partly dependent on induction of dual specificity phosphatase 1. *The Journal of experimental medicine*, Vol.203, No.8, (August 2006), pp. 1883-1889, ISSN 0022-1007

Adcock, IM., Lane, SJ., Brown, CR., Lee, TH., & Barnes, PJ. (1896). Abnormal glucocorticoid receptor-activator protein 1 interaction in steroid-resistant asthma. *The Journal of experimental medicine*, Vol.182, No.6, (December 1995), pp. 1951-1958, ISSN 0022-1007

Akdis, M., Verhagen, J., Taaylor, A., Karamloo, F., Karagiannidis, C., Crameri, R., Thunberg, S., Deniz, G., Valenta, R., Fiebig, H., Kegel, C., Disch, R., Schmidt-Weber, CB., Blaser, K., & Adis, CA. (1896). Immune responses in healthy and allergic individuals are characterized by a fine balance between allergen-specific T regulatory 1 and T helper 2 cells. *The Journal of experimental medicine*, Vol.199, No.11, (June 2004), pp. 1567-1575, ISSN 0022-1007

Anderson, GP. (1823). Endotyping asthma: new insights into key pathogenic mechanisms in a complex, heterogeneous disease. *Lancet*, Vol.372, No.9643, (September 2008), pp. 1107-1119, ISSN 0140-6736

Banerjee, A., Damera, G., Bhandare, R., Gu, S., Lopez-Boado, Y., Panettieri, R. Jr., & Tliba, O. (1968). Vitamin D and glucocorticoids differentially modulate chemokine expression in human airway smooth muscle cells. *British journal of pharmacology*, Vol.155, No.1, (September 2008), pp. 84-92, ISSN 0007-1118

Bantel, H., Schmitz, ML., Raible, A., Gregor, M., & Schulze-Osthoff, K. (1987). Critical role of NF-kappaB and stress-activated protein kinases in steroid unresponsiveness. *The FASEB journal: official publication of the Federation of American Societies for Experimental Biology*, Vol.16, No.13, (November 2002), pp. 1832-1834, ISSN 0892-6638

Barnes, PJ. (2001). Role of GATA-3 in allergic diseases. *Current molecular medicine*, Vol.8, No.5, (August 2008), pp. 330-334 ISSN 1566-5240

Berry, MA., Hargadon, B., Shelley, M., Parker, D., Shaw, DE., Green, RH., Bradding, P., Brightling, CE., Wardlaw, AJ., & Pavord, ID. (1928). Evidence of a role of tumor necrosis factor alpha in refractory asthma. *The New England journal of medicine*, Vol.354, No.7, (February 2006), pp. 697-708, ISSN 0028-4793

Bhandare, R., Damera, G., Banerjee, A., Flammer, JR., Keslacy, S., Rogatsky, I., Panettieri, RA., Amrani, Y., & Tliba, O. (1989). Glucocorticoid receptor interacting protein-1 restores glucocorticoid responsiveness in steroid-resistant airway structural cells. *American journal of respiratory cell and molecular biology*, Vol.42, No.1, (January 2010), pp. 9-15, ISSN 1044-1549

Bhavsar, P., Hew, M., Khorasani, N., Torrego, A., Barnes, PJ., Adcock, I., & Chung, KF. (1946). Relative corticosteroid insensitivity of alveolar macrophages in severe asthma compared with non-severe asthma. *Thorax*, Vol.63, No.9, (September 2008), pp. 784-790 ISSN 0040-6376

Bhavsar, P., Khorasani, N., Hew, M., Johnson, M., & Chung, KF. (1988). Effect of p38 MAPK inhibition on corticosteroid suppression of cytokine release in severe asthma. *The European respiratory journal: official journal of the European Society for Clinical Respiratory Physiology*, Vol.35, No.4, (April 2010), pp. 750-756 ISSN 0903-1936

Borger, P., Matsumoto, H., Boustany, S., Gencay, MM., Burgess, JK., King, GG., Black, JL., Tamm, M., & Roth, M. (1971). Disease-specific expression and regulation of CCAAT/enhancer-binding proteins in asthma and chronic obstructive pulmonary disease. *The Journal of allergy and clinical immunology*, Vol.119, No.1, (January 2007), pp. 98-105, ISSN 0091-6749

Borger, P., Miglino, N., Baraket, M., Black, JL., Tamm, M., & Roth, M. (1971). Impaired translation of CCAAT/enhancer binding protein alpha mRNA in bronchial smooth muscle cells of asthmatic patients. *The Journal of allergy and clinical immunology*, Vol.123, No.3, (March 2009), pp. 639-645, ISSN 0091-6749

Borish, L., Aarons, A., Rumbyrt, J., Cvietusa, P., Negri, J., & Wenzel, S. (1971). Interleukin-10 regulation in normal subjects and patients with asthma. *The Journal of allergy and clinical immunology*, Vol.97, No.6, (June 1996), pp. 1288-1296, ISSN 0091-6749

Bullens, DM., Truyen, E., Coteur, L., Dilissen, E., Hellings, PW., Dupont, LJ., & Ceuppens, JL. (2000). IL-17 mRNA in sputum of asthmatic patients: linking T cell driven inflammation and granulocytic influx? *Respiratory research*, Vol.7, (November 2006), pp. 135, ISSN 1465-9921

Caramori, G., Oates, T., Nicholson, AG., Casolari, P., Ito, K., Barnes, PJ., Papi, A., Adcock, IM., & Chung, KF. (1977). Activation of NF-kappaB transcription factor in asthma death. *Histopathology* Vol.54, No.4, (March 2009), pp. 507-509 ISSN 0309-0167

Chakir, J., Shannon, J., Molet, S., Fukakusa, M., Elias, J., Laviolette, M., Boulet, LP., & Hamid, Q. (1971). Airway remodeling-associated mediators in moderate to severe asthma: effect of steroids on TGF-beta, IL-11, IL-17, and type I and type III collagen expression. *The Journal of allergy and clinical immunology*, Vol.111, No.6, (June 2003), pp. 1293-1298, ISSN 0091-6749

Chaudhuri, R., Livingston, E., McMahon, AD., Lafferty, J., Fraser, I., Spears, M., McSharry, CP., & Thomson, NC. (1994). Effects of smoking cessation on lung function and airway inflammation in smokers with asthma. *American journal of respiratory and critical care medicine*, Vol.174, No.2, (July 2006), pp. 127-133, ISSN 1073-449X

Clark, AR. (1939). MAP kinase phosphatase 1: a novel mediator of biological effects of glucocorticoids? *The Journal of endocrinology*, Vol.178, No.1, (July 2003), pp. 5-12, ISSN 0022-0795

Clarke, DL., Clifford, RL., Jindarat, S., Proud, D., Pang, L., Belvisi, M., & Knox, AJ. (1905). TNFα and IFNγ synergistically enhance transcriptional activation of CXCL10 in human airway smooth muscle cells via STAT-1, NF-κB, and the transcriptional coactivator CREB-binding protein. *The Journal of biological chemistry*, Vol.285, No.38, (September 2010), pp. 29101-29110, ISSN 0021-9258

Corrigan, CJ. & Loke, TK. (2005). Clinical and molecular aspects of glucocorticoid resistant asthma. *Therapeutics and clinical risk management*, Vol.3, No.5, (October 2007), pp. 771-787, ISSN 1176-6336

Cui, J., Pazdziorko, S., Miyashiro, JS., Thakker, P., Pelker, JW., Declercq, C., Jiao, A., Gunn, J., Mason, L., Leonard, JP., Williams, CM., & Marusic, S. (1971). TH1-mediated airway hyperresponsiveness independent of neutrophilic inflammation. *The Journal of allergy and clinical immunology*, Vol.115, No.2, (February 2005), pp. 309-315, ISSN 0091-6749

Cundall, M., Sun, Y., Miranda, C., Trudeau, JB., Barnes, S., & Wenzel, SE. (1971). Neutrophil-derived matrix metalloproteinase-9 is increased in severe asthma and poorly inhibited by glucocorticoids. *The Journal of allergy and clinical immunology*, Vol.112, No.6, (December 2003), pp. 1064-1071, ISSN 0091-6749

Dean, JL., Sully, G., Clark, AR., & Saklatvala, J. (1989). The involvement of AU-rich element-binding proteins in p38 mitogen-activated protein kinase pathway-mediated mRNA stabilisation. *Cellular signalling*, Vol.16, No.10, (October 2004), pp. 1113-1121, ISSN 0898-6568

Demoly, P., Basset-Seguin, N., Chanez, P., Campbell, AM., Gauthier-Rouvière, C., Godard, P., Michel, FB., & Bousquet, J. (1989). c-fos proto-oncogene expression in bronchial biopsies of asthmatics. *American journal of respiratory cell and molecular biology*, Vol.7, No.2, (August 1992), pp. 128-133, ISSN 1044-1549

Denny, WB., Prapapanich, V., Smith, DF., & Scammell, JG. (1917). Structure-function analysis of squirrel monkey FK506-binding protein 51, a potent inhibitor of glucocorticoid receptor activity. *Endocrinology*, Vol.146, No.7, (July 2005), pp. 3194-3201, ISSN 0013-7227

Denny, WB., Valentine, DL., Reynolds, PD., Smith, DF., & Scammell, JG. (1917). Squirrel monkey immunophilin FKBP51 is a potent inhibitor of glucocorticoid receptor binding. *Endocrinology*, Vol.141, No.11, (November 2000), pp. 4107-4113, ISSN 0013-7227

Douwes, J., Gibson, P., Pekkanen, J., & Pearce, N. (1946). Non-eosinophilic asthma: importance and possible mechanisms. *Thorax*, 57, No.7, (July 2002), pp. 643-648, ISSN 0040-6376

Flammer, JR., Dobrovolna, J., Kennedy, MA., Chinenov, Y., Glass, CK., Ivashkiv, LB., & Rogatsky, I. (1981). The type I interferon signaling pathway is a target for glucocorticoid inhibition. *Molecular and cellular biology*, Vol.30, No.19, (October 2010), pp. 4564-4574, ISSN 0270-7306

Franchimont, D., Martens, H., Hagelstein, MT., Louis, E., Dewe, W., Chrousos, GP., Belaiche, J., & Geenen, V. (1952). Tumor necrosis factor alpha decreases, and interleukin-10 increases, the sensitivity of human monocytes to dexamethasone: potential regulation of the glucocorticoid receptor. *The Journal of clinical endocrinology and metabolism*, Vol.84, No.8, (August 1999), pp. 2834-2839, ISSN 0021-972X

Gagliardo, R., Chanez, P., Mathieu, M., Bruno, A., Costanzo, G., Gougat, C., Vachier, I., Bousquet, J., Bonsignore, G., & Vignola, AM. (1994). Persistent activation of nuclear factor-kappaB signaling pathway in severe uncontrolled asthma. *American journal of respiratory and critical care medicine*, Vol.168, No.10, (November 2003), pp. 1190-1198 ISSN 1073-449X

Galliher-Beckley, AJ. & Cidlowski, JA. (1999). Emerging roles of glucocorticoid receptor phosphorylation in modulating glucocorticoid hormone action in health and disease. *IUBMB life*, Vol.61, No.10, (October 2009), pp. 979-986, ISSN 1521-6543

Galliher-Beckley, AJ., Williams, JG., Collins, JB., & Cidlowski, JA. (1981). Glycogen synthase kinase 3beta-mediated serine phosphorylation of the human glucocorticoid receptor redirects gene expression profiles. *Molecular and cellular biology*, Vol.28, No. 24, (December 2008), pp. 7309-7322, ISSN 0270-7306

Gibson, PG, Simpson, JL., & Saltos, N. (1970). Heterogeneity of airway inflammation in persistent asthma: evidence of neutrophilic inflammation and increased sputum interleukin-8. *Chest*, Vol.119, No.5, (May 2001), pp. 1329-1336, ISSN 0012-3692

Ginde, AA., Mansbach, JM., & Camargo, CA. Jr. (2001). Vitamin D, respiratory infections, and asthma. *Current allergy and asthma reports*, Vol.9, No.1, (January 2009), pp. 81-87, ISSN 1529-7322

Goleva, E., Hauk, PJ., Boguniewicz, J., Martin, RJ., & Leung, DY. (1971). Airway remodeling and lack of bronchodilator response in steroid-resistant asthma. *The Journal of allergy and clinical immunology*, Vol.120, No.5, (November 2007), pp. 1065-1072, ISSN 0091-6749

Goleva, E., Hauk, PJ., Hall, CF., Liu, AH., Riches, DW., Martin, RJ., & Leung, DY. (1971). Corticosteroid-resistant asthma is associated with classical antimicrobial activation of airway macrophages. *The Journal of allergy and clinical immunology*, Vol.122, No.3, (September 2008), pp. 550-559.e.3, ISSN 0091-6749

Goleva, E., Li, LB., & Leung, DY. (1989). IFN-gamma reverses IL-2- and IL-4-mediated T-cell steroid resistance. *American Journal of respiratory cell and molecular biology*, Vol.40, No.2, (February 2009), pp. 223-230, ISSN 1044-1549

Goleva, E., Li, LB., Eves, PT., Strand, MJ., Martin, RJ., & Leung, DY. (1994). Increased glucocorticoid receptor beta alters steroid response in glucocorticoid-insensitive asthma. *American journal of respiratory and critical care medicine*, Vol.173, No.6, (March 2006), pp. 607-616, ISSN 1073-449X

Green, RH., Brightling, CE., Woltmann, G., Parker, D., Wardlaw, AJ., & Pavord, ID. (1946). Analysis of induced sputum in adults with asthma: identification of subgroup with isolated sputum neutrophilia and poor response to inhaled corticosteroids. *Thorax*, Vol.57, No.10, (October 2002), pp. 875-879, ISSN 0040-6376

Hakonarson, H., Bjornsdottir, US., Halapi, E., Bradfield, J., Zink, F., Mouy, M., Helgadottir, H., Gudmundsdottir, AS., Andrason, H., Adalsteinsdottir, AE., Kristjansson K., Birkisson, I., Arnason, T., Andresdottir, M., Gislason, D., Gislason, T., Gulcher, JR., & Stefansson K. (1915). Profiling of genes expressed in peripheral blood mononuclear cells predicts glucocorticoid sensitivity in asthma patients. *Proceedings of the National Academy of Sciences of the United States of America*, Vol.102, No.41, (October 2005), pp. 14789-14794, ISSN 0027-8424

Hamid, QA., Wenzel, SE., Hauk, PJ., Tsicopoulos, A., Wallaert, B., Lafitte, JJ., Chrousos, GP., Szefler, SJ., & Leung, DY. (1994). Increased glucocorticoid receptor beta in airway cells of glucocorticoid-insensitive asthma. *American journal of respiratory and critical care medicine*, Vol.159, No.5 Pt 1, (May 1999), pp. 1600-1604, ISSN 1073-449X

Hamilton, LM., Puddicombe, SM., Dearman, RJ., Kimber, I., Sandström, T., Wallin, A., Howarth, PH., Holgate, ST., Wilson, SJ., & Davies, DE. (1988). Altered protein tyrosine phosphorylation in asthmatic bronchial epithelium. *The European respiratory journal: official journal of the European Society for Clinical Respiratory Physiology*, Vol.25, No.6, (June 2005), pp. 978-985, ISSN 0903-1936

Hamilton, LM., Torres-Lozano, C., Puddicombe, SM., Richter, A., Kimber, I., Dearman, RJ., Vrugt, B., Aalbers, R., Holgate, ST., Djukanović, R., Wilson, SJ., & Davies, DE. (1989). The role of the epidermal growth factor receptor in sustaining neutrophil inflammation in severe asthma. *Clinical and experimental allergy: journal of the British Society for Allergy and Clinical Immunology*, Vol.33, No.2, (February 2003), pp. 233-240, ISSN 0954-7894

Hansen, G., Berry, G., DeKruyff, RH., & Umetsu, DT. (1924). Allergen-specific Th1 cells fail to counterbalance Th2 cell-induced airway hyperreactivity but cause severe airway inflammation. *The Journal of clinical investigation*, Vol.103, No.2, (January 1999), pp. 175-183, ISSN 0021-9738

Hart, LA., Krishnan, VL., Adcock, IM., Barnes, PJ., & Chung, KF. (1994). Activation and localization of transcription factor, nuclear factor-kappaB, in asthma. *American journal of respiratory and critical care medicine*, Vol.158, No.5 Pt 1, (November 1998), pp. 1585-1592, ISSN 1073-449X

Hauk, PJ., Hamid, QA., Chrousos, GP., & Leung, DY. (1971). Induction of corticosteroid insensitivity in human PBMCs by microbial superantigens. *The Journal of allergy and clinical immunology*, Vol.105, No.4, (April 2000), pp. 782-787, ISSN 0091-6749

Hauk, PJ., Wenzel, SE., Trumble, AE., Szefler, SJ., & Leung, DY. (1971). Increased T-cell receptor vbeta8+ T cells in bronchoalveolar lavage fluid of subjects with poorly controlled asthma: a potential role for microbial superantigens. *The Journal of allergy and clinical immunology*, Vol.104, No.1, (July 1999), pp. 37-45, ISSN 0091-6749

Hawrylowicz, C., Richards, D., Loke, TK., Corrigan, C., & Lee, T. (1971). A defect in corticosteroid-induced IL-10 production in T lymphocytes from corticosteroid-resistant asthmatic patients. *The Journal of allergy and clinical immunology*, Vol.109, No.2, (February 2002), pp. 369-370, ISSN 0091-6749

Heaton T, Rowe, J., Turner, S., Aalbarse, RC., de Klerk, N., Suriyaarachchi, D., Serralha, M., Holt, BJ., Hollams, E., Yerkovich, S., Holt, K., Sly, PD., Goldblatt, J., Le Souef, P., & Holt, PG. (1823). An immunoepidemiological approach to asthma: identification of in-vitro T-cell response patterns associated with different wheezing phenotypes in children. *Lancet*, Vol.365, No.9454, (January 2005), pp. 142-149, ISSN 0140-6736

Hew, M., Bhavsar, P., Torrego, A., Meah, S., Khorasani, N., Barnes, PJ., Adcock, I., & Chung, KF. (1994). Relative corticosteroid insensitivity of peripheral blood mononuclear cells in severe asthma. *American journal of respiratory and critical care medicine*, Vol.174, No.2, (July 2006), pp. 134-141, ISSN 1073-449X

Hirasawa, N., Yashima, K., & Ishihara, K. (1973). Enhancement of ligand-dependent down-regulation of glucocorticoid receptor by lipopolysaccharide. *Life Sciences*, Vol.85, No.15-16, (October 2009), pp. 578-585, ISSN 0024-3205

Howarth, PH., Babu, KS., Arshad, HS., Lau, L., Buckley, M., McConnell, W., Beckett, P., Al Ali, M., Chauhan, A., Wilson, SJ., Reynolds, A., Davies, DE., & Holgate, ST. (1946). Tumour necrosis factor (TNFalpha) as a novel therapeutic target in symptomatic corticosteroid dependent asthma. *Thorax*, Vol.60, No.12, (December 2005), pp. 1012-1018. ISSN 0040-6376

Huang, Y., Zhao, JJ., Lv, YY., Ding, PS., & Liu, RY. (1973). Hypoxia down-regulates glucocorticoid receptor alpha and attenuates the anti-inflammatory actions of dexamethasone in human alveolar epithelial A549 cells. *Life Sciences*, Vol.85, No.3-4, (July 2009), pp. 107-112, ISSN 0024-3205

Irusen, E., Matthews, JG., Takahashi, A., Barnes, PJ., Chung, KF., & Adcock, IM. (1971). p38 Mitogen-activated protein kinase-induced glucocorticoid receptor phosphorylation reduces its activity: role in steroid-insensitive asthma. *The Journal of allergy and clinical immunology*, Vol.109, No.4, (April 2002), pp. 649-657, ISSN 0091-6749

Ismaili, N. & Garabedian, MJ. (1877). Modulation of glucocorticoid receptor function via phosphorylation. *Annals of the New York Academy of Sciences*, Vol.1024, (June 2004), pp. 86-101, ISSN 0077-8923

Ito, K., Caramori, G., & Adcock, IM. (1909). Therapeutic potential of phosphatidylinositol 3-kinase inhibitors in inflammatory respiratory disease. *The Journal of pharmacology and experimental therapeutics*, Vol.321, No.1, (April 2007), pp. 1-8, ISSN 0022-3565

Ito, K., Caramori, G., Lim, S., Oates, T., Chung, KF., Barnes, PJ., & Adcock, IM. (1994). Expression and activity of histone deacetylases in human asthmatic airways.

American journal of respiratory and critical care medicine, Vol.166, No.3, (August 2002a), pp. 392-396, ISSN 1073-449X

Ito, K., Herbert, C., Siegle, JS., Vuppusetty, C., Hansbro, N., Thomas, PS., Foster, PS., Barnes, PJ., & Kumar, RK. (1989). Steroid-resistant neutrophilic inflammation in a mouse model of an acute exacerbation of asthma. *American journal of respiratory cell and molecular biology*, Vol.39, No.5, (November 2008), pp. 543-550, ISSN 1044-1549

Ito, K., Lim, S., Caramori, G., Chung, KF., Barnes, PJ., & Adcock, IM. (1987). Cigarette smoking reduces histone deacetylase 2 expression, enhances cytokine expression, and inhibits glucocorticoid actions in alveolar macrophages. *The FASEB journal: official publication of the Federation of American Societies for Experimental Biology*, Vol.15, No.6, (April 2001), pp. 1110-1112, ISSN 0892-6638

Ito, K., Lim, S., Caramori, G., Cosio, B., Chung, KF., Adcock, IM., & Barnes, PJ. (1915). A molecular mechanism of action of theophylline: Induction of histone deacetylase activity to decrease inflammatory gene expression. *Proceedings of the National Academy of Sciences of the United States of America*, Vol.99, No.13, (June 2002b), pp. 8921-8926, ISSN 0027-8424

Ito, K., Yamamura, S., Essilfie-Quaye, S., Cosio, B., Ito, M., Barnes, PJ., & Adcock, IM. (1896). Histone deacetylase 2-mediated deacetylation of the glucocorticoid receptor enables NF-kappaB suppression. *The Journal of experimental medicine*, Vol.203, No.1, (January 2006), pp. 7-13, ISSN 0022-1007

Itoh, M., Adachi, M., Yasui, H., Takekawa, M., Tanaka, H., & Imai, K. (1987). Nuclear export of glucocorticoid receptor is enhanced by c-Jun N-terminal kinase-mediated phosphorylation. *Molecular endocrinology*, Vol.16, No.10, (October 2002), pp. 2382-2392, ISSN 0888-8809

Jacques, E., Semlali, A., Boulet, LP., & Chakir, J. (1989). AP-1 overexpression impairs corticosteroid inhibition of collagen production by fibroblasts isolated from asthmatic subjects. *American journal of physiology. Lung cellular and molecular physiology*, Vol.299, No.2, (August 2010), pp. L281-L287, ISSN 1040-0605

Kam, JC., Szefler, SJ., Surs, W., Sher, ER., & Leung, DY. (1950). Combination IL-2 and IL-4 reduces glucocorticoid receptor-binding affinity and T cell response to glucocorticoids. *Journal of immunology*, Vol.151, No.7, (October 1993), pp. 3460-3466 ISSN 0022-1767

Kasperska-Zajac A. (1975). Asthma and dehydroepiandrosterone (DHEA): facts and hypotheses. *Inflammation*, Vol.33, No.5, (October 2010), pp. 320-324, ISSN 0360-3997

Kawaguchi, M., Kokubu, F., Fujita, J., Huang, SK., & Hizawa, N. (2006). Role of interleukin-17F in asthma. *Inflammation and allergy drug targets*, Vol. 8, No.5, (December 2009), pp. 383-389, ISSN 1871-5281

Kelly, A., Bowen, H., Jee, YK., Mahfiche, N., Soh, C., Lee, T., Hawrylowicz, C., & Lavender, P. (1971). The glucocorticoid receptor beta isoform can mediate transcriptional repression by recruiting histone deacetylases. *The Journal of allergy and clinical immunology*, Vol.121, No.1, (January 2008), pp. 203-208, ISSN 0091-6749

Kröger, A., Köster, M., Schroeder, K., Hauser, H., & Mueller, PP. (1995). Activities of IRF-1. *Journal of interferon & cytokine research: the official journal of the International Society for Interferon and Cytokine Research*, Vol.22, No.1, (January 2002), pp. 5-14, ISSN 1079-9907

Lane, SJ., Adcock, IM., Richards, D., Hawrylowicz, C., Barnes, PJ., & Lee, TH. (1924). Corticosteroid-resistant bronchial asthma is associated with increased c-fos expression in monocytes and T lymphocytes. *The Journal of clinical investigation*, Vol.102, No.12, (December 1998), pp. 2156-2164, ISSN 0021-9738

Leung, DY., Martin, RJ., Szefler, SJ., Sher, ER., Ying, S., Kay, AB., & Hamid, Q. (1896). Dysregulation of interleukin 4, interleukin 5, and interferon gamma gene expression in steroid-resistant asthma. *The Journal of experimental medicine*, Vol.181, No.1, (January 1995), pp. 33-40, ISSN 0022-1007

Leung, DY., Spahn, JD., & Szefler, SJ. (1996). Immunologic basis and management of steroid-resistant asthma. *Allergy and asthma proceedings: the official journal of regional and state allergy societies*, Vol.20, No.1, (January-February 1999), pp. 9-14, ISSN 1088-5412

Li, LB., Goleva, E., Hall, CF., Ou, LS., & Leung, DY. (1971). Superantigen-induced corticosteroid resistance of human T cells occurs through activation of the mitogen-activated protein kinase kinase/extracellular signal-regulated kinase (MEK-ERK) pathway. *The Journal of allergy and clinical immunology*, Vol.114, No.5, (November 2004), pp. 1059-1069, ISSN 0091-6749

Li, LB., Leung, DY., Martin, RJ., & Goleva, E. (1994). Inhibition of histone deacetylase 2 expression by elevated glucocorticoid receptor beta in steroid-resistant asthma. *American journal of respiratory and critical care medicine*, Vol.182, No.7, (October 2010), pp. 877-883, ISSN 1073-449X

Lim, S., Crawley, E., Woo, P., & Barnes, PJ. (1823). Haplotype associated with low interleukin-10 production in patients with severe asthma. *Lancet*, Vol.352, No.9122, (July 1998), pp. 113, ISSN 0140-6736

Livingston, E., Chaudhuri, R., McMahon, AD., Fraser, I., McSharry, CP., & Thomson NC. (1988). Systemic sensitivity to corticosteroids in smokers with asthma. *The European respiratory journal: official journal of the European Society for Clinical Respiratory Physiology*, Vol.29, No.1, (January 2007), pp. 64-71, ISSN 0903-1936

Livingston, E., Darroch, CE., Chaudhuri, R., McPhee, I., McMahon, AD., Mackenzie, SJ., & Thomson, NC. (1971). Glucocorticoid receptor alpha:beta ratio in blood mononuclear cells is reduced in cigarette smokers. *The Journal of allergy and clinical immunology*, Vol.114, No.6, (December 2004), pp. 1475-1478, ISSN 0091-6749

Loke, TK., Mallett, KH., Ratoff, J., O'Connor, BJ., Ying, S., Meng, Q., Soh, C., Lee, TH., & Corrigan, CJ. (1971). Systemic glucocorticoid reduces bronchial mucosal activation of activator protein 1 components in glucocorticoid-sensitive but not glucocorticoid-resistant asthmatic patients. *The Journal of allergy and clinical immunology*, Vol.118, No.2, (August 2006), pp. 368-375, ISSN 0091-6749

Marwick, JA., Caramori, G., Stevenson, CS., Casolari, P., Jazrawi, E., Barnes, PJ., Ito, K., Adcock, IM., Kirkham, PA., & Papi, A. (1994). Inhibition of PI3Kdelta restores glucocorticoid function in smoking-induced airway inflammation in mice. *American journal of respiratory and critical care medicine*, Vol.179, No.7, (April 2009), pp. 542-548, ISSN 1073-449X

Marwick, JA., Chung, KF., & Adcock, IM. (2007). Phosphatidylinositol 3-kinase isoforms as targets in respiratory disease. *Therapeutic advances in respiratory disease*, Vol.4, No.1, (February 2010), pp. 19-34, ISSN 1753-4658

Matthews, JG., Ito, K., Barnes, PJ., & Adcock, IM. (1971). Defective glucocorticoid receptor nuclear translocation and altered histone acetylation patterns in glucocorticoid-resistant patients. *The Journal of allergy and clinical immunology*, Vol.113, No.6, (June 2004), pp. 1100-1108, ISSN 0091-6749

McKinley, L., Alcorn, JF., Peterson, A., Dupont, RB., Kapadia, S., Logar, A., Henry, A., Irvin, CG., Piganelli, JD., Ray, A., & Kolls, JK. (1950). TH17 cells mediate steroid-resistant airway inflammation and airway hyperresponsiveness in mice. *Journal of immunology*, Vol.181, No.6, (September 2008), pp. 4089-4097, ISSN 0022-1767

Moore, WC., Bleecker, ER., Curran-Everett, D., Erzurum, SC., Ameredes, BT., Bacharier, L., Calhoun, WJ., Castro, M., Chung, KF., Clark, MP., Dweik, RA., Fitzpatrick, AM., Gaston, B., Hew, M., Hussain, I., Jarjour, NN., Israel, E., Levy, BD., Murphy, JR., Peters, SP., Teague, WG., Meyers, DA., Busse, WW., Wenzel, SE; & National Heart, Lung, Blood Institute's Severe Asthma Research Program. (1971). Characterization of the severe asthma phenotype by the National Heart, Lung, and Blood Institute's Severe Asthma Research Program. *The Journal of allergy and clinical immunology*, Vol.119, No.2, (February 2007), pp. 405-413, ISSN 0091-6749

Morjaria, JB., Chauhan, AJ., Babu, KS., Polosa, R., Davies, DE., & Holgate, ST. (1946). The role of a soluble TNFalpha receptor fusion protein (etanercept) in corticosteroid refractory asthma: a double blind, randomised, placebo controlled trial. *Thorax*, Vol.63, No.7, (July 2008), pp. 584-591, ISSN 0040-6376

Okumura, S., Sagara, H., Fukuda, T., Saito, H., & Okayama, Y. (1971). FcepsilonRI-mediated amphiregulin production by human mast cells increases mucin gene expression in epithelial cells. *The Journal of allergy and clinical immunology*, Vol.115, No.2, (February 2005), pp. 272-279, ISSN 0091-6749

Papi, A. & Johnston, SL. (1905). Respiratory epithelial cell expression of vascular cell adhesion molecule-1 and its up-regulation by rhinovirus infection via NF-kappaB and GATA transcription factors. *The Journal of biological chemistry*, Vol.274, No.42, (October 1999), pp. 30041-30051, ISSN 0021-9258

Pavord, ID. (1946). Non-eosinophilic asthma and the innate immune response. *Thorax*, Vol.62, No.3, (March 2007), pp. 193-194, ISSN 0040-6376

Pavord, ID., Brightling, CE., Woltmann, G., & Wardlaw, AJ. (1823). Non-eosinophilic corticosteroid unresponsive asthma. *Lancet*, Vol.353, No.9171, (June 1999), pp. 2213-2214, ISSN 0140-6736

Pène, J., Chevalier, S., Preisser, L., Vénéreau, E., Guilleux, MH., Ghannam, S., Molès, JP., Danger, Y., Ravon, E., Lesaux, S., Yssel, H., & Gascan, H. (1950). Chronically inflamed human tissues are infiltrated by highly differentiated Th17 lymphocytes. *Journal of immunology*, Vol.180, No.11, (June 2008), pp. 7423-7430, ISSN 0022-1767

Préfontaine, D., Lajoie-Kadoch, S., Foley, S., Audusseau, S., Olivenstein, R., Halayko, AJ., Lemière, C., Martin, JG., & Hamid, Q. (1950). Increased expression of IL-33 in severe asthma: evidence of expression by airway smooth muscle cells. *Journal of immunology*, Vol.183, No.8, (October 2009), pp. 5094-5103, ISSN 0022-1767

Puddicombe, SM., Polosa, R., Richter, A., Krishna, MT., Howarth, PH., Holgate, ST., & Davies, DE. (1987). Involvement of the epidermal growth factor receptor in epithelial repair in asthma. *The FASEB journal: official publication of the Federation of American Societies for Experimental Biology*, Vol.14, No.10, (July 2000), pp. 1362-1374, ISSN 0892-6638

Pujols, L., Mullol, J., Pérez, M., Roca-Ferrer, J., Juan, M., Xaubet, A., Cidlowski, JA., & Picado, C. (1989). Expression of the human glucocorticoid receptor alpha and beta isoforms in human respiratory epithelial cells and their regulation by dexamethasone. *American journal of respiratory cell and molecular biology* Vol.24, No.1, (January 2001), pp. 49-57, ISSN 1044-1549

Ray, A. & Cohn, L. (1924). Th2 cells and GATA-3 in asthma: new insights into the regulation of airway inflammation. *The Journal of clinical investigation*, Vol.104, No.8, (October 1999), pp. 985-993, ISSN 0021-9738

Reynolds, PD., Ruan, Y., Smith, DF., & Scammell, JG. (1952). Glucocorticoid resistance in the squirrel monkey is associated with overexpression of the immunophilin FKBP51. *The journal of clinical endocrinology and metabolism*, Vol.84, No.2, (February 1999), pp. 663-669, ISSN 0021-972X

Robins, S., Roussel, L., Schachter, A., Risse, PA., Mogas, AK., Olivenstein, R., Martin, JG., Hamid, Q., & Rousseau, S. (1989). Steroid-insensitive ERK1/2-activity drives CXCL8 synthesis and neutrophilia by airway smooth muscle. *American journal of respiratory cell and molecular biology*, (Apr 2011), [Epub ahead of print], ISSN 1044-1549

Rogatsky, I., Logan, SK., & Garabedian, MJ. (1915). Antagonism of glucocorticoid receptor transcriptional activation by the c-Jun N-terminal kinase. *Proceedings of the National Academy of Sciences of the United States of America*, Vol.95, No.5, (March 1998), pp. 2050-2055, ISSN 0027-8424

Rogatsky, I., Wang, JC., Derynck, MK., Nonaka, DF., Khodabakhsh, DB., Haqq, CM., Darimont, BD., Garabedian, MJ., & Yamamoto, KR. (1915). Target-specific utilization of transcriptional regulatory surfaces by the glucocorticoid receptor. *Proceedings of the National Academy of Sciences of the United States of America*, Vol.100, No.24, (November 2003), pp. 13845-13850, ISSN 0027-8424

Roth, M. & Black, JL. An imbalance in C/EBPs and increased mitochondrial activity in asthmatic airway smooth muscle cells: novel targets in asthma therapy? *British journal of pharmacology*, Vol.157, No.3, (June 2009), pp. 334-341, ISSN 0007-1188

Roth, M., Johnson, PR., Borger, P., Bihl, MP., Rüdiger, JJ., King, GG., Ge, Q., Hostettler, K., Burgess, JK., Black, JL., & Tamm, M. (1928). Dysfunctional interaction of C/EBPalpha and the glucocorticoid receptor in asthmatic bronchial smooth-muscle cells. *The New England journal of medicine*, Vol.351, No.6, (August 2004), pp. 560-574, ISSN 0028-4793

Roth, M., Johnson, PR., Rüdiger, JJ., King, GG., Ge, Q., Burgess, JK., Anderson, G., Tamm, M., & Black, JL. (1823). Interaction between glucocorticoids and beta2 agonists on bronchial airway smooth muscle cells through synchronised cellular signalling. *Lancet*, Vol.360, No.9342, (October 2002), pp. 1293-1299, ISSN 0140-6736

Schmitz, J., Owyang, A., Oldham, E., Song, Y., Murphy, E., McClanahan, TK., Zurawski, G., Moshrefi, M., Qin, J., Li, X., Gorman, DM., Bazan, JF., & Kastelein, RA. (1994). IL-33, an interleukin-1-like cytokine that signals via the IL-1 receptor-related protein ST2 and induces T helper type 2-associated cytokines. *Immunity*, Vol.23, No.5, (November 2005), pp. 479-490, ISSN 1074-7613

Shannon, J., Ernst, P., Yamauchi, Y., Olivenstein, R., Lemiere, C., Foley, S., Cicora, L., Ludwig, M., Hamid, Q., & Martin, JG. (1970). Differences in airway cytokine profile in severe asthma compared to moderate asthma. *Chest*, Vol.133, No.2, (February 2008), pp. 420-426, ISSN 0012-3692

Sher, ER., Leung, DY., Surs, W., Kam, JC., Zieg, G., Kamada, AK., & Szefler, SJ. (1924). Steroid-resistant asthma. Cellular mechanisms contributing to inadequate response to glucocorticoid therapy. *The Journal of clinical investigation,* Vol.93, No.1, (January 1994), pp. 33-39, ISSN 0021-9738

Simpson, JL., Scott, RJ., Boyle, MJ., & Gibson, PG. (1994). Differential proteolytic enzyme activity in eosinophilic and neutrophilic asthma. *American journal of respiratory and critical care medicine,* Vol.172, No.5, (September 2005), pp. 559-565, ISSN 1073-449X

Sin, DD. & Sutherland, ER. (1946). Obesity and the lung: 4. Obesity and asthma. *Thorax,* Vol.63, No.11, (November 2008), pp. 1018-1023, ISSN 0040-6376

Sousa, AR., Lane, SJ., Cidlowski, JA., Staynov, DZ., & Lee, TH. (1971). Glucocorticoid resistance in asthma is associated with elevated in vivo expression of the glucocorticoid receptor beta-isoform. *The Journal of allergy and clinical immunology,* Vol.105, No.5, (May 2000), pp. 943-950, ISSN 0091-6749

Sousa, AR., Lane, SJ., Soh, C., & Lee, TH. (1971). In vivo resistance to corticosteroids in bronchial asthma is associated with enhanced phosphorylation of JUN N-terminal kinase and failure of prednisolone to inhibit JUN N-terminal kinase phosphorylation. *The Journal of allergy and clinical immunology,* Vol.104, No.3 Pt 1, (September 1999), pp. 565-574, ISSN 0091-6749

Sukkar, MB., Issa, R., Xie, S., Oltmanns, U., Newton, R., & Chung, KF. (1989). Fractalkine/CX3CL1 production by human airway smooth muscle cells: induction by IFN-gamma and TNF-alpha and regulation by TGF-beta and corticosteroids. *American journal of physiology. Lung cellular and molecular physiology,* Vol.287, No.6, (December 2004), pp. L1230-L1240, ISSN 1040-0605

Sullivan, DE., Ferris, M., Pociask, D., & Brody, AR. (1989). Tumor necrosis factor-alpha induces transforming growth factor-beta1 expression in lung fibroblasts through the extracellular signal-regulated kinase pathway. *American journal of respiratory cell and molecular biology,* Vol.32, No.4, (April 2005), pp. 342-349, ISSN 1044-1549

Sutherland, ER., Goleva, E., Jackson, LP., Stevens, AD., & Leung, DY. (1994). Vitamin D levels, lung function and steroid response in adult asthma. *American journal of respiratory and critical care medicine,* Vol.181, No.7, (April 2010), pp. 699-704, ISSN 1073-449X

Sutherland, ER., Goleva, E., Strand, M., Beuther, DA., & Leung, DY. (1994). Body mass and glucocorticoid response in asthma. *American journal of respiratory and critical care medicine,* Vol.178, No.7, (October 2008), pp. 682-687, ISSN 1073-449X

Szatmáry, Z., Garabedian, MJ., & Vilcek, J. (1905). Inhibition of glucocorticoid receptor-mediated transcriptional activation by p38 mitogen-activated protein (MAP) kinase. *The Journal of biological chemistry,* Vol.279, No.42, (October 2004), pp. 43708-43715, ISSN 0021-9258

Szefler, SJ. & Leung, DY. (1988). Glucocorticoid-resistant asthma: pathogenesis and clinical implications for management. *The European respiratory journal: official journal of the European Society for Clinical Respiratory Physiology,* Vol.10, No.7, (July 1997), pp. 1640-1647, ISSN 0903-1936

Takahashi, E., Onda, K., Hirano, T., Oka, K., Maruoka, N., Tsuyuguchi, M., Matsumura, Y., Niitsuma, T., & Hayashi, T. (2001). Expression of c-fos, rather than c-jun or glucocorticoid-receptor mRNA, correlates with decreased glucocorticoid response of peripheral blood mononuclear cells in asthma. *International immunopharmacology*, Vol.2, No.10 (September 2002), pp. 1419-1427, ISSN 1567-5769

Thomson, NC., Chaudhuri, R., & Livingston, E. (1988). Asthma and cigarette smoking. *The European respiratory journal: official journal of the European Society for Clinical Respiratory Physiology*, Vol.24, No.5, (November 2004), pp. 822-833, ISSN 0903-1936

Tliba, O., Cidlowski, JA., & Amrani, Y. (1965). CD38 expression is insensitive to steroid action in cells treated with tumor necrosis factor-alpha and interferon-gamma by a mechanism involving the up-regulation of the glucocorticoid receptor beta isoform. *Molecular Pharmacology*, Vol.69, No.2, (February 2006), pp. 588-596, ISSN 0026-895X

Tliba, O., Damera, G., Banerjee, A., Gu, S., Baidouri, H., Keslacy, S., & Amrani, Y. (1989). Cytokines induce an early steroid resistance in airway smooth muscle cells: novel role of interferon regulatory factor-1. *American journal of respiratory cell and molecular biology*, Vol.38, No.4, (April 2008), pp. 463-472, ISSN 1044-1549

Truyen, E., Coteur, L., Dilissen, E., Overbergh, L., Dupont, LJ., Ceuppens, JL., & Bullens, DM. (1946). Evaluation of airway inflammation by quantitative Th1/Th2 cytokine mRNA measurement in sputum of asthma patients. *Thorax*, Vol.61, No.3, (March 2006), pp. 202-208, ISSN 0040-6376

Tsitoura, DC. & Rothman, PB. (1924). Enhancement of MEK/ERK signaling promotes glucocorticoid resistance in CD4+ T cells. *The Journal of clinical investigation*, Vol.113, No.4, (February 2004), pp. 619-627, ISSN 0021-9738

Urbach, V., Verriere, V., Grumbach, Y., Bousquet, J., & Harvey, BJ. (1963). Rapid anti-secretory effects of glucocorticoids in human airway epithelium. *Steroids*, Vol.71, No.4, (April 2006), pp. 323-328, ISSN 0039-128X

Vasavda, N., Eichholtz, T., Takahashi, A., Affleck, K., Matthews, JG., Barnes, PJ., & Adcock, IM. (1971). Expression of nonmuscle cofilin-1 and steroid responsiveness in severe asthma. *The Journal of allergy and clinical immunology*, Vol.118, No.5, (November 2006), pp. 1090-1096, ISSN 0091-6749

Vermeer, H., Hendriks-Stegeman, BI., van der Burg, B., van Buul-Offers, SC., & Jansen, M. (1952). Glucocorticoid-induced increase in lymphocytic FKBP51 messenger ribonucleic acid expression: a potential marker for glucocorticoid sensitivity, potency, and bioavailability. *The Journal of clinical endocrinology and metabolism*, Vol.88, No.1, (January 2003), pp. 277-284, ISSN 0021-972X

Vermeer, H., Hendriks-Stegeman, BI., van Suylekom, D., Rijkers, GT., van Buul-Offers, SC., & Jansen, M. (1974). An in vitro bioassay to determine individual sensitivity to glucocorticoids: induction of FKBP51 mRNA in peripheral blood mononuclear cells. *Molecular and cellular endocrinology*, Vol.218, No.1-2, (April 2004a) pp. 49-55, ISSN 0303-7207

Vermeer, H., Hendriks-Stegeman, BI., Verrijn Stuart, AA., van Buul-Offers, SC., & Jansen, M. (1994). A comparison of in vitro bioassays to determine cellular glucocorticoid sensitivity. *European journal of endocrinology*, Vol.150, No.1, (January 2004b), pp. 41-47, ISSN 0804-4643

Vianna, EO., Westcott, J., & Martin RJ. (1971). The effects of upper respiratory infection on T-cell proliferation and steroid sensitivity of asthmatics. *The Journal of allergy and clinical immunology*, Vol.102, No.4 Pt 1, (October 1998), pp. 592-597, ISSN 0091-6749

Vignola, AM., Chiappara, G., Siena, L., Bruno, A., Gagliardo, R., Merendino, AM., Polla, BS., Arrigo, AP., Bonsignore, G., Bousquet, J., & Chanez, P. (1971). Proliferation and activation of bronchial epithelial cells in corticosteroid-dependent asthma. *The Journal of allergy and clinical immunology*, Vol.108, No.5, (November 2001), pp. 738-746, ISSN0091-6749

Wang, X., Wu, H., & Miller, AH. (1996). Interleukin 1alpha (IL-1alpha) induced activation of p38 mitogen-activated protein kinase inhibits glucocorticoid receptor function. *Molecular psychiatry*, Vol.9, No.1, (January 2004), pp. 65-75, ISSN 1359-4184

Wenzel SE. Eosinophils in asthma–Closing the loop or opening the door? (1928). *The New England journal of medicine*, Vol.360, No.10, (March 2009), pp. 1026-1028, ISSN 0028-4793

Wenzel, SE., Schwartz, LB., Langmack, EL., Halliday, JL., Trudeau, JB., Gibbs, RL., & Chu, HW. (1994). Evidence that severe asthma can be divided pathologically into two inflammatory subtypes with distinct physiologic and clinical characteristics. *American journal of respiratory and critical care medicine*, Vol.160, No.3, (September 1998), pp. 1001-1008, ISSN 1073-449X

Wochnik, GM., Rüegg, J., Abel, GA., Schmidt, U., Holsboer, F., & Rein, T. (1905). FK506-binding proteins 51 and 52 differentially regulate dynein interaction and nuclear translocation of the glucocorticoid receptor in mammalian cells. *The Journal of biological chemistry*, Vol.280, No.6, (February 2005), pp. 4609-16. ISSN 0021-9258

Woodruff, PG., Boushey, HA., Dolganov, GM., Barker, CS., Yang, YH., Donnelly, S., Ellwanger, A., Sidhu, SS., Dao-Pick, TP., Pantoja, C., Erle, DJ., Yamamoto, KR., & Fahy, JV. (1915). Genome-wide profiling identifies epithelial cell genes associated with asthma and with treatment response to corticosteroids. *Proceedings of the National Academy of Sciences of the United States of America*, Vol.104, No.40 (October 2007), pp. 15858-15863, ISSN 0027-8424

Woolcock, AJ. Corticosteroid-resistant asthma. Definitions. (1994). *American journal of respiratory and critical care medicine*, Vol.154, No.2 Pt 2, (August 1996), pp. S45-S48, ISSN 1073-449X

Xystrakis, E., Kusumakar, S., Boswell, S., Peek, E., Urry, Z., Richards, DF., Adikibi, T., Pridgeon, C., Dallman, M., Loke, TK., Robinson, DS., Barrat, FJ., O'Garra, A., Lavender, P., Lee, TH., Corrigan, C., & Hawrylowicz, CM. (1924). Reversing the defective induction of IL-10-secreting regulatory T cells in glucocorticoid-resistant asthma patients. *The journal of clinical investigation*, Vol.116, No.1, (January 2006), pp. 146-155, ISSN 0021-9738

Yamada, K., Elliott, WM., Hayashi, S., Brattsand, R., Roberts, C., Vitalis, TZ., & Hogg, JC. (1971). Latent adenoviral infection modifies the steroid response in allergic lung inflammation. *The Journal of allergy and clinical immunology*, Vol.106, No.5, (November 2000), pp. 844-851, ISSN 0091-6749

Yang, M., Kumar, RK., & Foster, PS. (1950). Pathogenesis of steroid-resistant airway hyperresponsiveness: interaction between IFN-gamma and TLR4/MyD88 pathways. *Journal of immunology*, Vol.182, No.8, (April 2009), pp. 5107-5115, ISSN 0022-1767

Zhu, J., Yamane, H., Cote-Sierra, J., Guo, L., & Paul, WE. (1990). GATA-3 promotes Th2 responses through three different mechanisms: induction of Th2 cytokine production, selective growth of Th2 cells and inhibition of Th1 cell-specific factors. *Cell research*, Vol.16, No.1, (January 2006), pp. 3-10 ISSN 1001-0602

Zhu, Z., Tang, W., Gwaltney, JM. Jr., Wu, Y., & Elias, JA. (1898). Rhinovirus stimulation of interleukin-8 in vivo and in vitro: role of NF-kappaB. *The American journal of physiology*, Vol.273, No.4 Pt 1, (October 1997), pp. L814-L824, ISSN 0002-9513

Zhu, Z., Tang, W., Ray, A., Wu, Y., Einarsson, O., Landry, ML., Gwaltney, J. Jr., & Elias, JA. (1924). Rhinovirus stimulation of interleukin-6 in vivo and in vitro. Evidence for nuclear factor kappa B-dependent transcriptional activation. *The Journal of clinical investigation*, Vol.97, No.2, (January 1996), pp. 421-430, ISSN 0021-9738

10

Antioxidant Strategies in the Treatment of Bronchial Asthma

Martin Joyce-Brady, William W. Cruikshank and Susan R. Doctrow
The Pulmonary Center at Boston University School of Medicine, Boston, MA, USA

1. Introduction

The oxidant-antioxidant hypothesis and asthma: The pathogenesis of asthma is unknown but imbalances between oxidants and antioxidants are believed to play a fundamental role. One key component of the oxidant-antioxidant hypothesis centers on the huge burden of oxidants derived from inflammatory cell infiltration into the lung. The eosinophil, in particular, is implicated as a major source of oxidative injury, including protein nitration [1]. Dysfunctional mitochondria in lung cells are another potential source of oxidants. Mitochondrial injury to airway epithelium occurs in murine models of allergic asthma [2, 3]. There is evidence to support its role in human asthma as well including increased oxidative injury to mitochondrial epithelial cell superoxide dismutase (SOD) [4], enhanced mitochondrial proliferation in bronchial smooth muscle [5], and mutations in mitochondrial DNA [6]. Overall, this oxidative burden, generated by both inflammatory and lung cells, can overwhelm antioxidant defense to cause oxidant stress during asthma. This stress can alter or inactivate the function of essential proteins, lipids and nucleic acids culminating in severe cell injury, dysfunction and death.

An accumulating body of literature suggests that oxidant stress is an important factor in asthma pathogenesis [7-11]. Oxidant stress can impact the function of a number of different cell types in the lung, and new research has drawn attention to immune cells and airway epithelial cells for the following reasons. First, immune cells are located within the lung and are directly exposed to inhaled allergens so that the local antioxidant milieu of the lung may impact the magnitude of oxidant stress in these cells. Second, antioxidant supplements, including glutathione precursors [12, 13] have been shown to alter the cellular redox milieu of immune cells and effect pro-inflammatory cytokine production and inflammatory load in the lung **(Figure 1)**. Third, as described above, the airway epithelium appears to be one cellular target that is subject to mitochondrial injury in asthma and in murine asthma models. Fourth, studies from the author's laboratory suggest that extracellular glutathione within the lung lining fluid has a robust impact on airway epithelial cell responses to inflammation and the development of airway hyperreactivity (AHR). AHR may be related to airway epithelial cell integrity and maintenance of barrier function [14]. These data suggest that the source and the location of oxidative stress, as well as the nature of the oxidant(s) to be targeted, are likely to impact the success of an antioxidant intervention. Nonetheless, broader based interventions have also shown some success in animal models, as discussed below.

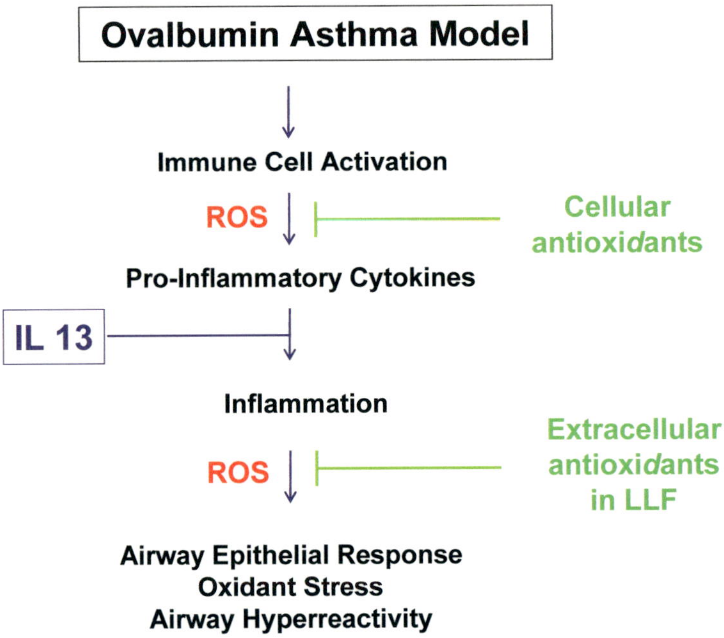

Fig. 1. **Murine Models of Allergic Asthma**. Two general models are driven by ovalbumin as allergen, or IL13 as pro-inflammatory cytokine. Cellular antioxidants, such as glutathione, can affect the redox milieu of immune cells to attenuate pro-inflammatory cytokine induction (12). Extracellular antioxidants, such as lung lining fluid (LLF) glutathione, can buffer reactive oxygen species (ROS) from inflammatory cells, protect airway epithelial cells against oxidant stress and prevent airway hyperreactivity (14).

Oxidant stress, transcription factor NF-E2 related factor 2 (Nrf2) and asthma: Cellular antioxidants effectively buffer oxidants generated by metabolism or inhaled during ventilation in the normal lung. Oxidant stress results when the oxidant burden exceeds antioxidant defense and this elicits a cellular response to increase antioxidant capacity and restore balance. Recent studies have identified a central component of this endogenous antioxidant response pathway as transcription factor NF-E2 related factor 2, also known as Nrf2 [15, 16]. Nrf2 is a basic leucine zipper transcription factor and a member of the cap-n-collar family of transcription factors. It recognizes a core promoter DNA sequence known as the "antioxidant responsive element" (ARE) and up-regulates several antioxidant and phase 2 detoxifying genes in cells. Targeted deletion of Nrf2 in mice produces no obvious phenotype under normal conditions [17]. But Nrf2 null mice exhibit increased susceptibility to oxidant stress from pro-oxidant agents such as acetaminophen, which causes liver failure [18], and butylated hydroxytoluene, which causes respiratory failure [19]. Nrf2 deficient mice are also sensitive to several oxidant-mediated injuries in the lung, including exposure to hyperoxia [20] and bleomycin [21]. A common theme in this susceptibility centers on uncompensated oxidant stress which causes excess inflammation along with extensive cell injury leading to cell death and organ failure. An expanding literature now supports Nrf2 as a general regulator of the ARE-mediated cellular antioxidant defense system that enables cell to survive under oxidant stress [15, 22]. The biological relevance of the Nrf2 pathway continues to expand with recent descriptions of its interaction with the notch1 signaling pathway during tissue regeneration [23] and the p53/p21 pathway during cell cycle control in response to oxidant-mediated DNA damage [24]. In fact, the known susceptibility of the p21 deficient lung to oxidant stress may result from lack of the p21 protein-protein interaction that liberates Nrf2 from its cytoplasmic inhibitor Keap1 [25]. Previous studies have documented induction of p21 protein in airway epithelial cells with asthma. This novel interaction with Nrf2 suggests a biological couple between cell cycle arrest and antioxidant activation that enables cell survival under oxidant stress [26].

The relevance of Nrf2 to oxidant stress and asthma stems from the fact that Nrf2 null mice are more susceptible to asthma than normal mice using ovalbumin to model experimental allergic airway disease [11]. Oxidant stress, inflammation, airway hyperreactivity and mucus induction are magnified in the lungs of Nrf2 null mice compared to normal mice [27]. Oxidant stress was quantified by total lung glutathione which rose in the normal lung, largely as reduced glutathione (GSH), but not in the Nrf2 null lung. The genes for glutathione synthesis were identified as Nrf2-targets in asthma, as well as in a variety of other oxidant-stress related murine models of lung injury in these mice. In addition, glutathione signaling was shown to be differentially utilized as an effector to regulate gene expression in Nrf2 dependent and independent pathways [28]. These studies added further support to the central biologic role of the glutathione tripeptide in cellular redox homeostasis [28, 29].

These studies in the Nrf2 null mouse models of increased susceptibility to oxidant stress suggested that oxidant stress is causal in various forms of lung injury, including asthma. They supported epidemiologic studies that linked antioxidant intake with decreased risk of asthma severity [30, 31], and reinvigorated a search for antioxidant therapeutics to treat asthma despite the fact that single antioxidant agents were largely ineffective in clinical trials. In adition, studies using a mouse model of impaired glutathione metabolism together with those using glutathione precursors to manipulate glutathione homeostasis raised the possibility that antioxidants from separate intracellular or extracellular pools may be relevant for different cell types during asthma pathogenesis, such as immune cells during sensitization and epithelial cells in response to inflammation [12, 14].

Taken altogether, these studies suggest different strategies that could be explored to develop novel antioxidant therapeutics for asthma. The first is a broad-based approach using activators of the Nrf2 pathway to induce an array of antioxidant genes to widely augment cellular antioxidant defense [15]. One caveat, however, is that the therapeutic benefits of this broad-based approach cannot exclusively be attributed to an "antioxidant" mechanism of action. Nrf2 controls many cytoprotective genes in addition to known antioxidants, and these genes are also expressed at much lower levels in Nrf2 null versus normal mice [11, 28, 32]. In addition, the more severe asthmatic phenotype in Nrf2 null mice is associated not only with increased oxidative stress, but also with increased inflammation. Since loss of Nrf2 does not appear to control production of Th2 cytokines directly, the increased inflammation is attributable to an oxidative stress-mediated activation of pro-inflammatory transcription factors, such as NF-κB [33]. Nonetheless, such observations make it difficult to dissociate antioxidant from anti-inflammatory effects, or from effects on cytoprotective pathways other than those involving antioxidant enzymes, in strategies involving Nrf2 modulation.

A second and more specific therapeutic approach could be designed around more localized, or ROS-specific, interventions using synthetic antioxidant compounds, or agents that otherwise modulate levels of downstream effects of oxidants. Examples of this include glutathione selective approaches to augment content in extracellular pools by targeting glutathione metabolism in lung lining fluid [14, 34] or intracellular pools using glutathione precursors [12]. Other approaches that have been suggested include mitochondria-targeted antioxidants [6] or synthetic catalytic ROS scavengers [35, 36] that can gain intracellular access, in some cases mitochondrial access [37, 38].

2. Therapeutic approaches

Broad-based strategy based on Nrf2 pathway activation. Characterization and design of compounds that can activate the Nrf2 pathway are an active focus of research for inflammatory disease and cancer chemoprevention [39-41] (also www.reatapharma.com). A group of synthetic triterpenoids are now known to exhibit cytoprotective, antioxidant and anti-inflammatory activity largely thru activation of the Nrf2 pathway and are under intense characterization and development as potent Nrf2 activators [42]. CDDO-Im is a well characterized compound that can be delivered enterally and has shown therapeutic benefits in mouse models of hyperoxic acute lung injury [43], cystic fibrosis-like lung disease [44] and lung cancer [45]. There are no reports, as of yet, on the usage of an Nrf2 activator in allergic asthma. But the synthetic triterpenoid CDDO-Im has been shown to induce Nrf2-mediated activity and protection through its action in normal mice exposed to cigarette smoke as a model of chronic obstructive pulmonary disease, COPD, as compared to Nrf2 null mice. These results are instructive with regard to oxidant stress and airway function [46]. The oxidant burden in COPD results not only from infiltration of the lung with inflammatory cells (which are mainly neutrophils in contrast to eosinophils in allergic asthma), but also from cigarette smoke itself and markers of oxidant stress have been consistently demonstrated in the lung and the blood of smoke-exposed mammals [47, 48]. Certain COPD phenotypes include lung cell injury and death, enlargement of alveoli and eventually right heart failure. All of these changes were modeled in normal mice exposed to cigarette smoke and all were attenuated by concomitant delivery of CDDO-Im as measured by decreased levels of oxidant stress, cellular apoptosis, alveolar destruction and pulmonary hypertension. Furthermore, when Nrf2 null mice were exposed to cigarette smoke, these changes were all magnified, compared to normal mice, and protection by CDDO-Im was absent, supporting the notion that this compound requires Nrf2 for much of its activity [46].

Interestingly, oxidant stress was assessed by total glutathione content of the lung which decreased acutely with exposure to cigarette smoke and increased over time in normal mice but not in Nrf2 null mice. Treatment with CDDO-Im increased lung glutathione even in normal mice exposed to air as a control, given that this compound is an electrophile itself, but again not in Nrf2 null mice. The genes for glutathione synthesis, γ-glutamyl cysteine ligase and glutathione synthetase, are known Nrf2 targets. The former is the rate limiting enzyme for glutathione synthesis, and its activity is regulated by glutathione levels thru feedback inhibition [49]. Hence increasing content of this synthetic enzyme is permissive to an increase in glutathione content to reset feedback inhibition anew. This stimulation has the potential to be developed for increased protection of an "at risk" population exposed to primary or second-hand smoke [46]. Even though single candidate association studies have not implicated these glutathione synthetic genes in asthma or COPD, they have implicated the glutathione-S-tranferase genes GSTM1 and GSTP1, suggesting a role for glutathione derivatives with airway inflammation [50]. Lastly, treatment with CDDO-Im did increase lung glutathione weakly in Nrf2 null mice exposed to cigarette smoke. This suggests an Nrf2-

independent mediator for some CDDO-Im activity that may be fulfilled by an Nrf2-related gene, such as Nrf1 [51] or an Nrf2-independent pathway [39, 40].

Regarding lung inflammation in this mouse model of COPD, the inflammatory load, assessed thru broncho-alveolar lavage, was similar in cigarette smoke-exposed normal mice regardless of treatment with CDDO-Im [46]. Hence induction of Nrf2-regulated genes was sufficient to protect against cell injury and death in the cigarette smoke exposed lung despite a similar degree of inflammation. The array of antioxidant and detoxifying genes may have provided a much broader level of protection than that afforded by any single antioxidant therapy. The findings in COPD models suggest that CDDO-Im and similar agents should also be investigated as potential asthma treatments. Since inflammation is a prominent feature of established asthma, even in remission, it is possible that this treatment may have to be continued on a chronic basis to prevent future exacerbations. In this regard, CDDO-Im can attenuate cytokine and chemokine expression in LPS-stimulated neutrophils [52] and thereby decrease the inflammatory response. If CDDO-Im can produce similar results in models of allergic inflammation, it could be used to prevent severe exacerbations of asthma. Such as approach is warranted as it has recently been reported that Nrf2 protein itself is susceptible to suppression and inactivation in children with severe asthma when oxidant stress is intense [53]. In adult atopic asthmatics, allergen-provoked airway inflammation also suppresses Nrf2 protein function and this can be attenuated by larger than usual dosing of Vitamin E [54]. The ultimate ability of Vitamin E to rescue Nrf2 function under intense oxidant stress is not yet known.

Selective strategies based on ROS-scavenging or other antioxidant-modulating compounds. These strategies would, in contrast to the very broad Nrf2-modulating approach described above, administer compounds with their own antioxidant properties, or others that specifically modulate endogenous antioxidants. As an example of the latter approach, genetic or pharmacological modulation of endogenous pools of glutathione (GSH) has beneficial effects in asthma models [12,13,14].

Glutathione Modulating Reagents: The central role of glutathione in antioxidant defense and signal transduction, was described previously in the literature [55-57] and largely reinforced by studies with Nrf2 [28, 29]. Studies with the Nrf2 null mice demonstrated that loss of the Nrf2 pathway perturbed lung glutathione homeostasis in the ovalbumin model of asthma [11]. And recent literature demonstrated that glutathione alone can serve a direct role in asthma. In one example from the author's laboratory, genetic loss of glutathione metabolism in lung lining fluid was shown to augment the concentration of the extracellular glutathione pool and prevent EGF receptor activation, airway epithelial cell mucin gene induction and airway hyperreactivity in a cytokine-driven model of asthma **(Figure 1)** [14]. Loss of glutathione metabolism resulted from the genetic absence of the regulatory enzyme γ-glutamyltranferase (GGT) [58, 59]. Furthermore, asthma could be limited in normal mice by inhibiting their lung lining fluid GGT pharmacologically with the compound acivicin. A second example of pharmacologically modulating GSH pools involved the glutathione precursor γ-glutamylcysteinylethyl ester (γ-GCE) which was shown to effectively augment reduced cellular glutathione content (GSH) and redox ratio (GSH/GSSG) in antigen presenting cells to limit pro-inflammatory gene induction and attenuate lung inflammation in the ovalbumin model of asthma [12]. Previous studies with cysteine precursors produced similar results but difference in cell permeability were hypothesized to limit overall effectiveness [13, 60, 61]. A potential advantage of these two strategies is that their therapeutic targets are more selective and focused on glutathione homeostasis itself as compared to the broad array of antioxidant and other cytoprotective genes activated by Nrf2.

Our finding that loss of glutathione metabolism in lung lining fluid could actually attenuate asthma was rather unexpected. Lung lining fluid (LLF) is a continuous but very thin layer of fluid that bathes the epithelial surface of the lung [62] and shields alveolar cells against environmental and endogenous toxins, including oxidants. LLF contains an abundance of antioxidants, including reduced glutathione [63]. This extracellular pool of glutathione buffers hypohalous acid, a potent oxidant from inflammatory cells [64] and inhaled chlorine gas [65], limits hydrogen peroxides and lipid peroxide accumulation in conjunction with extracellular glutathione peroxidase [66], and maintains bioavailability of other small antioxidant molecules, such as nitric oxide [67], ascorbic acid [68], and alpha-tocopherol [69]. In humans with asthma, the abundance of LLF glutathione content is increased beyond the normal level and the magnitude of this increase is inversely related to asthma severity [70].

Metabolism of LLF glutathione is regulated by a single extracellular enzyme, GGT, that is associated with surfactant phospholipid [71]. Glutathione metabolism supplies cells with cysteine, the rate-limiting amino acid for glutathione biosynthesis. In the presence of oxidant stress, cells in the lung induce GGT [72] via Nrf2 signaling [73, 74] to maintain cysteine availability for enhanced glutathione synthesis. In the absence of GGT, cells becomes starved for cysteine and glutathione deficiency results [58, 75]. Indeed in the GGT^{enu1} mouse model of GGT deficiency, lung cells are glutathione deficient and under oxidant stress even in normoxia, and this is magnified in hyperoxia [76]. The presence of oxidant stress at baseline suggested that the GGT^{enu1} mouse would be more susceptible to asthma, which could then be attenuated by restoring cellular glutathione with a cysteine precursor [75, 77, 78]. However, in a cytokine-driven model of allergic inflammation, cellular glutathione deficiency did not predispose the GGT^{enu1} mouse to asthma. Rather, in the absence of metabolism, LLF glutathione content in the GGT^{enu1} mouse increased well beyond its mildly elevated baseline level, buffered oxidant stress and shielded the GGT^{enu1} mouse lung against asthma, even though the level of inflammation matched that of the asthma-susceptible normal mouse lung [14]. Moreover, asthma susceptibility in the normal mouse lung could be attenuated by inhibiting normal LLF GGT activity with the irreversible GGT inhibitor acivicin. To do this effectively, however, acivicin had to be delivered thru the airway (inhaled), as opposed to the systemic circulation [14].

These studies provided several insights about asthma and oxidant stress. First, the extracellular LLF glutathione pool can shield lung epithelial cells against oxidant-mediated induction of mucin gene expression and preserve barrier function despite cellular glutathione deficiency. Second, not all cellular sites of oxidant stress are directly casual in asthma. Endothelial, bronchial epithelial and alveolar macrophages of GGT^{enu1} lung exhibit oxidant stress at baseline, but methacholine-induced airway hyperreactivity is absent. Third, the LLF glutathione pool serves a dual role in antioxidant defense and cysteine supply with glutathione metabolism regulating the balance. As the key regulator of this metabolism, GGT is a novel target to treat asthma as it is accessible to inhibition thru the airway via its presence in lung surfactant and its modulation can augment the antioxidant capacity within LLF. Although acivicin can irreversibly inhibit GGT, there is a critical problem associated with its usage from a pharmaceutical point of view and that is CNS toxicity *in vivo* and inhibition of several glutamine-dependent biosynthetic enzymes. The recent design and synthesis of a series of γ-phosphono diester analogues of glutamate as GGT inhibitors helped overcome this concern [79]. The lead compound in this class of compounds is currently the most promising candidate for pharmaceuticals to chemically inactivate GGT activity *in vivo*. This compound does inhibit lung GGT activity and its advantages include greater specificity, potency, and lack of toxicity [34]. Lastly, cellular glutathione deficiency can be averted by providing a cysteine precursor or the glutathione precursor γ-glutamylcysteinylester (γ-GCE). Esterification of glutathione as a means to increase its membrane permeability was described by Alton Meister [80]. γ-glutamylcysteinyl ester uptake appears to be even more efficient than glutathione and it is directly converted to glutathione by glutathione synthetase which bypasses the rate-limiting enzyme γ-GCS. Hence it is feasible to augment both cellular and extracellular glutathione content using a combination of these reagents.

Synthetic catalytic antioxidant mimetic compounds: Superoxide dismutases (SOD) are key endogenous antioxidant defense enzymes, converting superoxide to hydrogen peroxide. There are three forms of SOD, cytosolic (SOD1), extracellular (ECSOD or SOD3) and mitochondrial (SOD2) and various studies have implicated one or more of the SOD enzymes in lung disease [81]. Compared to other tissues, the lung has very high levels of ECSOD, localized in the vasculature and airways. Its localization, as well as its upregulation during inflammation and the increased SOD activity detected in BAL from asthma patients, makes it attractive to speculate that ECSOD plays a role in asthma. However, the relatively mild phenotype shown by mice lacking ECSOD in asthma models leaves the involvement of ECSOD unclear [82]. The mitochondrial form of SOD (MnSOD or SOD2) is oxidatively inactivated in asthmatic airway samples [4], suggesting that impairment of mitochondrial oxidative defenses might contribute to the asthmatic phenotype. Evidence for mitochondrial injury in murine asthma models [2, 3], discussed earlier, is consistent with this hypothesis, though the mechanism(s) of mitochondrial damage have not been elucidated. SOD2 polymorphisms are also associated with bronchial hyperresponsivenss in humans [83]. The product of SOD, hydrogen peroxide, is neutralized by several different enzymes, including not only catalase but also various peroxidases including glutathione peroxidase, using glutathione as a substrate [81, 84]. Along with SOD, hydrogen peroxide scavenging enzymes have also been detected in the lung lining fluid [85], and may also contribute to defense against asthmatic responses. Such findings, overall, do imply that supplementation of the right antioxidant enzyme(s) at the right location(s) could be a viable therapeutic approach for asthma. To avoid the many pharmaceutical challenges, including stability, intracellular accessibility, and expense, associated with therapeutic use of proteins, some investigators have developed low molecular weight synthetic compounds with antioxidant activities. In particular three classes of Mn complex have been studied as *catalytic* antioxidant enzyme mimetics with efficacy in various disease models, including those involving the lung [81, 85]. Porphyrin Mn complexes [36] and salen Mn complexes [35] are multifunctional catalytic antioxidant compounds, acting on superoxide, hydrogen peroxide, and certain reactive nitrogen species. Macrocyclic Mn complexes, such as M40403, are a class of compounds reported to have SOD activity, with no hydrogen peroxide scavenging properties [86]. Chang and Crapo [87] reported that the Mn porphyrin AEOL-10150 suppressed inflammation and improved airway physiology in a murine allergic asthma model. M40403, a lead macrocyclic complex, was shown to be similarly effective in a guinea pig ovalbumin-induced asthma model [88]. While there have not yet been reports of their effects in asthma models, salen Mn complexes, exemplified by compounds such as EUK-189 and a newer cyclized analog EUK-207, are also of potential interest. These compounds have efficacy in other lung injury models, such as a porcine ARDS [89] and pulmonary radiation injury [90, 91] models. As compared to several other agents tested, salen Mn complexes were effective at preventing severe oxidative pathologies in mice lacking SOD2, implying that these compounds have the ability to protect the mitochondria [38]. Certain Mn porphryin compounds have also shown efficacy in mitochondrial injury models [37, 92], while M40403 did not rescue mice lacking SOD2 [93]. If, indeed, mitochondrial injury is important in asthma, then the effects of such multifunctional ROS/RNS scavenging compounds deserve further study as potential asthma therapeutics. Unlike these Mn complexes, which have broader effects, certain other antioxidant compounds were designed to specifically target the mitochondria [6, 94, 95]. While there has been no report yet testing such agents in asthma models, it seems likely that, because of the multiple potential sites of oxidative injury in asthma, an approach targeted only at the mitochondrial would not be optimally effective. It is worth noting, as well, that both Mn complexes that improved airway physiology in asthma models also suppressed inflammation. As was the case for the Nrf2 null mouse, this makes it difficult to sort out whether their therapeutic benefit is due primarily to their anti-oxidant properties, or is secondary to their anti-inflammatory effects. This is in contrast to the approaches aimed specifically at lung lining fluid GSH, where airway physiology and oxidative stress were improved in the absence of any suppression of inflammation. Certainly, a better understanding of the mechanism(s) and site(s) of action of a given agent will help to facilitate its successful use as an asthma drug. And potentially, for a disease as complex as asthma, combination therapies consisting of both anti-inflammatory and selected antioxidant compounds would be more effective than any agent given alone.

3. Summary

Oxidant stress induced by the accumulation of oxidants in excess of antioxidant defense plays a causal role in asthma. Recent studies in mouse models of asthma have drawn attention to the roles of oxidant stress and antioxidant defense in cellular and extracellular sites of the lung. Cellular sites of oxidant stress during immune cell activation and extracellular sites of oxidant stress in lung lining fluid may play distinct roles during the early phase of sensitization to allergens and the late phase of lung response to inflammation, respectively. It also appears that not all sites of oxidant stress are necessarily directly related to the development of AHR. Novel strategies to treat asthma may involve activation of the Nrf2 pathway and its array of antioxidant and cytoprotective genes, although the necessity of all of the genes is not yet clear, nor are the long term effects of deactivation of this pathway on normal cell function and asthma progression. Alternative strategies designed to modulate lung cell or lung lining fluid glutathione or to administer synthetic antioxidants with more specific ROS targets or other properties may (as compared to the broad panel of Nrf2-regulated antioxidants) provide a more focused approach to control pro-inflammatory stimuli and lung antioxidant defense. Of further interest would be whether the strategy, while acting against oxidative stress, is also anti-inflammatory (e.g. Nrf2 activation) or whether it appears to act downstream of inflammation (e.g. GGT inhibition to increase extracellular GSH). Communication of epithelial cell injury to the adaptive immune system and activation of airway inflammation are common themes identified in human genome-wide association studies (GWAS) to date, although genes with known antioxidant functions are not readily apparent in susceptibility loci [96]. GWAS studies have also confirmed the genetic heterogeneity of asthma [96-98]. The causal mechanisms underlying any of these gene associations, however, are yet to be defined. Overall these data suggest that combinations of multiple agents are likely to be more effective than any agent alone. These might be agents that combat oxidative stress, through the various mechanisms discussed here, in combination with other treatments acting by distinct mechanisms to modulate anti-cytokine or anti-inflammatory pathways.

Abbreviations: SOD, superoxide dismutase; Nrf2, NF-E2 related factor 2; ARE, antioxidant response element; GSH, glutathione; GSSG, glutathione disulfide; GGT, gamma-glutamyl transferase; ROS, reactive oxygen species; LLF, lung lining fluid; BAL, bronch-alveolar lavage; CDDO-Im, 1-[2-cyano-3-,12-dioxooleana-1,9(11)-dien-28-oyl]imidazole; GWAS, genome-wide association study.

4. Acknowledgement

Martin Joyce-Brady is a recipient of an Ignition Award from the Boston University Office of Technology Development.

5. References

[1] MacPherson JC, Comhair SA, Erzurum SC et al. Eosinophils are a major source of nitric oxide-derived oxidants in severe asthma: characterization of pathways available to eosinophils for generating reactive nitrogen species. J Immunol 2001; 166(9):5763-5772.

[2] Aguilera-Aguirre L, Bacsi A, Saavedra-Molina A, Kurosky A, Sur S, Boldogh I. Mitochondrial dysfunction increases allergic airway inflammation. J Immunol 2009; 183(8):5379-5387.

[3] Mabalirajan U, Dinda AK, Kumar S et al. Mitochondrial structural changes and dysfunction are associated with experimental allergic asthma. J Immunol 2008; 181(5):3540-3548.

[4] Comhair SA, Xu W, Ghosh S et al. Superoxide dismutase inactivation in pathophysiology of asthmatic airway remodeling and reactivity. Am J Pathol 2005; 166(3):663-674.

[5] Trian T, Benard G, Begueret H et al. Bronchial smooth muscle remodeling involves calcium-dependent enhanced mitochondrial biogenesis in asthma. J Exp Med 2007; 204(13):3173-3181.

[6] Reddy PH. Mitochondrial Dysfunction and Oxidative Stress in Asthma: Implications for Mitochondria-Targeted Antioxidant Therapeutics. Pharmaceuticals (Basel) 2011; 4(3):429-456.

[7] Caramori G, Papi A. Oxidants and asthma. Thorax 2004; 59(2):170-3.

[8] Kelly FJ, Mudway I, Blomberg A, Frew A, Sandstrom T. Altered lung antioxidant status in patients with mild asthma. Lancet 1999; 354(9177):482-3.

[9] Gaston B, Drazen JM, Loscalzo J, Stamler JS. The biology of nitrogen oxides in the airways. Am J Respir Crit Care Med 1994; 149(2 Pt 1):538-51.

[10] Fitzpatrick AM, Teague WG, Holguin F, Yeh M, Brown LA. Airway glutathione homeostasis is altered in children with severe asthma: evidence for oxidant stress. J Allergy Clin Immunol 2009; 123(1):146-152.

[11] Rangasamy T, Guo J, Mitzner WA et al. Disruption of Nrf2 enhances susceptibility to severe airway inflammation and asthma in mice. J Exp Med 2005; 202(1):47-59.

[12] Koike Y, Hisada T, Utsugi M et al. Glutathione redox regulates airway hyperresponsiveness and airway inflammation in mice. Am J Respir Cell Mol Biol 2007; 37(3):322-329.

[13] Lee YC, Lee KS, Park SJ et al. Blockade of airway hyperresponsiveness and inflammation in a murine model of asthma by a prodrug of cysteine, L-2-oxothiazolidine-4-carboxylic acid. FASEB J 2004; 18(15):1917-1919.

[14] Lowry MH, McAllister BP, Jean JC et al. Lung lining fluid glutathione attenuates IL-13-induced asthma. Am J Respir Cell Mol Biol 2008; 38(5):509-516.

[15] Kensler TW, Wakabayashi N, Biswal S. Cell survival responses to environmental stresses via the Keap1-Nrf2-ARE pathway. Annu Rev Pharmacol Toxicol 2007; 47:89-116.

[16] Motohashi H, Yamamoto M. Nrf2-Keap1 defines a physiologically important stress response mechanism. Trends Mol Med 2004; 10(11):549-557.

[17] Chan K, Lu R., Chang JC, Kan YW. NRF2, a member of the NFE2 family of transcription factors, is not essential for murine erythropoiesis, growth, and development. Proc Natl Acad Sci USA 1992; 93:13943-13948.

[18] Chan K, Han XD, Kan YW. An important function of Nrf2 in combating oxidative stress: detoxification of acetaminophen. Proc Natl Acad Sci USA 2001; 98(8):4611-6.

[19] Chan K, Kan YW. Nrf2 is essential for protection against acute pulmonary injury in mice. Proc Natl Acad Sci U S A 1999; 96(22):12731-12736.

[20] Cho HY, Jedlicka AE, Reddy SP et al. Role of NRF2 in protection against hyperoxic lung injury in mice. Am J Respir Cell Mol Biol 2002; 26(2):175-182.

[21] Cho H, Reddy SP, Yamamoto M., Kleeberger SR. The transcription factor NRF2 protects against pulmonary fibrosis. FASEB J 2004; 18(11):1258-60.

[22] Cho HY, Reddy SP, Kleeberger SR. Nrf2 defends the lung from oxidative stress. Antioxid Redox Signal 2006; 8(1-2):76-87.

[23] Wakabayashi N, Shin S, Slocum SL et al. Regulation of notch1 signaling by nrf2: implications for tissue regeneration. Sci Signal 2010; 3(130):ra52.

[24] Chen W, Sun Z, Wang XJ et al. Direct interaction between Nrf2 and p21(Cip1/WAF1) upregulates the Nrf2-mediated antioxidant response. Mol Cell 2009; 34(6):663-673.

[25] Toledano MB. The guardian recruits cops: the p53-p21 axis delegates prosurvival duties to the Keap1-Nrf2 stress pathway. Mol Cell 2009; 34(6):637-639.

[26] Puddicombe SM, Torres-Lozano C, Richter A et al. Increased expression of p21(waf) cyclin-dependent kinase inhibitor in asthmatic bronchial epithelium. Am J Respir Cell Mol Biol 2003; 28(1):61-68.

[27] Pyrgos G, Fahey J, Talalay P, Reynolds C, Brown R. Restoration of Bronchoprotection and Bronchodilation in Asthma Through Stimulation of the Nrf2 Pathway. Am J Respir Crit Care Med 2010; 181:A4986.

[28] Reddy NM, Kleeberger SR, Yamamoto M et al. Genetic dissection of the Nrf2-dependent redox signaling-regulated transcriptional programs of cell proliferation and cytoprotection. Physiol Genomics 2007; 32(1):74-81.

[29] Malhotra D, Portales-Casamar E, Singh A et al. Global mapping of binding sites for Nrf2 identifies novel targets in cell survival response through ChIP-Seq profiling and network analysis. Nucleic Acids Res 2010; 38(17):5718-5734.

[30] Wood LG, Gibson PG, Garg ML. Biomarkers of lipid peroxidation, airway inflammation and asthma. Eur Respir J 2003; 21(1):177-86.

[31] Wood LG, Gibson PG. Reduced circulating antioxidant defences are associated with airway hyper-responsiveness, poor control and severe disease pattern in asthma. Br J Nutr 2010; 103(5):735-741.

[32] Rangasamy T, Cho CY, Thimmulappa RK et al. Genetic ablation of Nrf2 enhances susceptibility to cigarette smoke-induced emphysema in mice. J Clin Invest 2004; 114(9):1248-1259.

[33] Sarada S, Himadri P, Mishra C, Geetali P, Ram MS, Ilavazhagan G. Role of oxidative stress and NFkB in hypoxia-induced pulmonary edema. Exp Biol Med (Maywood) 2008; 233(9):1088-1098.

[34] Joyce-Brady M, Hiratake J. Inhibiting Glutathione Metabolism in Lung Lining Fluid as a Strategy to Augment Antioxidant Defense. Current Enzyme Inhibition 2011; 7:71-78.

[35] Doctrow SR, Huffman K, Marcus CB et al. Salen-manganese complexes as catalytic scavengers of hydrogen peroxide and cytoprotective agents: structure-activity relationship studies. J Med Chem 2002; 45(20):4549-4558.

[36] Patel M, Day BJ. Metalloporphyrin class of therapeutic catalytic antioxidants. Trends Pharmacol Sci 1999; 20(9):359-364.

[37] Melov S, Schneider JA, Day BJ et al. A novel neurological phenotype in mice lacking mitochondrial manganese superoxide dismutase. Nat Genet 1998; 18(2):159-163.

[38] Melov S, Doctrow SR, Schneider JA et al. Lifespan extension and rescue of spongiform encephalopathy in superoxide dismutase 2 nullizygous mice treated with superoxide dismutase-catalase mimetics. J Neurosci 2001; 21(21):8348-8353.

[39] Liby KT, Yore MM, Sporn MB. Triterpenoids and rexinoids as multifunctional agents for the prevention and treatment of cancer. Nat Rev Cancer 2007; 7(5):357-369.

[40] Sporn MB, Liby KT, Yore MM, Fu L, Lopchuk JM, Gribble GW. New synthetic triterpenoids: potent agents for prevention and treatment of tissue injury caused by inflammatory and oxidative stress. J Nat Prod 2011; 74(3):537-545.

[41] Zhang Y, Gordon GB. A strategy for cancer prevention: stimulation of the Nrf2-ARE signaling pathway. Mol Cancer Ther 2004; 3(7):885-893.

[42] Yates MS, Tauchi M, Katsuoka F et al. Pharmacodynamic characterization of chemopreventive triterpenoids as exceptionally potent inducers of Nrf2-regulated genes. Mol Cancer Ther 2007; 6(1):154-162.

[43] Reddy NM, Suryanaraya V, Yates MS et al. The triterpenoid CDDO-imidazolide confers potent protection against hyperoxic acute lung injury in mice. Am J Respir Crit Care Med 2009; 180(9):867-874.

[44] Nichols DP, Ziady AG, Shank SL, Eastman JF, Davis PB. The triterpenoid CDDO limits inflammation in preclinical models of cystic fibrosis lung disease. Am J Physiol Lung Cell Mol Physiol 2009; 297(5):L828-L836.

[45] Liby K, Risingsong R, Royce DB et al. Triterpenoids CDDO-methyl ester or CDDO-ethyl amide and rexinoids LG100268 or NRX194204 for prevention and treatment of lung cancer in mice. Cancer Prev Res (Phila) 2009; 2(12):1050-1058.

[46] Sussan TE, Rangasamy T, Blake DJ et al. Targeting Nrf2 with the triterpenoid CDDO-imidazolide attenuates cigarette smoke-induced emphysema and cardiac dysfunction in mice. Proc Natl Acad Sci U S A 2009; 106(1):250-255.

[47] MacNee W. Pulmonary and Systemic Oxidant/Antioxidant Imbalance in Chronic Obstructive Pulmonary Disease. The Proceedings of the American Thoracic Society 2005; 2:50-60.

[48] Rahman I, MacNee W. Lung glutathione and oxidative stress: implications in cigarette smoke-induced airway disease. Am J Physiol 1999; 277(6 Pt 1):L1067-L1088.

[49] Dalton TP, Chen Y, Schneider SN, Nebert DW, Shertzer HG. Genetically altered mice to evaluate glutathione homeostasis in health and disease. Free Radic Biol Med 2004; 37(10):1511-1526.
[50] Postma DS, Kerkhof M, Boezen HM, Koppelman GH. Asthma and chronic obstructive pulmonary disease: common genes, common environments? Am J Respir Crit Care Med 2011; 183(12):1588-1594.
[51] Yang H, Magilnick N, Lee C et al. Nrf1 and Nrf2 regulate rat glutamate-cysteine ligase catalytic subunit transcription indirectly via NF-kappaB and AP-1. Mol Cell Biol 2005; 25(14):5933-5946.
[52] Thimmulappa RK, Scollick C, Traore K et al. Nrf2-dependent protection from LPS induced inflammatory response and mortality by CDDO-Imidazolide. Biochem Biophys Res Commun 2006; 351(4):883-889.
[53] Fitzpatrick AM, Stephenson ST, Hadley GR et al. Thiol redox disturbances in children with severe asthma are associated with posttranslational modification of the transcription factor nuclear factor (erythroid-derived 2)-like 2. J Allergy Clin Immunol 2011; 127(6):1604-1611.
[54] Dworski R, Han W, Blackwell TS, Hoskins A, Freeman ML. Vitamin E prevents NRF2 suppression by allergens in asthmatic alveolar macrophages in vivo. Free Radic Biol Med 2011; 51(2):516-521.
[55] Meister A. Glutathione, ascorbate, and cellular protection. Cancer Res 1994; 54(7 Suppl):1969s-1975s.
[56] Schafer FQ, Buettner GR. Redox environment of the cell as viewed through the redox state of the glutathione disulfide/glutathione couple. Free Radic Biol Med 2001; 30(11):1191-1212.
[57] Biswas SK, Rahman I. Environmental toxicity, redox signaling and lung inflammation: the role of glutathione. Mol Aspects Med 2009; 30(1-2):60-76.
[58] Harding CO, Williams P, Wagner E et al. Mice with genetic gamma-glutamyl transpeptidase deficiency exhibit glutathionuria, severe growth failure, reduced life spans, and infertility. J Biol Chem 1997; 272(19):12560-12567.
[59] Jean JC, Harding CO, Oakes SM, Yu Q, Held PK, Joyce-Brady M. gamma-Glutamyl transferase (GGT) deficiency in the GGTenu1 mouse results from a single point mutation that leads to a stop codon in the first coding exon of GGT mRNA. Mutagenesis 1999; 14(1):31-36.
[60] Blesa S, Cortijo J, Mata M et al. Oral N-acetylcysteine attenuates the rat pulmonary inflammatory response to antigen. Eur Respir J 2003; 21(3):394-400.
[61] Whitekus MJ, Li N, Zhang M et al. Thiol antioxidants inhibit the adjuvant effects of aerosolized diesel exhaust particles in a murine model for ovalbumin sensitization. J Immunol 2002; 168(5):2560-2567.
[62] Bastacky J, Lee CY, Goerke J et al. Alveolar lining layer is thin and continuous: low-temperature scanning electron microscopy of rat lung. J Appl Physiol 1995; 79(5):1615-1628.
[63] Cantin AM, North SL, Hubbard RC, Crystal RG. Normal Alveolar Epithelial Lining Fluid Contains High-Levels of Glutathione. Journal of Applied Physiology 1987; 63(1):152-157.
[64] Venglarik CJ, Giron-Calle J, Wigley AF, Malle E, Watanabe N, Forman HJ. Hypochlorous acid alters bronchial epithelial cell membrane properties and prevention by extracellular glutathione. J Appl Physiol 2003; 95(6):2444-52.
[65] Zhu L, Pi J, Wachi S, Andersen ME, Wu R, Chen Y. Identification of Nrf2-dependent airway epithelial adaptive response to proinflammatory oxidant-hypochlorous acid

challenge by transcription profiling. Am J Physiol Lung Cell Mol Physiol 2008; 294(3):L469-L477.
[66] Avissar N, Finkelstein JN, Horowitz S et al. Extracellular glutathione peroxidase in human lung epithelial lining fluid and in lung cells. Am J Physiol 1996; 270(2 Pt 1):L173-L182.
[67] Klings ES, Lowry MH, Li G et al. Hyperoxia-induced lung injury in gamma-glutamyl transferase deficiency is associated with alterations in nitrosative and nitrative stress. Am J Pathol 2009; 175(6):2309-2318.
[68] Meister A. Glutathione-ascorbic acid antioxidant system in animals. J Biol Chem 1994; 269(13):9397-9400.
[69] Leedle RA, Aust SD. The effect of glutathione on the vitamin E requirement for inhibition of liver microsomal lipid peroxidation. Lipids 1990; 25(5):241-245.
[70] Smith LJ, Houston M, Anderson J. Increased levels of glutathione in bronchoalveolar lavage fluid from patients with asthma. Am Rev Respir Dis 1993; 147(6 Pt 1):1461-4.
[71] Joyce-Brady M, Takahashi Y, Oakes SM et al. Synthesis and release of amphipathic gamma-glutamyl transferase by the pulmonary alveolar type 2 cell. Its redistribution throughout the gas exchange portion of the lung indicates a new role for surfactant. J Biol Chem 1994; 269:14219-26.
[72] Takahashi Y, Oakes SM, Williams MC, Takahashi S, Miura T, Joyce-Brady M. Nitrogen dioxide exposure activates gamma-glutamyl transferase gene expression in rat lung. Toxicol Appl Pharmacol 1997; 143(2):388-396.
[73] Zhang H, Liu H, Dickinson DA et al. gamma-Glutamyl transpeptidase is induced by 4-hydroxynonenal via EpRE/Nrf2 signaling in rat epithelial type II cells. Free Radic Biol Med 2006; 40(8):1281-1292.
[74] Zhang H, Liu H, Iles KE et al. 4-Hydroxynonenal induces rat gamma-glutamyl transpeptidase through mitogen-activated protein kinase-mediated electrophile response element/nuclear factor erythroid 2-related factor 2 signaling. Am J Respir Cell Mol Biol 2006; 34(2):174-181.
[75] Lieberman MW, Wiseman AL, Shi ZZ et al. Growth retardation and cysteine deficiency in gamma-glutamyl transpeptidase-deficient mice. Proc Natl Acad Sci U S A 1996; 93(15):7923-7926.
[76] Jean JC, Liu Y, Brown LA, Marc RE, Klings E, Joyce-Brady M. Gamma-glutamyl transferase deficiency results in lung oxidant stress in normoxia. Am J Physiol Lung Cell Mol Physiol 2002; 283(4):L766-L776.
[77] Barrios R, Shi ZZ, Kala SV et al. Oxygen-induced pulmonary injury in gamma-glutamyl transpeptidase-deficient mice. Lung 2001; 179(5):319-330.
[78] Held P, Harding CO. L-2-oxothiazolidine-4-carboxylate supplementation in murine gamma-GT deficiency. Free Radical Biology and Medicine 2003; 34(11):1482-1487.
[79] Han L, Hiratake J, Kamiyama A, Sakata K. Design, synthesis, and evaluation of gamma-phosphono diester analogues of glutamate as highly potent inhibitors and active site probes of gamma-glutamyl transpeptidase. Biochemistry 2007; 46(5):1432-1447.
[80] Meister A. Glutathione deficiency produced by inhibition of its synthesis, and its reversal; applications in research and therapy. Pharmacol Ther 1991; 51(2):155-194.
[81] Kinnula VL, Crapo JD. Superoxide dismutases in the lung and human lung diseases. Am J Respir Crit Care Med 2003; 167(12):1600-1619.
[82] Bowler RP, Crapo JD. Oxidative stress in airways: is there a role for extracellular superoxide dismutase? Am J Respir Crit Care Med 2002; 166(12 Pt 2):S38-S43.

[83] Siedlinski M, van Diemen CC, Postma DS, Vonk JM, Boezen HM. Superoxide dismutases, lung function and bronchial responsiveness in a general population. Eur Respir J 2009; 33(5):986-992.
[84] Halliwell B. Free radicals, antioxidants and human disease: Curiosity, cause or consequence. Lancet 1994; 344:721-4.
[85] Andreadis AA, Hazen SL, Comhair SA, Erzurum SC. Oxidative and nitrosative events in asthma. Free Radic Biol Med 2003; 35(3):213-225.
[86] Salvemini D, Wang ZQ, Zweier JL et al. A nonpeptidyl mimic of superoxide dismutase with therapeutic activity in rats. Science 1999; 286(5438):304-306.
[87] Chang LY, Crapo JD. Inhibition of airway inflammation and hyperreactivity by an antioxidant mimetic. Free Radic Biol Med 2002; 33(3):379-386.
[88] Masini E, Bani D, Vannacci A et al. Reduction of antigen-induced respiratory abnormalities and airway inflammation in sensitized guinea pigs by a superoxide dismutase mimetic. Free Radic Biol Med 2005; 39(4):520-531.
[89] Gonzalez PK, Zhuang J, Doctrow SR et al. EUK-8, a synthetic superoxide dismutase and catalase mimetic, ameliorates acute lung injury in endotoxemic swine. J Pharm Exp Ther 1995; 275:798-806.
[90] Mahmood J, Jelveh S, Calveley V, Zaidi A, Doctrow SR, Hill RP. Mitigation of radiation-induced lung injury by genistein and EUK-207. Int J Radiat Biol 2011; 87(8):889-901.
[91] Rosenthal RA, Fish B, Hill RP et al. Salen Mn complexes mitigate radiation injury in normal tissues. Anticancer Agents Med Chem 2011; 11(4):359-372.
[92] Liang LP, Huang J, Fulton R, Day BJ, Patel M. An orally active catalytic metalloporphyrin protects against 1-methyl-4-phenyl-1,2,3,6-tetrahydropyridine neurotoxicity in vivo. J Neurosci 2007; 27(16):4326-4333.
[93] Doctrow SR, Baudry M, Huffman K, Malfroy B, Melov S. Medicinal Inorganic Chemistry. New York: American Chemical Society and Oxford University Press; 2005.
[94] Kagan VE, Wipf P, Stoyanovsky D et al. Mitochondrial targeting of electron scavenging antioxidants: Regulation of selective oxidation vs random chain reactions. Adv Drug Deliv Rev 2009; 61(14):1375-1385.
[95] Tauskela JS. MitoQ--a mitochondria-targeted antioxidant. IDrugs 2007; 10(6):399-412.
[96] Akhabir L, Sandford AJ. Genome-wide association studies for discovery of genes involved in asthma. Respirology 2011; 16(3):396-406.
[97] Hirota T, Takahashi A, Kubo M et al. Genome-wide association study identifies three new susceptibility loci for adult asthma in the Japanese population. Nat Genet 2011.
[98] Torgerson DG, Ampleford EJ, Chiu GY et al. Meta-analysis of genome-wide association studies of asthma in ethnically diverse North American populations. Nat Genet 2011.

11

Rehabilitation and Its Concern

Ganesan Kathiresan[1,2]
[1]La Trobe University,
[2]Masterskill University College,
[1]Australia
[2]Malaysia

1. Introduction

Researchers have investigated a variety of rehabilitative modes of training in an attempt to ascertain the appropriate mode of exercise, dose, and work load, number of repetitions and order and number of exercises in order to bring about favourable improvements in asthmatic symptomology. However, the research regarding the effects of exercise training on asthmatics is sparse and there has continually been a self-inflicted restriction of physical and sporting activities in asthmatics. This is so despite clinicians having advised that exercise can take place when asthmatics use beta-agonists prior to exercise, avoid conditions that are likely to produce exercise- induced asthma and participate in swimming which is deemed less asthmogenic than other forms of exercise (Cochrane & Clark, 1990). Asthmatics can safely and successfully exercise with the correct interventions (Nagel, 2008) as seen when 41 medals were won (albeit controversially due to the stimulant effects of asthma medication) at the 1984 Olympic Games by American athletes with a history of asthma or exercise-induced asthma (EIA) in high-respiratory events such as cycling and swimming (Haas et al., 1987). The number of patients with chronic obstructive pulmonary diseases and asthma are on the rise over the entire world. Education, environmental control and drug therapy are the corner stone's in the management of asthma. Nowadays pulmonary rehabilitation is a recognised discipline for stabilisation and improvement of asthma and chronic obstructive pulmonary diseases. Pulmonary rehabilitation program (PRP) could improve the quality of life, pulmonary functions, exercise tolerance, reduce the symptoms and anxiety of patients and decrease frequency and duration of hospitalisation (Frownfelter, 1987; Cambach, 1999).

The concept of rehabilitation, involving holistic efforts to restore patients with debilitating and disabling disease to an optimally functioning state, is a relatively recent practice in pulmonary medicine. In 1974, a committee of the American College of Chest Physicians defined pulmonary rehabilitation as "an art of medical practice wherein an individually tailored, multidisciplinary program is formulated which through accurate diagnosis, therapy, emotional support and education stabilizes or reverses both physiopathological and psychopathological manifestations of pulmonary diseases and attempts to return the patients to the highest possible functional capacity allowed by his handicap and overall life situation"(Petty,1975). More recent definitions were formulated by the NIH and by a task force of the European Respiratory Society (ERS). According to the NIH, pulmonary rehabilitation has to be defined as a multidimensional continuum of services directed to persons with pulmonary disease and their families, usually by an interdisciplinary team of specialists, with the goal of achieving and maintaining the individual's maximum level of independence and functioning in the community (Fishman, 1994). According to the ERS task force, pulmonary rehabilitation is a process which systematically uses scientifically based diagnostic management and evaluation options, to achieve the optimal daily functioning and health-related quality of life of individual patients suffering from impairment and disability, due to chronic respiratory diseases as measured by clinically and/or physiologically relevant outcome measures (Donner et al., 1997). Although both definitions are primarily applied to patients with COPD, they are clearly also applicable to other patients suffering from chronic respiratory diseases. The new official statement of the ATS on pulmonary rehabilitation, published in 1999, supports this approach by defining pulmonary rehabilitation as a multidisciplinary program of care for patients with chronic respiratory impairment that is individually tailored and designed to optimize physical and social performance and autonomy(American Thoracic Society, 1999).These definitions refer to the philosophical concept of rehabilitation as the restoration of the individual to the fullest medical, mental, emotional, social and vocational potential of which the person is capable. From the beginning it has been clear that the goals of rehabilitation were multifactorial and included the following:

- Decreasing respiratory symptoms and complications
- Encouraging self-management and control over daily functioning
- Improving physical conditioning and exercise performance
- Improving emotional well-being
- Reducing hospitalizations

These goals are nowadays considered as outcome parameters for asthma management in general. Therefore, pulmonary rehabilitation as the application of the whole spectrum of scientifically evaluated non-pharmacological treatment options has to be considered as an integrated part of optimal management of both disease conditions especially for the patients with persistent physiological deficit after optimal pharmacological treatment or persistent impact on psychological functioning or health status. Present insights in determining factors on daily life functioning and health status, related to the systemic effects of the disease process of Bronchial Asthma, strengthen this approach to consider this intervention as part of an integrated management process.

2. Eligibility criterion

Any patient with symptomatic severe asthma, who is disabled either by the underlying disease, or by related therapy or by complications or by the systemic effects of the disease process, should be considered for pulmonary rehabilitation. The ATS statement considers pulmonary rehabilitation indicated for patients with chronic respiratory impairment who despite optimal medical management, are dyspneic, have reduced exercise tolerance, or experience a restriction in activities (American Thoracic Society, 1999). In fact, based on the defined goals of COPD and Asthma management by the ATS as well as by the ERS, pulmonary rehabilitation can no longer be considered as a separate intervention but as part of an integrated medical approach for the disabled COPD and Asthma patient (American Thoracic Society, 1999; Siafakas et al., 1995). Improvement in health status, functional capacity and reduction of symptoms, which are defined treatment goals for COPD and Asthma should not be restricted to these specific conditions, and instead should be considered as outcome parameters for all chronic respiratory diseases including severe asthma.

Furthermore, it is important as part of the selection procedure that the patient is not distracted or limited by other serious or unstable medical conditions, that he/she is willing and able to learn about his disease and is motivated to devote the time and effort necessary to benefit from a comprehensive care program (Ries, 1995). Most of these rehabilitation programs can be completed in an outpatient setting. An ERS task force also defined specific selection criteria for in-hospital treatment (Donner et al., 1997). In-hospital management allows comprehensive diurnal assessment of the individual patient outside the habitual home environment. In-hospital rehabilitation can also be considered for specific intervention strategies or facilitates training of the most disabled patients, e.g. those with supplemental oxygen or patients receiving noninvasive mechanical ventilation. Post-intensive care patients with either disabling respiratory problems or weaning failure after acute respiratory support are also candidates for a comprehensive management program. Selection criteria for inpatient programs according the ERS are summarized in **Table 1**. Asthma is generally considered as one of the non-COPD indications for pulmonary rehabilitation (Donner et al., 1997). A survey of clinical control of asthma in Europe highlighted that a considerable percentage of children, as well as of adults, is markedly limited in daily life, as well as in social activities (Rabe et al., 2000).However, most asthma management programs largely rely on pharmacological intervention by administration of bronchodilating and anti-inflammatory agents in a stepwise manner (WHO,1995). Nonpharmacological intervention strategies are largely overlooked in asthma management plans.

	Selection criteria for inpatient programs according the ERS
1	Need for an integrated 24-hour supervised monitoring management plan, including training, teaching of coping skills, and other aspects of daily life functioning
2	Behavioral intervention to correct psychosocial problems
3	Need for specific intervention strategies, such as nutritional therapy
4	Participation in pre-operative and post-operative rehabilitation programs
5	Post-intensive care patients with either disabling respiratory problems or weaning failure after acute respiratory support
6	Identification and assessment of patients for long term oxygen therapy or long-term home mechanical Ventilation
7	Logistic aspects when outpatient rehabilitation is not available and the traveling distance does not allow the patient to participate in intensive rehabilitation

Table 1. Selection criteria for inpatient programs according the ERS

3. Components of rehabilitation

Based on the historically defined approach of pulmonary rehabilitation, each patient enrolled in a rehabilitation program has to be considered as a unique individual with specific physio and psychopathological impairment caused by the underlying disease. Therefore, pulmonary rehabilitation incorporated many different therapeutic modalities applied as a comprehensive, multidisciplinary care program including pharmacological treatment. Specific components in this Physical Therapy approach of patients with asthma are supported by scientific data supporting the efficacy and effectiveness of the applied intervention procedure. In order to improve quality of life or to promote self-management behavior of chronically ill patients with asthma, it is also important to consider the different dimensions of the rehabilitation program. In general, a distinction has to be made between:

- Aim of the intervention;
- Level on which the intervention is focused;
- Directness of the intervention (Maes, 1993).

For pulmonary rehabilitation (PR) in general, these dimensions are described in **Table 2**.

PR dimensions		
1	**Aim of the intervention**	Reduction and control of respiratory symptoms
		Improvement in physical functioning
		Improvement in quality of life
		Reduction of the number of acute exacerbations
		Promotion of self-management behavior
		Improvement of cognition and behavior
		Reduction of psychological impact of physical impairment and disability
		Improvement of survival
2	**Level of focusing of the intervention**	Individual
		Group
		Environment
3	**Directness of the intervention**	Direct
		Indirect
		Supported by educational material

Table 2. PR dimensions

Based on this approach, interventions directed at improvement, for example quality of life, have to be focused on improvement of general psychological, social, practical and physical well-being of the patient. Dependent upon the aim and the phase the patient is in, the interventions can involve physical exercise programs as well as stress-management programs, social skills training or different kinds of counseling and support. The level of focusing of the intervention has to be decided depending on the aim of the intervention and the expected efficiency. Group-directed programs are preferable and programs have to be directed at the environment of the patient (Van den Broek, 2005). Psychological group interventions directed at patients and partners can increase efficiency in order to get management goals (Wouters, 2007). Furthermore, interventions can be directed at changing or adaptation of the environment of the asthma patient. These interventions are often specified by the term "social engineering", because these interventions are directed at modification of living-, work-, or leisure-time situations and healthy life-styles of the patient from a social or patient perspective (Van den Broek, 1995). Finally, the directness of intervention has to be considered. As part of a comprehensive intervention, indirect interventions can be considered in order to improve social support for the patient or to train other professionals in intervention skills. This theoretical approach of intervention programs is still largely unattainable in most rehabilitation programs, based on the limited resources still now spent on non pharmacological intervention strategies in asthma. In this approach, components of a rehabilitation program are individualized based on a careful assessment of the patient, not limited to lung function testing, but addressing physical and emotional deficits, knowledge of the disease, cognitive and psychosocial functioning, as well as nutritional assessment. Furthermore, this assessment must be an ongoing process during the whole rehabilitation process. Education, exercise training, vocational therapy, physical therapy, psychosocial support and nutritional intervention are now generally applied modalities in pulmonary rehabilitation.

4. Patient education

Patient education is generally used as an "umbrella term for various forms of goal-directed and systematically applied communication processes, directed at the improvement of cognition, understanding and motivation, and the improvement of action- and decision-making possibilities of a patient to improve the coping with and recovery of the disease"(Damoiseaux, 1984). Ideally, patient education is more than provision of information to the patient, but is a "planned learning experience using a combination of methods such as teaching, counseling and behavior modification techniques which influence patient knowledge and health behavior" (Jones et al., 1990). Promotion of self management behavior in asthma can be directed to improve adherence to medical advice with respect to medication and healthy life-style, directed at the stabilization or retardation of the progression of the clinical picture or at the avoidance of undesirable consequences and complications. Medical advice to chronically ill patients can also be directed at various aspects of cognition and behavior. In asthma, studies concerning patient education are directed on improvement of self-management, are restricted to medical outcome measures and are conducted by a wide variety of health care workers not explicitly trained to provide educational intervention (Green et al., 1977). The outcome variables as measured in different studies are generally restricted to number of attacks, emergency room visits, visits to the physician, knowledge, re-hospitalization rate and use of drugs while in most studies no psychosocial outcome variables are included. Therefore, it is very important that an effective educational program in asthma directed at improvement of self-management and quality of life provides information in a structured way and those both psychological as well as medical parameters are included. To involve several dimensions of the multiple problems of the asthmatic patient, a multidisciplinary program is preferred and follow-up sessions seem to be helpful in the prevention of re-hospitalization or relapse. Group-directed programs are preferable and programs have to be directed at the environment of the patient (Van den Broek, 1995).In asthma, most educational programs are conducted by various professionals, the environment of the patient is generally not involved and most of the studies do not pay attention to the problems of partners. Characteristics like depression, anxiety and optimism, wellbeing, the number and length of hospital admissions and use of health services can be influenced positively by patient education programs. Most of these studies have only short term effects. Van den Broek (1995) reported the effects of a patient education group intervention program as part of a pulmonary rehabilitation program. Patients were randomly assigned to an experimental group and a control group. Partners participated in the study. Patients in the control group received medical advice and standard clinical care. The experimental group followed a structured educational program consisting of two components: an informative part and an educational part. The total program was directed at teaching self-management skills. Patients were followed for 12 months after the end of the rehabilitation program. The characteristics of an optimal education program for patients with asthma are described in Table 3 (Van den Broek, 1995).

Characteristics of an optimal education program
• The program should be conducted by experts specially trained in techniques to change behavioral or irrational cognitions
• Information should be provided in a structured way
• A group-program is preferable from a health economical perspective, but a combination of an individualized program and a group-program may be most effective
• Both participation of the social environment and attention to the problems of the partners should have a high priority to maintain newly acquired skills and cognitions in the home-situation
• Both medical and psychosocial parameters have to be emphasized
• The responsibility of the patient for his own health must be emphasized
• In order to promote the patient's self-activity and to support the maintenance of behavioral changes in the home-situation, additional materials should be made available to the patient to be used at home
• Follow-up sessions are necessary to support the patient and his or her partner in the home-situation
• Specific patient education interventions should be implemented in a multidisciplinary program, in addition to standard care to improve physical and psychological functioning
• Short- and long-term effects have to be evaluated by valid measurements.

Table 3. Characteristics of an optimal education program

Stabilization or reversal of disease-related psychopathology was one of the initially defined goals of pulmonary rehabilitation. Personality traits and intrapsychic conflicts, as well as acute pschychological states as panic, anxiety or depression, are widely recognized problem categories in patients with asthma and COPD. Specific psychosocial intervention strategies are usually required in order to modify these problems. Kaptein and Dekker (2000) recently reviewed the nature of psychosocial support in different rehabilitation programs. They concluded that relaxation techniques as a predominantly passive form of intervention were the most frequently applied type of psychosocial support, aimed at more controlled and efficient breathing. The authors concluded that future research is needed to assess the outcome of more specific psychosocial intervention strategies, as well as to delineate the contribution of psychosocial intervention itself over and above pulmonary rehabilitation programs.

5. Motivation

Motivation is the best predictor of the success of rehabilitation (Brannon et al., 1998). Over 70% of patients with Asthma and COPD do not adhere to treatment (Mellins et al.1992), which may be because of inadequate information or depression. Motivation is essential if participants are to practise at home. A twice-a-week programme of structured exercise is not enough by itself to improve exercise tolerance (Ringbaek, 2000). Participants are unlikely to ignore their own beliefs and goals in order to follow a prescriptive approach, and education is not achieved by simply feeding information into an empty vessel and pressing the right buttons. The hierarchical hospital environment may encourage some patients to take up the sick role and assume that the experts know best. This apparent compliance is counterproductive in the rehabilitation process. Motivation is enhanced by participants taking responsibility for their own management (Hough, 1996).

Factors that increase and decrease motivation are:

Increase motivation	Decrease motivation
• Clear advance information in large print • Realistic expectations • Active participation, e.g. self-monitoring, invitations to question, comment, design programmes, contribute ideas • Verbal commitment from participants • Praise, warmth, humour, honesty and responsiveness from the rehabilitation team • Family involvement • Focus on health rather than disease • Short simple regimes (Mellins et al., 1992) • Understanding the rationale of each component • Early success, reinforced by progress charts • Access to notes (McLaren,1991) • Continuity o f personnel • Certificate of completion.	• Fatigue • Fear of failure • Anxiety or depression • Advice that is inconvenient or difficult to follow • Embarrassment • Boredom, e.g. repetitive exercise, 12-minute walking test, waiting for transport. • Lack of recognition of the individual as a whole.

6. Exercise training

Impaired exercise tolerance is a prominent feature especially in patients suffering from Asthma and COPD. Exercise limitation especially in patients with Asthma is the result of complex changes including a wide spectrum of variables:

- Reduced expiratory airflow as a consequence of poor elastic recoil
- Increased airways resistance leading to increased work of breathing and increased ventilatory drive
- Reduced pulmonary vascular bed and increased pulmonary vascular resistance contributing to exercise induced hypoxemia
- Impaired cardiac output by impediment of right heart filling and left ventricular systolic function and skeletal muscle dysfunction.

Leg fatigue attributable to peripheral muscle weakness has now been generally recognized as a common limiting symptom during exercise in Asthma and COPD (Killian et al., 1992). Several factors have been suggested to explain the occurrence of skeletal muscle dysfunction in Asthma and COPD: chronic inactivity and deconditioning, systemic inflammation, systemic corticosteroid administration, hypoxemia, electrolyte disturbances and muscle depletion as a consequence of a chronic process of tissue wasting. Asthma and COPD-related changes in structure and metabolism of the skeletal muscles are furthermore reported:

- Decreased oxidative capacity(Maltais et al.,1996),
- Greater proportion of fatigue-susceptible fibers as a consequence of shifts from type 1 fibers to type 2 fibers (Satta et al.,1997),
- Changes in energy rich phosphagen metabolism (Pouw et al., 1998).

Lower capacity for muscle aerobic metabolism is related to an increased lactic acidosis for a given exercise work rate and enhances ventilator needs by increasing non aerobic carbon dioxide production. This requirement imposes an additional burden on the respiratory muscles already facing increased impedance to breathing. Exercise in Asthma and COPD is also related to an earlyonset of muscle intracellular acidosis (Wuyam et al., 1992). Remarkably, opposite changes in diaphragmatic fiber composition are now reported especially in more severe Asthma and COPD patients towards a higher proportion of fatigue-resistant fibers (Levine et al., 1997). Besides these changes in intrinsic diaphragmatic muscle structure, mechanical disadvantages and altered muscle fiber length mainly as a consequence of static and dynamic hyperinflation, as well as an altered muscle environment contribute to a dysfunction of inspiratory muscles and especially of the diaphragm in Asthma and COPD.A possible imbalance between inspiratory muscle function and increased muscle load related to the increased resistive and elastic load is an important determinant of dyspnea, susceptibility to inspiratory muscle fatigue, drive on the respiratory muscles and hypercapnia (O'Donnell DE & Webb KA, 1993).Towards this complexity in pathophysiological and metabolic changes especially in Asthma patients, the outcome of exercise training as part of a rehabilitation program has to be interpreted.

Indeed, pulmonary rehabilitation programs almost include a measure of exercise training, generally based on transfer of standard recommendations for exercise training from healthy subjects to these disabled pulmonary patients frequently ignoring the complexity of bodily changes related to or a consequence of the disease state. Therefore, exercise testing before a training program is generally advised in order to determine the nature of exercise limitation, e.g. cardio circulatory, ventilatory, diffusion limitation, limitation in the pulmonary circulation, or peripheral muscle limitation. Subsequent exercise training can be prescribed based on the individual limitations of the patient.

Pulmonary rehabilitation could improve the quality of life and pulmonary functions. Cambach et al had reported that quality of life and exercise capacity improved after the rehabilitation program. Field et al also had demonstrated that children with asthma had improved pulmonary function after the daily relaxation and massage therapy. They found best improvement in FEF25-75 values (in common with our findings) which reflects small airway obstruction. These results mean PRP could lead improvement in airway obstruction and control of asthma. In another study carried out by Cox et al it was shown that pulmonary rehabilitation had beneficial effects on endurance, psychological variables, quality of life, skills, coordination, smoking habits, airway obstruction and dyspnea . However bronchial hyperresponsiveness, need of pulmonary drugs and complaint of cough did not change. They followed patients for two years and long term effects of PRP were evaluated. Kathiresan G et al shown that there is a beneficial effect on quality of life (Table 4) and pulmonary functions (Table 5) pulmonary rehabilitation should be placed as a component of management in childhood asthma.

	First visit	Second visit	p
Rehabilitation group			
Symptom score	0.63 ± 0.71	0.19 ± 0.40	0.01
	(median: 0.5)	(median: 0)	
Medication score	4.40 ± 1.70	3.50 ± 0.80	0.007
Quality of life Index	6.02 ± 0.5	6.40 ± 0.40	0.009
Control Group			
Symptom score	0.67 ± 0.57	0.49 ± 1.40	0.16
		(median: 0)	
Medication score	4.09 ± 0.79	4.06 ± 0.93	0.32
Quality of life Index	6.15 ± 0.29	6.27 ± 0.49	0.16

Table 4. Symptom and medication score and quality of life index of rehabilitation group and control group

	First visit	Second visit	p
Rehabilitation group			
VC	76.62 ± 8.64	83.12 ± 12.38	0.05
FVC	78.00 ± 8.83	84.75 ± 10.76	0.02
FEV_1	74.23 ± 11.67	80.62 ± 12.27	0.009
PEF	65.62 ± 8.50	73.43 ± 7.32	0.001
FEF_{25-75}	75.73 ± 11.12	85.31 ± 14.45	0.006
Control group			
VC	78.66 ± 10.39	80.25 ± 6.25	0.75
FVC	79.67 ± 8.64	81.41 ± 7.07	0.36
FEV_1	73.75 ± 7.12	75.91 ± 5.43	0.15
PEF	6.33 ± 7.22	68.91 ± 9.16	0.21
FEF_{25-75}	74.54 ± 11.96	76.66 ± 10.37	0.37

Table 5. Pulmonary functions (% predicted values for age and height) of rehabilitation group and control group

7. Exercise prescription

In general, exercise training can be divided into two types: aerobic or endurance training and strength training. The majority of the studies of exercise training in Asthma and COPD have focused on endurance training. However, no clear recommendations for Asthma and COPD are yet available. However, in normal subjects, clear recommendations are available about duration, intensity and frequency for aerobic training (Casaburi, 1993). According to these recommendations, aerobic training calls for rhythmical, dynamic activity of large muscles, performed three to four times a week for 20–30 min per session at an intensity of at least 50% of maximal oxygen consumption. Such a program of aerobic training is capable of inducing structural and physiological adaptations that provide the trained individual with improved endurance for performance of high-intensity activity. Most of the rehabilitation programs include exercise sessions of at least 30 min, three to five times a week. Although no ideal duration has been established, duration in many programs is around 8 weeks. Limited information is also available regarding physiological outcome of different types of exercise testing. Continuous training especially seems to be related to physiological improvement while interval training (Coppoolse et al., 1999).

	Mode	Intensity	Protocol	Duration	Frequency
Lower limb **1) endurance training Ground walking Treadmill walking Stationary Cycle or a combination of the above with a total duration of 30 minutes**	Walking training Ground-based	80% average speed on 6MWT 75% peak speed on ISWT Dyspnoea rating of 3 (moderate)	Continuous or interval	30 minutes	4 or 5 times a week that includes 2 or 3 supervised sessions and home exercise training
	Walking training Treadmill	As for ground-based walking training but reduce speed by 0.5 to 1 kph until familiar with treadmill	Continuous or interval	30 minutes	4 or 5 days a week that includes 2 or 3 supervised sessions and home exercise training
	Stationary cycle training (if possible)	Dyspnoea rating of 3 (moderate)	Continuous or interval	30 minutes	4 or 5 days a week that includes 2 or 3 supervised sessions and home exercise training
2) strength training	Strength training with weights (Leg press, Quadriceps extension). Strength training without weights(Squats, Straight leg raise, Step-ups or stair climbing, Sit-to-stand from progressively lower chairs)	10 RM (repetition maximum)		10 repetitions (1 set)	2 or 3 times a week with at least 1 day rest between sessions
Upper limb **1) endurance training**	supported arm training and Unsupported arm Training	Determine the weight that the patient can only lift 15 times Dyspnoea rating of 2 or 3 (slight or moderate)		15 repetitions (1 set)	4 or 5 times a week that includes 2 or 3 supervised sessions and home exercise training
2) strength training	Strength training for the upper limbs should focused on the accessory muscles of inspiration and muscle groups used in everyday functional tasks	10 RM (repetition maximum)		10 repetitions (1 set)	2 or 3 times a week with at least 1 day rest between sessions

Table 6. Individual exercise prescription

In healthy subjects training is normally targeted by means of percentage of maximal heart rate (60–90% of predicted) or the percentage of maximal oxygen uptake (50–80% predicted) achieved (American College of Sports Medicine (ACSM), 1990). However, principles of exercise training intensity derived from normals are often not applicable to pulmonary patients who are limited by breathing capacity and dyspnea. Indeed, Casaburi et al. compared high work rate training versus low work rate training and concluded that physiologic training effects were much less marked in patients who trained at low work rate, even though the total amount of work involved in the training regimen was the same irrespective of the training group to which the patient was assigned.

An exercise training program requires an individual prescription (Table 6) in terms of:

- Intensity.
- Duration.
- Frequency.
- Type (interval or continuous).
- Mode (e.g. walking, cycling, arm exercise).
- Progression.

8. Callisthenic training

Perez et al. (2003) found that callisthenics before exercise training resulted in maximal expiratory flow rate diminishment. This diminishment is significant in that it can act as a preventative method in the development of exercise induced asthma and as such allows the asthmatic to optimally benefit from training. Similarly, Fitch et al. (1986) and Bungaard et al. (1982) used callisthenics as part of their exercise prescription and found improvements in asthma symptomology.

9. Postural retraining

Postural exercises have been recommended since the posture of an asthmatic is typically pronounced by thoracic kyphosis and the flattening of the sacrolumbar portion. These postural misalignments can lead to a decrease respiratory capacity and can severely affect visceral functioning. However, these postural abnormalities have been found to be improved following postural retraining that includes postural, breathing and abdominal strengthening exercises (Goyeche et al., 1980). Possible reasons why postural retraining is implicated is since an asthmatic's posture is affected by changes in the contractile (i.e. muscles) and non-contractile units (i.e. bone, ligaments, tendons, cartilage and connective tissue), and since asthmatics' have a decreased general mobility which can lead to degenerative changes and as such possibly altering afferent impulses and decreasing the lung's reflexogenic efficiency. Futher, since asthmatics have a loss of midcervical lordosis more weight and tension is exerted at the cervical-thoracic junction which can lead to an increase in thoracic kyphosis that abducts the scapulae which shortens the pectoralis major and pectoralis minor, lengthens the rhomboids and lowers the trapezius I and II and shortens the serratus anterior, latissimus dorsi, subscapularis and teres major, all of which affect normal breathing (Ayub, 1987). Strunk et al. (1991) also pointed out that postural retraining can correct thoracic kyphosis and improve breathing in asthmatics especially in severe asthmatics that are more likely to suffer from such postural abnormalities when the pectoral and intercostal muscles are stretched. Ayub (1987) stated that postural retraining in asthmatics should focus on the facilitation of correcting righting, equilibrium and protective reactions with normal tactile, proprioceptive and kinesthetic input.

10. Breathing training

Diaphragmatic breathing exercises could benefit an asthmatic's condition since they compress the abdominal contents which increase intra-abdominal pressure that causes lateral transmission of pressure to the lower ribs laterally, upward and outward motion of the lower ribs and anterior/posterior motion of the upper ribs. This then results in an increase in thoracic volume that decreases intrathoracic pressure which facilitates inspiration (Cahalin et al., 2002). Breathing retraining is essential to an asthmatic since, breathing in an asthmatic is of the thoracic type and since dyspnea can cause the asthmatic to increase inspiration further leading to further overextension of the already over-inflated lungs. This is then worsened by the increased dead-space ventilation, metabolic requirements and a tendency to maintain a low arterial partial pressure of oxygen.

Asthmatics can have a decreased chest expansion and chest deformity as a result of a shortened diaphragm, intercostals and accessory muscles from prolonged spasm. With asthma, the accessory respiratory muscles are fully contracted and the diaphragm is maximally depressed. The accessory muscles are overactive during inspiration which causes stenosis of the major airways leading to an abnormal respiratory pattern. During an asthma attack, the diaphragm is maximally extended and either contracts spasmodically or not at all. This poor excursion of the diaphragm can negatively affect airway reserve, vital capacity (VC) and alveolar gas exchange (Goyeche et al., 1980).

The physiological effects of diaphragmatic breathing are varied and it is claimed that diaphragmatic breathing can correct abdominal chest wall motion, decrease the work of breathing and dyspnea and improve ventilation distribution (Vitacca et al., 1998). The purpose of breathing exercises is to empty the lungs by prolonging the expiratory phase, retrain normal breathing patterns, increase expansile forces in hypoventilated areas, increase lung volume, dilate airways, force mucus into larger airways, re-educate the autonomic diaphragmatic movements, reduce the thoracic type breathing, relax spasmodic muscle contractions, mobilise the ribs and chest wall and correct kyphosis (Goyeche et al., 1980). These benefits are achieved by shortening inspiration and lengthening expiration (Bouchard et al., 1993), by performing expiration via the pulling in of the abdominal muscles dorsally towards the spine while relaxing the abdominal, intercostals and neck musculature (Cahalin et al., 2002). This is achieved by using special weights or belts to increase intra-abdominal pressure, by applying compression to the lower ribs to facilitate expiratory ascent of the diaphragm during expiration which can increase the movement of secretions from the small bronchi into the respiratory passages, by exhaling through a resistive breathing device or by breathing while creating a hissing noise in order to reduce bronchial constriction. These techniques have led to symptom-free and medication-free asthma, an improved ability to halt an imminent attack, improved loosening and expulsion of mucus, enlargement of the diaphragm excursion, improved chest expansion at the epigastrium, improved aximum breathing capacity and VC (Cahalin et al., 2002). Patients with elevated respiratory rates, low tidal volumes and abnormal arterial blood gases have been identified as those who will benefit the most from diaphragmatic breathing exercises (Cahalin et al., 2002).

Diaphragmatic breathing exercises have also been proven to reduce patients' anxiety levels and to alter their attitude towards work (Lustig et al., 1972) while breathing retraining has been shown to decrease bronchodilator use and acute exacerbations and to improve quality of life(Holloway & Ram, 2004). Ambrosino et al (1981) in turn, have found that deep diaphragmatic breathing and pursed lip breathing can increase a lung patient's maximal exercise tolerance. Diaphragmatic breathing can also lead to an increase in alveolar ventilation due to the changes in breathing pattern via decreases in breathing frequency and increases in tidal volume resulting in increases minute ventilation (Vitacca et al., 1998). Additional benefits of breathing exercises are to correct deviant posture, strengthen abdominal muscles, teach diaphragmatic and lower costal breathing and increase chest expansion (Lustig et al., 1972). Fluge et al. (2004) demonstrated that breathing exercises have been found to increase FEV1, VC and to reduce RV significantly while Strunk et al. (1991) also indicated that breathing exercises can decrease the work of breathing, improve ventilation, decrease oxygen consumption and decrease psychological anxiety.

Yoga is a preferred method of training in older adults and the active or fitness-based yoga that emphasises cardiovascular fitness, resistance training, flexibility and relaxation is an effective treatment for asthmatics (Tummers & Hendrick, 2004). Nagarathna and Nagendra (1985) pointed out that yoga techniques can benefit asthmatics by reducing psychological over activity and emotional instability and thereby reducing efferent vagal discharge while decreasing vagal outflow to the lung which can cause bronchodilation and a small decrease in bronchial reactivity. Yoga can also increase endogenous corticosteroid release, possibly decreasing bronchial reactivity (Udupa & Singh, 1972). Breathing exercises have been found to decrease anxiety during an asthma attack and also prevent the onset of an attack (Sly et al., 1972). Breathing exercises have resulted in clinical improvements which translated into improved school attendance, exercise tolerance, asthma control and self-confidence. Improvements have also been observed in breathing capacity, VC, but not FEV1 (Millman et al., 1965). However, Sly et al. (1972), found that a combination of physical conditioning and breathing exercises can improve VC, reduce the severity of asthma attacks and the need for symptomatic medication, but no change in psychological adjustment and subjectively was there a change in independence, outgoingness, getting along with others, feelings of acceptance, enthusiasm and capability to be a follower (McElhenny & Peterson, 1963). Up to eight month of breathing exercises have resulted in improved pulmonary function, decreased absenteeism and improved sociability, self-assertion and peer relationships. Subjectively, the subjects reported an improvement in their control of asthma, exercise tolerance and emotional stability (McElhenny & Peterson, 1963). Girodo et al. (1992) also found reductions in medication usage and in the intensity of asthmatic symptoms of 32 asthmatic patients utilising breathing training making use of a physical corset. One of the problems with prescribing breathing exercises is that although eagerly accepted by asthma patients, they are just as easily found boring and soon forgotten (Strunk et al.,

1991). Therefore, the structure and setting of the exercises are important since it has been established that breathing exercises have resulted in thousands of asthma suffers reducing their medication intake and experiencing a sense of control even though this breathing technique does not alter the disease process (Cooper et al., 2003). This is notable in that improvements in subjective attributes and perceptions in asthmatic patients may have major effects on their quality of life and the ability to cope with their disease.

11. Inspiratory resistive breathing training

The purpose of inspiratory resistive breathing training is to enhance respiratory muscle function and in doing so possibly reduce the severity of breathlessness and improve exercise tolerance. This may benefit the asthmatic patients, especially those with severe asthma, since asthmatics could suffer from respiratory muscle dysfunction due to the loss in respiratory muscle bulk and resultant respiratory muscle strength. The use of inspiratory resistive breathing training in asthmatic patients could possibly result in improvements in inspiratory muscle coordination, improvements in inspiratory muscle strength and endurance and the correction of inappropriate respiratory muscle effort (Kim et al., 1993). These improvements and corrections then possibly result in improvements in spirometry variables, a desensitisation to dyspnea, lessening of asthma symptoms, reduced hospitalisations, less emergency room contacts, absences from school and work and/or the decreased use of medication (Ram et al., 2004). According to Ram et al. (2004), despite the possible benefits of inspiratory resistive breathing training, this mode of exercise's current use in asthmatics is presently insufficient and its clinical benefits not yet justified.

12. Aerobic training programme

Kathiresan et al. (2010) evaluated the effect of a supervised aerobic training programme on the cardio respiratory fitness and clinical indicators of control in a group of children with moderate to severe but stable asthma. The degree of response to training and the positive effect on the clinical management were strongly influenced by the level of fitness in the initial evaluation; beneficial effects were shown only in the less fit patients. The results suggest that exercise therapy for the most untrained children can have a role, at least in the short term, in reducing the minimal medication needed for control of moderate to severe asthma. Previous studies in normal and asthmatic patients have shown that the initial grade of fitness and motivation is an important predictor of aerobic improvement after training (Brodal et al., 1977). Cochrane and Clark,(1990) for example, found that the relative gain in $\tilde{V}O2max$ after training in asthmatic subjects was negatively related to symptom score on the training day and the baseline level of fitness, and positively to motivation . Thus, the improvement after training in muscular capillarisation, oxidative capacity, muscular strength, and cardio circulatory adjustments is likely to occur in motivated subjects with worse baseline aerobic conditions. However, it should be recognised that the so called "regression to the mean" effect cannot be ruled out by this finding; the random longitudinal variation tends to increase the lower values of a given distribution or, alternatively, the higher values tend to randomly decrease with time. Children's with moderate to severe asthma showed significant degree of improvement after aerobic fitness training **(Figure 1)**. Nevertheless, as previously noted, this higher potential for improvement in the most unfit individuals is a well known phenomenon and it seems highly improbable that such a statistical artifact would be consistently related to another measurable biological effect such as the reduction in inhaled steroids (**Figures 2** and **3**). In this context, there is now growing evidence to show that the systemic effects of inhaled beclomethasone in children are dose dependent (Hanania et al., 1995; Yiallourds et al., 1997) and medication usage seems to be a particularly useful index of overall asthma control. Although the respiratory system is usually considered to be largely insensitive to training effects per se (with the possible exception of muscle ventilator strength and endurance), a cause-effect relationship could explain this association. Thus, one can speculate that a possibly lower occurrence of EIB after training would induce a lower chronic release of inflammatory mediators and therefore reduce the need for inhaled steroids. However, we did not find a significant reduction in the prevalence of a positive EIB test with training, regardless of whether or not there was a positive response (**Figure 2**). Another more plausible hypothesis is that the improvement was related to a higher degree of acceptance and level of self-care in the least fit patients who usually have negative attitudes toward their disease and exertion (Strunk et al., 1989). Thus, Strunk et al. (1989) showed that the wide variability in aerobic performance in a group of 90 children with moderate and severe asthma was mainly related to the degree of social and disease adjustment Engström et al. (1991) in a group of 10 severely asthmatic children submitted to physical training showed that only psychological modifications correlated significantly with aerobic improvement. Thus, individual variations in acceptance and knowledge of the disease seem to influence the usual level of physical activity in asthmatic children, and therefore their degree of fitness. In this context, exercise training may induce a more decided posture in relation to the disease, with consequences in the minimum medication required for clinical control. Results are consistent with those of Thio et al. (1996) who were not able to find a lower prevalence of EIB after dynamic exercise training, although in a previous cross sectional study we found an association between a reduction in $\tilde{V}O2AT$ and a higher prevalence of EIB in asthmatic children (Nery et al., 1994). While one can predict a reduction in EIB with aerobic improvement (secondary to training induced lower submaximal ventilation) (Bungaard et al., 1981), in our study this enhancement alone was probably not sufficient to reduce the EIB, at least when assessed in a formal challenge test. A particularly notable finding was the relative inefficacy of the training programme in improving the maximal aerobic parameters in almost 60% of the children. However, one should recognise that maximal incremental testing is not representative of the daily pattern of exercise activities in the paediatric group (which is better characterised by short bursts of activity); new submaximal protocols have been suggested to be more suitable for evaluating training responses in children (Cooper, 1995). In addition, the degree of fitness in the initial evaluation was above that expected for asthmatic children and the low pre-intervention prevalence of unfit children could have induced a type II error. This finding is consistent, however, with the suggestion that secular trends do not reduce the average aerobic fitness of westernized children (Santuz et al., 1997). Kathiresan et al. (2010) shown that the less fit asthmatic children were able to normalize their aerobic fitness with a supervised training programme without clinical complications. Their ability to improve aerobic capacity was not related to clinical and spirometric severity before training. Interestingly, we found a significant association between aerobic improvement and reduction in use of both inhaled and oral steroids.

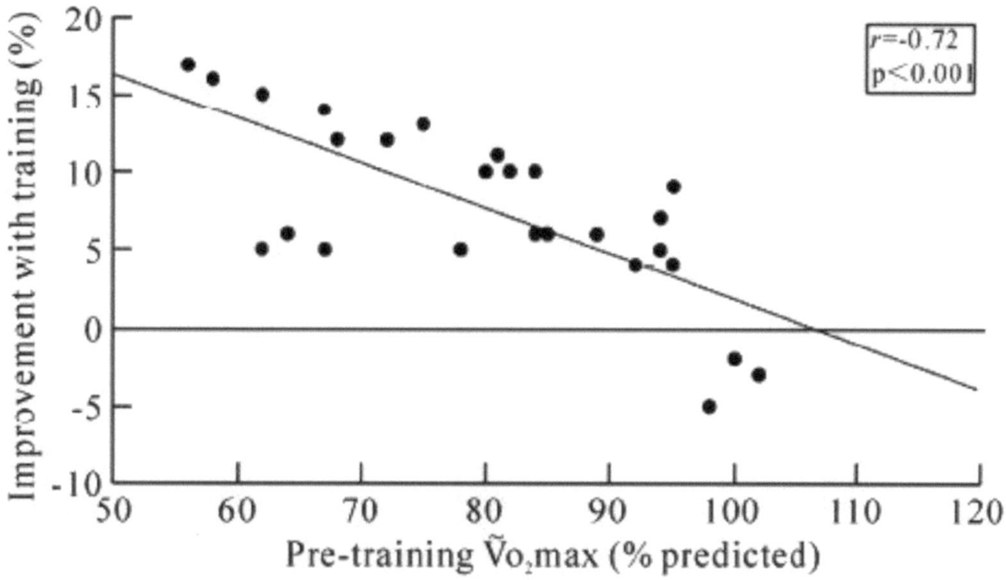

Fig. 1. Relationship between baseline maximal aerobic fitness and degree of improvement after training in 26 children with moderate to severe asthma.

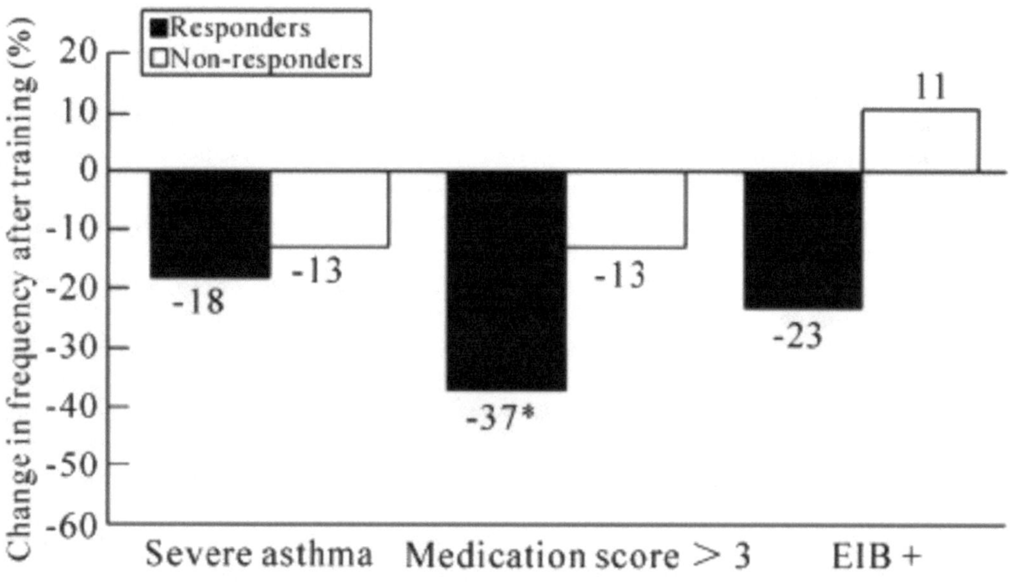

Fig. 2. Association between changes in clinical indicators of asthma severity and positive (responders) or negative (nonresponders) response to aerobic training. *p < 0.05 (Fisher's exact test).

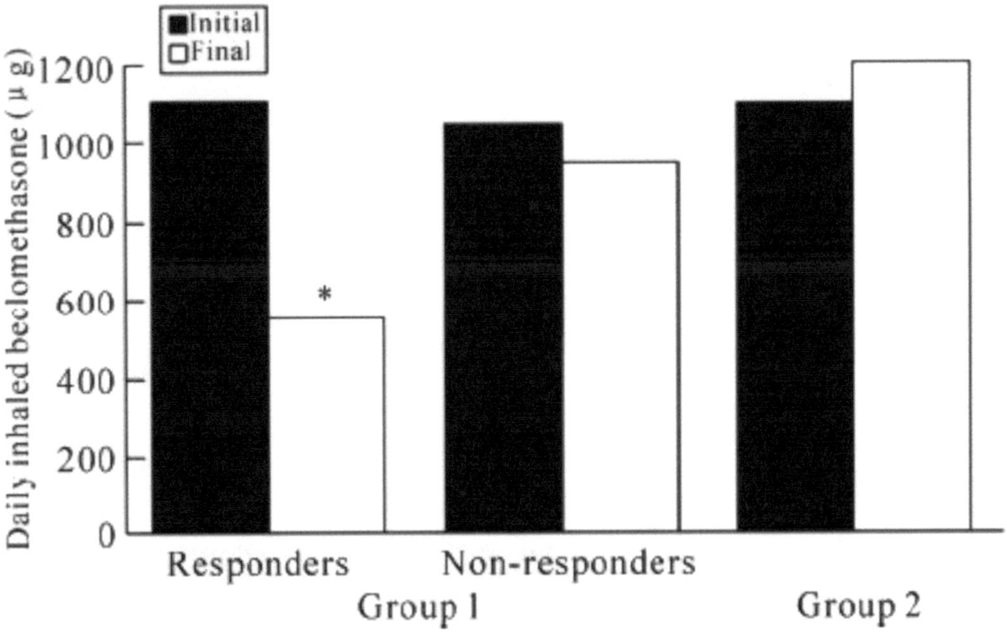

Fig. 3. Mean values of daily inhaled beclomethasone in the initial and final evaluations. Group 1 = trained children with (responders) and without (non-responders) aerobic improvement after training; group 2 = untrained children.*p < 0.05 (paired t test).

13. Anaerobic or lactate threshold training

The anaerobic component of physical conditioning may be important in the overall physiologic profile of the individual with asthma (Council et al., 2003). Council et al. (2003) propose that asthmatics should participate in brief, intense bouts of muscle work alternating with rest periods since this mode of training is less likely to induce EIA and reduces the risk of asthma exacerbations while allowing the asthmatic patient to train optimally for longer periods. The importance of improving lactic acid metabolism and tolerance in EIA patients and exercising at or above lactate threshold is of critical importance since, this intensity is not only less likely to induce EIA, it is sufficient to increase aerobic capacity while minimising the amount of water loss from hyperventilation during exercise thus suppressing the onset of EIA. A benefit of lactate threshold training is that this training can increase the anaerobic threshold, reduce the onset of EIA and reduce hyperpnoea which often occurs when lactate threshold is passed (Matsumoto et al., 1999). Council et al. (2003) found that a work: rest ratio of 1: 4 for a total of 45 minutes at lactate threshold can significantly improve VO2max, decrease ventilatory reserve and increase exercise VE in asthmatics. Neder et al. (1999) also found that 30 minutes of exercise at lactate threshold significantly improved pulmonary function, decreased EIA symptoms and reduced medication intake. In light of the above, the present author supports the view of (Council et al., 2003) who indicated that the training effect of a combination of aerobic and lactate threshold training is unfounded in asthmatics and should be used with caution until further research has been conducted. This is so since few studies have been completed to determine the effect of lactate threshold training programme on the pulmonary and gas exchange parameters of asthmatics. Also, this mode of exercise training may prove dangerous in the untrained and elderly and in an unsupervised environment due to the intensity and effort required. It is essential that further research be undertaken to determine the effectiveness of lactate threshold training on asthmatics especially those with EIA since as stated previously, exercising at or above lactate threshold is less likely to induce EIA but is sufficient to increase aerobic capacity and minimise the amount of water loss from hyperventilation during exercise.

14. Aerobic and combined anaerobic or lactate threshold training

When aerobic and resistance training is combined in the form of circuit training, the effects on the majority of asthma severity measures seem unaffected (Robinson et al., 1992). Also circuit training resulted in no improvements in bronchial responsiveness to histamine, medication usage and symptom scores which included wheezing, coughing, breathlessness, medication use and peak expiratory flow (PEF) (Robinson et al., 1992). However, this exercise training programme did result in significant increases in VO2peak and reduced VE at high workloads. Robinson et al. [49] also found that this mode of training had other benefits on asthmatics other than those on disease severity. These included an increase in self-confidence in undertaking physical activity and an increase in daily physical activity. Additionally, Fitch et al. (1986) found no significant relationship between anaerobic circuit training and PEF, VO2max, VE and VT. However, when aerobic training was combined with anaerobic training, Council et al. (2003) found an increased usage of ventilatory reserves, increased anaerobic threshold and an increased VO2max. Since few studies have been completed on the various forms of combination training, this type of exercise treatment should be used with caution until further research has been conducted.

15. Peripheral muscle training

Patients with Asthma and COPD frequently report disabling dyspnea for daily activities involving the upper extremities such as combing hair, brushing teeth or shaving. It is known that even in healthy persons, arm exercise is relatively more demanding than leg exercise. Some studies have demonstrated that arm elevation is related to a disproportionate increase in the diaphragmatic contribution to the generation of ventilatory pressures (Couser et al., 1992) and that arm elevation is a fatiguing task for the muscles involved as assessed by electromyographic data Therefore, exercise training of the upper extremities may be beneficial for these patients also from the point of view that exercise training is specific to the muscles and tasks involved in the training. However, relatively few data exist assessing outcomes of upper extremity (UE) training compared with those available for lower extremity training. Studies have demonstrated that UE training leads to improved arm muscle endurance during isotonic arm ergometry (Ries et al., 1988) and that arm training conducted during a pulmonary rehabilitation program led to a reduced metabolic demand associated with arm exercise (Couser et al., 1992). Based on present findings, it can be concluded that strength and endurance training of the UE improves arm function and that these exercises are safe and should be included in rehabilitation programs for patients with pulmonary diseases. Further studies are needed to explore the effects of arm training on functional outcomes, to evaluate different forms of arm exercise training programs and to determine the effect of arm exercise training on respiratory muscle function.

Randomized, controlled trials have at present demonstrated that lower extremity training of several types and undertaken in several settings is a critical component of a pulmonary rehabilitation program. Pulmonary rehabilitation consisted of 12 4-hour sessions which included education, physical and respiratory care instruction, and psychosocial support and supervised exercise training, followed by monthly reinforcement sessions for 1 year. The education group received 2- hour sessions which included videotapes, lectures and discussions. This comprehensive rehabilitation program produced a significantly greater increase in maximal exercise tolerance, maximal oxygen uptake, exercise endurance, self efficacy of walking and these effects were associated with a marked reduction of the symptoms of perceived breathlessness, muscle fatigue and shortness of breath. These positive effects of rehabilitation on dyspnea were confirmed by the results of O'Donnell et al. (1993) who demonstrated that after rehabilitation there was a significant shift of the relationship between dyspnea and workload downwards, indicating that at any given workload, dyspnea was less. Similar results were reported by Goldstein et al. (1994) They performed a prospective randomized controlled trial of respiratory rehabilitation in 89 subjects.

Exercise activities included interval training, treadmill, upper-extremity training and leisure walking as part of an 8-week inpatient rehabilitation program. Significant improvements in exercise tolerance, measured by submaximal cycle time and walking distance were demonstrated and sustained for 6 months in the rehabilitation group. There were also significant differences in questionnaire assessment of dyspnea and dyspnea index. These and other results provide convincing evidence that lower extremity training is beneficial in patients with chronic airflow limitation and exercise limitation. Lower extremity training can be recommended on evidence-based scientific criteria to be included in the rehabilitation of patients with asthma and COPD.

16. Health-related quality of life (HRQoL)

Pulmonary rehabilitation plays a key role in the management of Asthma and COPD. Although the American Thoracic Society recently provided a grade of 1A for evidence of health-related quality of life (HRQoL) benefits related to pulmonary rehabilitation, knowledge about the psychological and behavioral processes explaining the impact of pulmonary rehabilitation on HRQoL in Asthma and COPD patients remains limited.

HRQoL outcomes related to pulmonary rehabilitation explores five themes:

- Optimizing pulmonary rehabilitation components to improve HRQoL;
- Characterization of a responder phenotype;
- Suitability of pulmonary rehabilitation following acute exacerbations;
- Exploration of psychological and behavioral mechanisms explaining pulmonary rehabilitation benefits;
- Long-term maintenance of HRQoL benefits after pulmonary rehabilitation.

Evidence supports the use of pulmonary rehabilitation to improve HRQoL in patients with Asthma and COPD. However, it is unclear how pulmonary rehabilitation improves HRQoL and which characteristics confer the greatest HRQoL benefits. Moreover, most studies failed to provide a compelling theoretical rationale for the intervention employed. Some studies have analyzed the long-term outcome of rehabilitation on quality of life. Ketelaars et al. (1997) evaluated the long-term effect of rehabilitation on HRQL. She reported that patients with moderate HRQL scores upon admission had the greatest decline after 9 months of followup, despite having made substantial gains in HRQL by the end of the initial rehabilitation program. Otherwise, patients with poorer baseline HRQL scores showed very little improvement during the rehabilitation program and remained severely impaired in HRQL long term. These authors suggested that differentiated aftercare programs may be indicated in order to maintain initial gains in HRQL. Wijkstra et al. (1996) reported that rehabilitation at home for 3 months followed by once-monthly physiotherapy sessions improves HRQL. Future research should focus on improving the understanding of the psychological mechanisms implicated in the adoption and maintenance of healthy behavior.

17. Case study

History/Chart note

A 20-year-old female was transported on a stretcher to the medical and physiotherapy facility at a national track meet. Her teammates report that she collapsed at the end of the 4 x 800 M. They stated that she does this all the time and has done so after other 800-M heats and practices. She becomes grey and extremely short of breath and usually is not able to speak during the first 5 minutes after the race. It usually takes approximately 25 minutes before she recovers. To their knowledge, she has never received medication or treatment for this but it has been described as "panic attacks." You are the only physiotherapist in the facility. The physician has gone across the track to deal with another injury. The woman is still very out of breath but her teammates state that she is doing better.

Questions

1. What assessment parameters should you monitor?
2. What factors would be indicative of worsening or improvement of her respiratory and cardiovascular status? Her PEFR is 3.81 L/sec. The age predicted PEFR for a person the same age and height is 8.87 L/sec. Do you think this person is having a panic attack?

Auscultation

What are the breath sounds and adventitious sounds that you would expect to hear on auscultation?

Chest X-ray

After a similar event, she went to Emergency Room and had a chest x-ray (Figure 8). Identify the characteristic features of this x-ray. What do you think it will look like when the patient is feeling well and her pulmonary function is near normal?

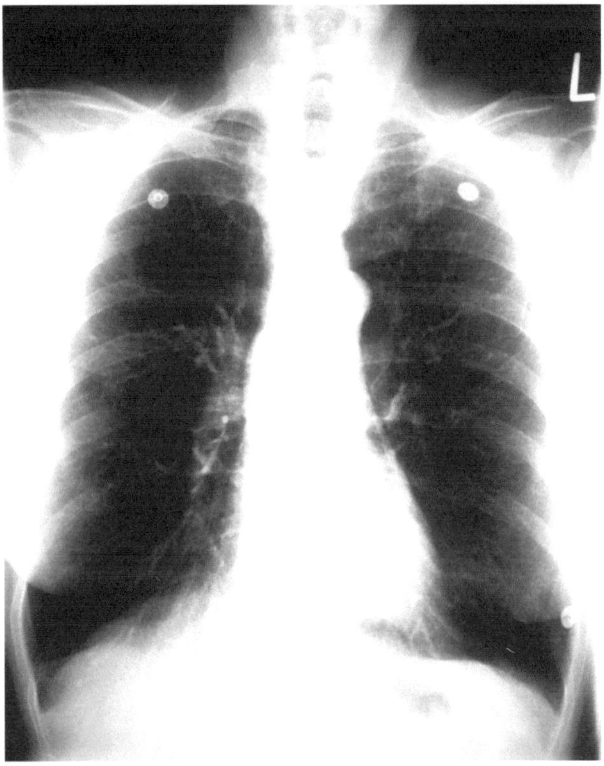

Arterial blood gases

Her arterial blood gases at the Emergency Room were

pH: 7.25 PaCO2: 59 HCO3:- 26 PaO2 : 60

What is the primary acid-base disturbance? Is compensation present? Is the patient hypoxemic? If so, is the hypoxemia due to hypoventilation or other causes?

Spirometry and expiratory flow rates

Her spirometry and PEFR before and after the use of bronchodilators are shown in Table 7. Her height is 180 cm. Interpret the spirometric values. What pattern of lung pathology is shown? Complete the table and calculate the % predicted values and the % improvement after bronchodilator administration.

	Pre BD	Pred	% Predicted	Post BD	% Improvement
FEV1	1.8	3.8L		3.0	
FVC	3.2	4.7		4.2	
FEV1/FVC	56%	80%		71%	
PEFR	3.81	8.87			

Table 7. Spirometry and Peak Expiratory Flow Rates

Physical therapy management

What health professionals would you advise this woman to see?

17.1 Answer guide

History/Chart NOTES

1. What assessment parameters would you monitor?
   - Vitals: HR, RR, BP, SpO2 if oximeter available but this device is not usually available in this situation
   - Cyanosis
   - Dyspnea; difficulty with speaking because of shortness of breath; indrawing (supra clavicular, intercostal, diaphragmatic)
   - Posture
   - Is the patient barrel chested?
   - Accessory muscle use
   - Abnormal auscultatory findings
   - PEFR but unlikely to have peak flow meter
2. What factors would be indicative of worsening or improvement of her respiratory and cardiovascular status?
   - Worsening of condition would include vitals moving further away from normal range, increased cyanosis, increased dyspnea, increased indrawing, worsening of auscultatory findings
   - Improvement would include vitals moving toward the normal range, and the patient attaining some level of composure, decreased dyspnea, and improved auscultatory findings

Auscultation

In a patient with acute asthma, one would expect to hear:

- Most commonly, high- or medium-pitched wheezes in both inspiratory and expiratory phases. The wheezes may also be polyphonic.

Chest X-ray

- Chest x-ray findings consistent with acute asthma are:
- Large lung fields
- Horizontal ribs
- Elongated mediastinum and small cardiothoracic index
- Flattening of hemidiaphragms

Other features of interest are:

- EKG electrodes
- Breast shadows bilaterally

Often, the chest x-ray of people with asthma can appear normal when they are not having an acute exacerbation.

Arterial blood gases

pH :7.25 PaCO2 :59 HCO3:– 25 PaO2 : 60

PaCO2 and pH indicate a respiratory acidosis.

The PaCO2 has increased 19 and no large change in HCO3– has occurred. The HCO3– may have increased 2 mEq/L if the patient's HCO3– was usually 23 mEq/L. Regardless,the HCO3– is well within the normal range and is consistent with an acute respiratory acidosis.

The PaCO2 has an increased 19 for a decrease in PaO2 of 20 to 40 mmHg consistent with hypoventilation and other causes contributing to hypoxemia.

Spirometry and peak expiratory flow rates

Interpret the spirometric values.

This person's FEV1, FVC, and the PEFR are reduced compared to the predicated values provided for a sample of healthy people of similar age, gender, and height. A more precise estimate of how abnormal these results are can be determined by calculating the percent-predicted values (see below).

What pattern of lung pathology is shown?

The pattern is consistent with an obstructive pattern because both the FEV1 and FVC are reduced.

Complete the table and calculate the % Predicted values and the % improvement after bronchodilator administration.

The % predicted values are calculated from: patient's result ÷ predicted value X 100 = % predicted

There is a significant bronchodilator response as shown by large improvement in the FEV1. The percent change post bronchodilator for the FEV1 can be calculated from:

$$= (\text{Post} - \text{Pre}) \div \text{Pre X100}$$
$$= (3.0 - 1.8) \div 1.8 \text{ X100} = 67\% \text{ change}$$

A change in the FEV1 after a bronchodilator of 14% to 15% or more is considered to be clinically significant.

Calculated values for spirometry and peak expiratory flow rate:

	Pre BD(L)	Pred	% Predicted	Post BD(L)	% Improvement
FEV1	1.8	3.8L	47	3.0	67
FVC	3.2	4.7	68	4.2	
FEV1/FVC	56%	80%	70	71%	
PEFR	3.81	8.87	43		

Abbreviations: Pre BD: before bronchodilator; Pred: predicted; Post BD: after bronchodilator.

Physical therapy management

What health professionals would you advise this woman to see?

The women should see a physician so that her asthma can be specifically diagnosed and managed optimally from a medical perspective. This could be a general practitioner, pulmonologist, and/or sports medicine physician. The patient may need specific advice on the medications that she is able to take to manage her asthma while she is competing. Some prescription drugs register positively when the athletes are drug tested.

18. References

Ambrosino, N., Paggiaro, PL., Macchi, M. (1981). A study of short-term effect of rehabilitative therapy in chronic obstructive pulmonary disease. *Respiration*, 41, 1, 40-44

American College of Sports Medicine. (1990). The recommended quantity and quality of exercise for developing and maintaining cardio respiratory and muscular fitness in healthy adults. *Med. Sci. Sports Exerc.*, 23,265–74

American Thoracic Society. (1981). Pulmonary rehabilitation: official American Thoracic Society Position Statement. *Am. Rev. Respir. Dis.*, 124, 663.

ATS statement. (1995). Standards for the diagnosis and care of patients with chronic obstructive pulmonary disease. *Am. J. Respir. Crit.Care Med.*, 152, S77–120.

Ayub, E. (1987) Posture and the upper quarter. In: Donatelli R, editor. *Physical Therapy of the Shoulder*. Churchill Livingstone: New York.

Barnes, P., Drazen J., Rennard P., Thomson N. (2008).*Asthma and COPD- Basic Mechanisms and Clinical Management* Margaret MacDonald and Simon Crump of Academic Press, http://www.sciencedirect.com/science/book/ 9780123740014

Bouchard, C., Shephard, RJ., Stephens, T.,(1993). Physical activity, fitness and health: A consensus statement. Champaign, IL: *Human Kinetics*.

Brannon, F. J., Foley, M. W. and Starr, J. A. (1998). Cardiopulmonary Rehabilitation: Basic Theory and Application, F. A. Davis, Philadelphia, PA.

Brodal, P., Ingjer, F. & Hermansen, L. (1977). Capillary supply of skeletal muscle fibers in untrained and endurance-trained men. *American Journal of Physiology*, 232, H705-H712.

Bungaard, A., Ingemann-Hansen, T., Schimdt, A. (1981). The importance of ventilation in exercise induced-asthma. Allergy, 36, pp. 385–389

Bungaard, A., Ingemann-Hansen, T., Schmidt, A. (1982). Exercise-induced asthma after walking, running and cycling. *Scand J Clin Lab Inv.*, 42, 15-18

Cahalin, LP., Braga, M., Matsuo, Y. (2002) Efficacy of diaphragmatic breathing in persons with chronic obstructive pulmonary disease: A review of the literature. *J Cardiopulm Rehab.*, 22, 1, 7-21

Cambach, W., Chadwick-Straver, RVM., Wagenaar, RC. (1997). The effects of a community-based pulmonary rehabilitation programme on exercise tolerance and quality of life: a randomized controlled trial. *Eur. Respir. J.*, 10, 104–13.

Cambach, W., Wagenaar, RC., Koelman, TW. (1999). The long term effects of pulmonary rehabilitation in patients with asthma and chronic obstructive pulmonary diseases: a research synthesis. *Arch Phys Med Rehabil*, 80, 103-11.

Casaburi, R. (1993). Exercise training in chronic obstructive lung disease. In: Casaburi R, Petty TL (eds). *Principles and Practice of Pulmonary Rehabilitation*, pp. 204–24. Philadelphia: WB Saunders

Casaburi, R., Patessio, A., Ioli, F. (1991). Reductions in exercise lactic acidosis and ventilation as a result of exercise training in patients with obstructive lung disease. *Am. Rev. Respir. Dis.*, 143, 9.

Cochrane, L.M. and Clark, C.J. (1990). Benefits and problems of a physical training programme for asthmatic patients. *Thorax*, 45, 5, 345-351.

Cooper, D.M. (1995). Rethinking exercise testing in children: A challenge. *American Journal of Respiratory and Critical Care Medicine*, 152, 1154-1157.

Cooper, S., Oborne, J., Newton, S., (2003). Effect of two breathing exercises (Buteyko and Pranayama) in asthma: A randomized controlled trail. *Thorax*, 58, 674-679

Coppoolse, R., Schols, A., Baarends, E. (1999). Interval versus continuous training in patients with severe COPD. *Eur. Respir. J.*, 14, 258–63.

Council, F., Varray, A., Matecki, S. (2003). Training of aerobic and anaerobic fitness in children with asthma. J Pediatr, 142, 2, 179-184.

Couser, JI., Maryinez, FJ., Celli, BR. (1992). Respiratory response and ventilatory muscle recruitment during arm elevation in normal subjects. *Chest*, 101, 336–40.

Cox, NJ., Hendricks, JC., Binkhorts, RA. (1993). A pulmonary rehabilitation program for patients with asthma and chronic obstructive pulmonary diseases (COPD). *Lung*, 171, 235-44.

Damoiseaux, V. (1984). Patiëntenvoorlichting: een terreinverkenning. [Patient education: an exploration]. Symposiumbundel patiëntenvoorlichting. GVO cahiers, University of Maastricht.

Donna L. Frownfelter. (1987). *Chest Physical Therapy and Pulmonary Rehabilitation*, 2ª ed. Chicago: Year Book Medical Publishers

Donner, CF., & Muir, JF. (1997). Rehabilitation and chronic care scientific group of the European Respiratory Society: ERSTask Force position paper selection criteria and programmes for pulmonary rehabilitation in COPD patients. *Eur. Respir. J.*, 10, 744–57.

Engstrom, I., Falstrom, K. & Karlborg, E. (1991) Psychological and respiratory physiological effects of a physical exercise programme on boys with severe asthma. *Acta Paediatr Scand*, 80, 1058-1062.

Field, T., Hanteleff, BS., Reif, MH. (1998). Children with asthma have improved pulmonary functions after massage therapy. *J Pediatr.*, 132, 854-8.

Fishman, AP. (1994). Pulmonary rehabilitation research: NIH workshop summary. *Am. J. Respir. Crit.Care Med.*, 149, 825–33.

Fitch, KD., Blitvich, JD., Morton, AR. (1986). The effect of running training on exercise-induced asthma. *Ann Allergy*, 57, 89-94

Fluge, T., Richter, J., Fabel, H., Zysno, E., Weller, E., Wagner, TO. (1994). Long-term effects of breathing exercises and yoga in patients with bronchial asthma. *Pneumologie*, 48, 7, 484-490. Hyperlink *[http://www.ncbi.nlm.nih.gov./Pubmed/]*. Retrieved: 21/10/2006

Girodo, M., Ekstrand, KA., Metivier, GJ. (1992). Deep diaphragmatic breathing techniques: Rehabilitation exercises for the asthmatic patient. *Arch Phys Med Rehab.*, 73, 8, 717-720

Global initiative for asthma.(1995). NHLB/WHO working group.

Goldstein, RS., Gort, EH., Stubbing, D. (1994). Randomised controlled trial of respiratory rehabilitation. *Lancet,* 344, 1394–7.

Goyeche, JRM., Ago, Y., Ikemi, Y. (1980). Asthma: The yoga perspective part I: The somato psychic imbalance in asthma: Towards a holistic therapy. *J Asthma,* 17, 3, 111-121

Green, LW., Werlin, SH., Schauffler, HH. (1977). Research and demonstration issues in self-care: measuring the decline of medicocentrism. *Health education monographs,* 5, 161–89.

Haas, F., Pasierski, S., Levine, N., Bishop, M., Axen, K.,Pineda, H. and Haas, A. (1987) Effect of aerobic training on forced expiratory airflow in exercising asthmatic humans. *Journal of Applied Physiology,* 63(3), 1230-1235.

Hanania, N.A., Chapman, K.R. and Kesten, S. (1995) Adverse effects of inhaled corticosteroids. *American Journal of Medicine,* 98(2), 196-208.

Holloway, E., & Ram, FSF. (2004). Breathing exercises for asthma (review). The cochrane database of systematic reviews, Issue 1. Art. No.: CD001277.pub2. DOI: 10.1002/14651858. CD001277.pub2. John Wiley & Sons.

Hough A. (2001). *Physiotherapy in Respiratory care,* 3rd ed. Glos.United Kindom : Nelson Thornes Medical Publishers

Jones, K., Tilford, S., Robinson, Y. (1990). Health education. Effectiveness and efficiency. India: Chapman and Hall.

Kaptein, AA., & Dekker, FW. Psychosocial support. *Eur. Respir. Mon.,* 5, 58–69.

Kathiresan, G., & Asokan, R. (2010). Effect of aerobic training on airflow obstruction, vo2 max, EIB in stable asthmatic children. *Health,* 2, 458-464.

Kathiresan, G., & Newens, AJ. (2011). Efficacy of home based pulmonary rehabilitation program on pulmonary functions and quality of life in asthmatic children. *Indian Journal of Physiotherapy and Occupational Therapy,* 5, 1, 140-141.

Ketelaars, CAJ., Abu-Saad, HH., Schlösser, MAG.(1997). Long-term outcome of pulmonary rehabilitation in patients with COPD. *Chest,* 112, 363–9.

Killian, KJ., Leblanc, P., Martin, DH. (1992). Exercise capacity and ventilatory, circulatory, and symptom limitation in patients with airflow limitation. *Am. Rev. Respir. Dis.,* 146, 935.

Kim, MJ., Larsom, JL., Covey, MK., Vitalo, CA., Alex, CG., Patel, M. (1993). Inspiratory muscle training in patients with chronic obstructive pulmonary disease. *Nurs Res.,* 42, 6, 356-362

Levine, S., Kaiser, L., Leferovich, J. (1997). Cellular adaptation in the diaphragm in chronic obstructive pulmonary disease. *N. Engl. J. Med.,* 337, 1799.

Lustig, FM., Haas, A., Castillo, R. (1972). Clinical and rehabilitation regime in patients with chronic obstructive pulmonary disease. *Arch Phys Med Rehab.,* 52, 315-322

Maes, S. (1993). Chronische ziekten. [Chronic illnesses]. In: *Handboek klinische psychologie.*

Maiman, LA., Green, LW., Gibson, G.(1979). Education for selftreatment by adult asthmatics. *JAMA,* 241, 1919–22.

Maltais, F., Simard, AA., Simard, C.(1996). Oxidative capacity of the skeletal muscle and lactic acid kinetics during exercise in normal subjects and in patients with COPD. *Am. J. Respir. Crit. Care Med.,* 153, 288.

Matsumoto, I., Araki, H., Tsuda, K., Odajima, H., Nishima, S., Higaki, Y., Tanaka, H., Tanaka, M., Shindo, M. (1999). Effects of swimming training on aerobic capacity and exercise induced bronchoconstriction in children with bronchial asthma. *Thorax*, 54, 196-201

McElhenny, TR., & Peterson, KH. (1963). Physical fitness for asthmatic boys. *J Am Med Assoc.*, 185, 142-149

Mellins, R. B., Zimmerman, B. and Clark, N. M. (1992) Patient compliance. Am. Rev. Respir. Dis. 146, 1376-1 3 77.

Millman, M., Grundon, WG., Kasch, F., Wilkerson, B., Headley, J.(1965). Controlled exercise in asthmatic children. *Ann Allergy*, 23, 220-225

Nagarathna, R., & Nagendra, HR. (1985). Yoga for bronchial asthma: A controlled study. *Brit Med J.*, 291, 1077-1079

Nagel, F. Asthma, sport, and exercise. http://www.asthma.co.za/articles/ref12.htm

Neder, AJ., Nert, LE., Silva, AC., Cabral, ALB., Fernandes, ALG.(1999). Short term effects of aerobic training in the clinical management of moderate to severe asthma in children. *Thorax*, 54, 202-206.

Nery, L.E., Silva, A.C., Neder, J.A., Cabral, A.L. and Fernandes, A.L. (1994) Exercise tolerance and anaerobic threshold (AT) in children with moderate to severe bronchial asthma. *American Journal of Respiratory and Critical Care Medicine*, 149, A786.

O'Donnell, DE., & Webb, KA.(1993). Exertional breathlessness in patients with chronic airflow limitation. The role of lung hyperinflation. *Am. Rev. Respir. Dis.*, 148, 1351–7.

O'Donnell, DE., Webb, KA., McGuire, MA.(1993). Older patients with COPD: benefits of exercise training. *Geriatrics*, 48, 59–66.

Perez, LJ., Rosas, VMA., del Rio, NBE., Sienra, MJJ.(2003). Calisthenics as a preventative measure against the decrease in maximum expiratory flow in asthmatic patients before and after a soccer game. *Rev Alerg Mex* , 50, 2, 37-42. Hyperlink [http://www.ncbi.nlm.nih. gov./Pubmed/]Retrieved: 28/11/2006.

Petty, TL. (1975). Pulmonary rehabilitation. In: *Basics of RD*. New York: American Thoracic Society.

Pouw, EM., Schols, AMWJ.,Van der Vusse, GJ. (1998). Elevated inosine monophosphate levels in resting muscle of patients with stable chronic obstructive pulmonary disease. *Am. J. Respir. Crit. Care Med.*, 157, 453.

Pulmonary Rehabilitation. (1997). Joint ACCP/AACVPR evidence-based guidelines. *Chest*, 112, 1363–96.

Pulmonary rehabilitation. (1999). Official statement of the American Thoracic Society. *Am. J. Respir. Crit. Care Med.*, 159, 1666–82.

Rabe, KF., Vermeire, PA., Soriano, JB.(2000). Clinical management of asthma in 1999: the Asthma Insights and Reality in Europe (AIRE) study. *Eur. Respir. J.*, 16, 802–7.

Ram, FSF., Wellington, SR., Barnes, NC. (2004). Inspiratory muscle training for asthma (review). The cochrane database of systematic reviews, Issue 3. Art. No.: CD003792. DOI: 10.1002/14651858. CD003792. John Wiley & Sons.

Ries, AL. (1995).What pulmonary rehabilitation can do for your patients. *J Respir. Dis.*,16, R16–24.

Ries, AL., Ellis, B., Hawkins, R. (1988). Upper extremity exercise training in chronic obstructive pulmonary disease. *Chest*, 93, 688–92.

Ringbaek, T. J. (2000) Rehabilitation of patients with COPD. Exercise twice a week is not sufficient! Respir. Med., 94, 150- 154.

Robinson, DM., Eggelstone, DM., Hill, PM., Rea, HH., Richards, GN., Robinson, SM.(1992). Effects of a physical conditioning programme on asthmatic patients. *New Zeal Med J.*, 105, 937, 253-256.

Santuz, P., Baraldi, E., Filippone, M. and Zacchello, F. (1997) Exercise performance in children with asthma: Is it different from that of healthy controls? *European Respiratory Journal*, 10(6), 1254-1260.

Satta, A., Migliori, GB., Spanevello, A. (1997). Fibre types in skeletal muscles of chronic obstructive pulmonary disease patients related to respiratory function and exercise tolerance. *Eur. Respir. J.*,10, 2853.

Shaw, I., Shaw, BS., Krasilshchikov, O. (2008).Exercise Training in the Treatment of Asthma: A Review. *institute sukan Negara, National Sports Institute of Malaysia*, 1, 2, 1-10

Siafakas, NM.,Vermeire, P., Pride, NB. (1995). Optimal assessment and management of chronic obstructive pulmonary disease. ERS consensus statement. *Eur. Respir. J.*, 8, 1398–420.

Sly, RM., Harper, RT., Rosselot, I. (1972). The effect of physical conditioning upon asthmatic children. *Ann Allergy*, 30, 86-93

Strunk, R.C., Mrazek, D.A., Fukuhara, J.T., Masterson, J., Ludwick, S.K. and LaBrecque, J.F. (1989) Cardio vascular fitness in children with asthma correlates with psychologic functioning of the child. *Pediatrics*, 84(3), 460-464.

Strunk, RC., Mascia, AV., Lipkowitz, MA., Wolf, SI. (1991). Rehabilitation of a patient with asthma in the outpatient setting. *J Allergy Clin Immun.*, 87, 3, 601-611.

Thio, B.J., Nagelkerke, A.F., Ketel, A.G., van Keeken, B.L. and Dankert-Roelse, J.E. (1996) Exercise-induced asthma and cardiovascular fitness in asthmatic children. *Thorax*, 51, 2, 207-209.

Tuberculosis and Health Association of Hennepin County. (1967) Physical conditioning program for asthmatic children. *J School Health*, 37, 2, 107-110

Tummers, N., & Hendrick, F. (2004). Older adults say yes to yoga. *Parks & Recreation*, 39, 3, 54-61

Udupa, KN., & Singh, RH. (1972). The scientific basis of yoga. *J Am Med Assoc.*, 220, 10, 1365

Van den Broek, AHS. (1995). Patient education and chronic obstructive pulmonary disease. Thesis University of Leiden. ISBN 90-802379-1-4.

Vitacca, M., Clini, E., Bianchi, N., Ambrosino, N. (1998). Acute effects of deep diaphragmatic breathing in COPD patients with chronic respiratory insufficiency. *Eur Respir J.*, 11, 408-415.

Weiner, MD., Azgad, Y., Ganam, R., Weiner, M. (1992). Inspiratory muscle training in patients with bronchial asthma. *Chest*, 102, 5, 1357-1361

Weisgerber, M., Guill, M., Weisgerber, J. and Butler, H. (2003) Benefits of swimming in asthma: Effect of a session of swimming lessons on symptoms and PFTS with review of the literature. *Journal of Asthma*, 40, 5, 453- 464.

Wijkstra, PJ.,Van der Mark, TW., Kraan, J. (1996). Long-term effects of home rehabilitation on physical performance in chronic obstructive pulmonary disease. *Am. J. Respir. Crit. Care Med.*, 153, 1234–41.

Wuyam, B., Payen, JF., Levy, P. (1992). Metabolism and aerobic capacity of skeletal muscle in chronic respiratory failure related to chronic obstructive pulmonary disease. *Eur. Respir.*, 5, 157.

Yiallourds, P.K., Milner, A.D. and Conway, E. (1997) Adrenal function and high dose inhaled corticosteroids for asthma. *Archives of Disease in Childhood*, 76, 5, 405-410.